The Friern Hospital Story

The history of a Victorian Lunatic Asylum

David Berguer

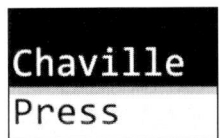

Published by:
Chaville Press
148 Friern Park
London
N12 9LU

First published 2012

© David Berguer

The right of David Berguer to be identified as the Author of this work has been asserted in accordance with the Copyrights, Designs and Patents Act 1988.

All rights reserved. No part of this book may be reprinted or reproduced or utilised in any form or by any electronic, mechanical or other means now known or hereafter invented including photocopying or recording, or in any information storage or retrieval system, without the permission in writing from the Publisher, nor otherwise be circulated in any form of binding or cover other than that in which it is published without similar condition including this condition being imposed on the subsequent purchaser.

A catalogue entry is available from the British Library

ISBN 978-0956934444

Front and back cover design by DesignbyCaroline.co.uk
Front cover photograph by Mark Wickwar

Printed and bound in Great Britain by Jellyfish Print Solutions

Also by David Berguer:
"Under the Wires at Tally Ho: Trams & Trolleybuses of North London 1905-1962"
ISBN 978 0 7524 5875 5

INTRODUCTION		i
CHRONOLOGY		ii
CHAPTER 1	MENTAL ILLNESS AND POVERTY	1
CHAPTER 2	CHOOSING THE SITE AT COLNEY HATCH	6
CHAPTER 3	DESIGN	9
CHAPTER 4	BUILDING THE ASYLUM	22
CHAPTER 5	PROBLEMS WITH SEWAGE	27
CHAPTER 6	GAS AND WATER	32
CHAPTER 7	THE EARLY DAYS	37
CHAPTER 8	HOUSEKEEPING	40
CHAPTER 9	PATIENTS	44
CHAPTER 10	TREATMENT	56
CHAPTER 11	WORK AND THERAPY	65
CHAPTER 12	TAKING CARE OF THE SOUL	70
CHAPTER 13	ENTERTAINMENT	78
CHAPTER 14	THE STAFF	85
CHAPTER 15	FIRE!	98
CHAPTER 16	WARTIME	106
CHAPTER 17	CHANGES & IMPROVEMENTS	111
CHAPTER 18	SANS EVERYTHING	124
CHAPTER 19	CARE IN THE COMMUNITY	130
CHAPTER 20	PREPARING FOR THE END	136
CHAPTER 21	DEVELOPMENT OF THE SITE	142
CHAPTER 22	PRINCESS PARK MANOR	149
CHAPTER 23	SEE YOU IN COURT	157
CHAPTER 24	FRIERN IN THE MEDIA	159
CHAPTER 25	REMINISCENCES	164
NOTES		169
INDEX		173

INTRODUCTION

When I started work on this book I knew I was letting myself in for a long but interesting task. There are so many strands to the story of a lunatic asylum – the social aspects, the financing, design and construction, the organisation and running, and treatment of patients and staff, the subsequent realisation that asylums had outlived their useful life and their eventual closure and redevelopment into more benign buildings.

The question was not so much what to include as what to leave out. Fortunately the London Metropolitan Archives have a large percentage of the documents relating to Colney Hatch Asylum, from minute books written in copperplate handwriting to photographs, plans and official reports. To look at all of them would take a lifetime, so I have tried to pick out the most relevant items to help to tell the story. Some future historian could doubtless throw a different light on the events from 1847 to the present day.

There had been a history of Friern, *Psychiatry for the Poor*, which was written by Richard Hunter and his mother Ida Macalpine, both of whom worked there as psychiatrists. It is an excellent work and is of great interest to anyone wishing to study the diagnosis and treatment of mental illness. It has one drawback, however, in that it was written in 1974 and therefore cannot cover the subsequent run down, closure and redevelopment of the asylum.

The task of researching the history of Friern was hugely enjoyable and gave a great insight into the Victorian way of going about things. Unfortunately, some things have not changed – in today's world, projects still come in over budget and are often curtailed through lack of money. The Care in the Community programme is a case in point. If enough money had been spent on it, it would have been a huge success but, alas, it has left mental patients and the public at risk and there are many today who think that it was a mistake to withdraw the kind of support that the Victorian asylums could offer. Perhaps their time will come again?

I would like to offer my thanks to the staff at the London Metropolitan Archives; the Royal Free Hospital Archives; the Barts and the London NHS Trust; the National Newspaper Library at Colindale, The Royal Society of Medicine; and the Wellcome Trust, to Yasmine Webb and Hugh Petrie at the London Borough of Barnet Local Studies and Archives, and particularly those who kindly agreed to be interviewed and who lent me their photographs. Every effort has been made to trace copyright holders; those overlooked are invited to get in touch with the publishers. A special thank you to my wife Patricia and my colleagues at the Friern Barnet & District Local History Society (FB&DLHS) for their support and encouragement and for checking the drafts and pointing out errors.

It was abundantly clear that everyone I spoke to who had worked at Friern took a real pride in their work and had the best interests of the patients at heart. I should like to dedicate this book to them and to the thousands of others who devoted their working lives to helping those less fortunate than themselves.

CHRONOLOGY

1831	The first Middlesex Pauper Lunatic Asylum is opened in Hanwell
1847	8 acres of land were sold by Mary Anne Curtis and her son William to the Great Northern Railway Company for the building of a line from King's Cross to the north. The GNR agreed to build a station at Colney Hatch
	On 27 January a committee is formed to select a site for the Second Middlesex County Pauper Lunatic Asylum. On 17 March a site at Colney Hatch is selected
1848	The site is surveyed and work commences on preparing the site
1849	On Tuesday 8 May the foundation stone is laid by the Prince Consort
1850	On Wednesday 7 August the railway line between Maiden Lane and Peterborough is opened to the public
1851	The first patients are received at Colney Hatch on Thursday 17 July
1852	The first fair in the grounds was held on Saturday 17 July
1857-59	An additional 700 beds are provided by the addition of 'B' and 'E' blocks and other wards, bringing the total beds to 1925
1860	Cooking by gas is introduced
1862	The original asphalt floors are replaced by wooden ones
1865	A two-storey convalescent home for females is opened. A Turkish bath for treatment of patients is opened on Wednesday 26 July
1866	Gas lighting is installed in the wards
1870	An additional 16 acres of land is purchased
1872	The cemetery is closed
1877	Middlesex opens its third Pauper Lunatic Asylum at Banstead in Surrey
1889	Colney Hatch becomes a London County Asylum under control of the London County Council
1890	The number of patients is 2248
1896	A temporary corrugated iron building is erected in the grounds to house 320 female patients
1903	On Tuesday 27 January the temporary building is destroyed by fire resulting in the death of 51 female patients. An operating theatre is built
1908-13	The asylum is enlarged by the building of seven villas in the grounds
1914	The number of patients is 2565
1929	The North Circular Road is built, resulting in the loss of 7 acres
1930	The Mental Treatment Act does away with the term "asylum". The name is changed to Colney Hatch Mental Hospital
1933	Electric lighting replaces gas
1937	The name is changed to Friern Mental Hospital. The patient population reaches 2654, an all time high

1939	The Ministry of Health denotes Friern as an Emergency Medical Hospital and units from St Bartholomew's are transferred there for the duration of the war. 770 beds are vacated by Friern patients
1940	On Saturday 28 September Villa 2 is completely destroyed by a bomb with the loss of 18 patients and 1 member of staff. On Saturday 5 October 1 patient is killed in Villa 6 when a bomb fell in the field opposite the villa. On Saturday 16 November a land mine destroys Villas 5 6 and 7 with the loss of 18 patients and 43 staff
1944	On Wednesday 23 February incendiaries destroy Villa 4
1948	In July the National Health Service is formed and takes over responsibility for running Friern
1958	Halliwick Hospital is built in the grounds
1959	The name is changed to Friern Hospital
1965	The farm closes
1970	The number of patients is now 1771
1974	The NHS is re-organised and Friern is now managed by Camden and Islington Area Health Authority under North East Thames Regional Health Authority
1982	A further reorganisation sees Friern now managed by Hampstead Health Authority under North East Thames Regional Health Authority
1983	Care in the Community is introduced
1988	Fairview Estate is built
1990	The number of patients is now 419
1992	The last Summer Fair takes place in July
1993	Friern Hospital closes on Wednesday 31 March
1995	Brookstream Corporation buys the site
1997	Regal Drive is built
1998	Friern Bridge Retail Park is opened in March. Halliwick Park Estate is built
2000	The first phase, the western half of the building, is completed and work starts on converting the eastern half. The development is named Princess Park Manor
2001	A public park is opened on Monday 30 April on 10 acres in front of the western half of the building
2003	The eastern half is now converted into apartments
2004	Work commences on a new extension at the eastern end designed in the same style as the original building
2009	The new extension at the eastern end is opened

CHAPTER ONE

Mental Illness and poverty

Mental illness has always posed problems for society. At its most basic, this is due to the recognition by everyone of the dark forces and strong emotions within themselves; dreams have been described as "the temporary insanity of everyday life." Because the dividing line between sanity and insanity is often very thin, the difference is magnified by the sane, in order to remove them as far as possible from the insane. With this attitude, it is clearly not easy for them to then feel sympathy with the afflicted.

For centuries, the causes of mental illness remained obscure and the insane were considered to be incurable, and so received no treatment. They did, however, receive punishment. The Greeks thought that they must have offended the Gods and in Roman times there were two schools of thought: either chain them up and keep them in total darkness, to frighten them back to normality, or treat them as comfortably as possible so that they would see the error of their ways. The level of ignorance and superstition in medieval times meant that anyone sleeping under moonlight would be driven mad, hence the term "lunatic".

Monks had traditionally looked after the body as well as the soul and they acted as medical men. However, even with the rise of the specialist lay physicians, monks continued to look after the insane. This often resulted in women being particularly badly treated by the inmates of monasteries; because they stirred men's passions, they were considered to be in league with the devil. When Henry VIII dissolved the monasteries, the mentally ill and the poor who had been given shelter and food by monks were left to roam the countryside, where they were subjected to being beaten and humiliated in public.

Early treatments for so-called madness could almost have been dreamed up by the mad themselves. An Anglo-Saxon remedy consisted of ground up herbs and roots mixed with ale and water and left overnight, then drunk from a church bell. A medieval cure for hallucinations consisted of eating well-sodden wolf's flesh, while melancholics were to be given a potion consisting of the head of a ram, with the horns removed but boiled 'skin and wool together' until soft. The brains were then removed, sprinkled with herbs and cooked on hot coals and given to the patient for three days. Even as late as 1852, it was thought that hysteria, 'a disease to which females are often subject', could be relieved by putting the feet at once into warm water.

Madness was often thought to be the work of the devil, so lunatics could be cured by lashing them to a cross for the night, which would scare the devil out of them, or they could be treated with holy water, or the devil could be exorcised from them by a priest. A protection against the devil consisted of putting lupins, wormwood, bishopwort and other herbs into a large pot and placing it under an altar where nine masses were being said. Salt was then added, along with sheep's grease and the mixture brought to the boil. The mixture was then spread on the eyes.[1] A more drastic treatment was trepanning which involved drilling holes in the skull, presumably to release the evil spirits. Archaeological investigations have uncovered examples of skulls thus affected, showing that the practice dated from pre-Christian times.

Strangely enough, in the 17th century where great advances in scientific knowledge took place, there was a revolt against such enlightenment, and witch hunts actually became more widespread. Confessions were forced out of those suspected of being witches by torture and they were put to death by hanging, burning or drowning. It has been estimated that around 12,000 so-called witches were put to death in Europe in the Middle

Ages, most of them women, and doubtless a good proportion of these would have been suffering from some form of mental illness. Joan of Arc was burned at the stake for claiming to hear the voices of saints.

Eventually things began to change, and in the early 1800s there was a growing concern about mental illness and for the way in which sufferers were treated. This was in some part due to the public awareness of the condition of King George III, who died in 1820 after suffering probably from porphyria, a chemical imbalance in the brain, for some twenty years. The treatments proposed for the King, however, give us an indication of the state of ignorance at the time; these ranged from having his intestines purged or his skull blistered, to listening to soothing music. Early nineteenth century doctors and quacks were fascinated with the magical powers of the newly discovered science of electricity and machines were invented which would give mild electric shocks to patients.

The long held tradition that those suffering from mental illness were like wild beasts who needed to be tamed was first challenged by William Battie who was a physician at St Luke's Asylum. In 1750 he suggested that only a small minority of patients were completely mad and that most of them were victims of circumstances that had somehow tipped them over the edge; in consequence he proposed that inmates should be treated individually according to their needs. The theme was "management does more than medicine" and the idea of physically restraining patients began to be seriously questioned. An example of the kind of restraint that was used can be found in a report by a House of Commons Committee which described the plight of a patient at Bethlem asylum:

> "A stout iron ring was riveted round his neck, from which a short chain passed through a ring made to slide upwards and downwards on an upright massive iron bar, more than six feet high, inserted into the wall. Round his body a strong iron bar about two inches wide was riveted; on each side of the bar was a circular projection which being fashioned to and enclosing each of his arms, pinioned them close to his sides."

The other disadvantaged group in society, the poor, had been a problem for centuries and there had been various attempts to deal with them, dating back as far as 1349 with the Statute of Labourers, but these were mainly concerned with punishing them. An Act of 1495 stated:

> "all such vagabonds, idle and suspected persons living suspiciously and then so taken and set in stocks, there to remain by the space of three days and three nights to have none other sustenance but bread and water, and there after the said three days and three nights, to be had out and set at large and then to be commanded to avoid the town."

The most important law to try and help them was the Poor Law of 1601 which classified the poor receiving relief as either the able bodied who were to be found work; the impotent or deserving poor and those who were unwilling to work. Every parish was made responsible for supporting the "deserving poor", in other words those who were too old or too ill to work or who had temporarily lost their job, and they would be provided with food and clothing. However this only applied to people born or permanently settled in the parish. It was therefore common for itinerant beggars to be sent to the next parish or back to the parish nearest to their place of birth.

It is important to recognise that attitudes to poverty were somewhat different during

Elizabethan times: poverty was generally considered necessary because the fear of it encouraged people to work. At various times in history vagrants who refused to work could be punished by whipping, by imprisonment, by branding with a "V", or, in persistent cases, death.

Workhouses were established in the late 17th century and by 1776 there were nearly 2000 in Britain, each holding an average of 50 people. Although workhouses were meant to provide temporary accommodation until people's positions improved, they increasingly became permanent resting places for those suffering from long term or incurable illnesses, including mental illness. The term workhouse was actually a misnomer, as many of the inmates were either unable or unwilling to work. By the 1830s the workhouse population was growing alarmingly and administrators were actively encouraged to make workhouses as unpleasant as possible in order to deter people from seeking relief.

The poor who suffered from mental illness, so-called "pauper lunatics", invariably ended up in workhouses but there was little attempt made to separate the 'idiots' or 'imbeciles' as they were called, from the poor and the destitute, and the former were then looked after by the latter, who were less than sympathetic to their charges. The less mentally disturbed posed few problems and would mix with the other inmates, but those with severe disturbances would be physically restrained. An idea of the prevailing conditions can be gleaned from a report in 1836[1] which read:

> "At Tiverton I found a female lunatic in the workhouse, who had been there for 28 years. She was confined in a small room, having neither furniture, fireplace nor bed; there was not anything in the room but a bundle of straws. She was without a single piece of clothing, perfectly naked, and had been confined in that state, during winter and summer for the last 28 years."

That may have been an extreme case, but a report in 1859[2] by the Commissioners in Lunacy highlighted the problems in workhouses:

> "A large proportion of the metropolitan workhouses are of great size, old, badly constructed, and placed in the midst of dense populations. The weak minded and insane patients are here crowded into small rooms, perhaps in an attic or a basement, and are sometimes associated with the worst characters. Seclusion and mechanical restraint would seem to follow of necessity. About a tenth of the workhouses in England and Wales have separate lunatic and idiot wards. The separate wards, however, are regarded as even more objectionable than the intermixture of inmates. And such wards themselves in old workhouses are exceedingly defective. The rooms are crowded; and the bedrooms are also used as day rooms; the ventilation is imperfect, and the yards are small and surrounded by high walls. Even where there are dayrooms, these are often gloomy and destitute of comforts."

There were asylums for the insane but these were privately run and few in number and the smaller ones, catering for one or two patients, were unregulated. They would not even necessarily house the insane: families would be tempted to commit those members of their families who did not conform to the standards of Victorian society, thus an unmarried mother could spend the rest of her life locked away; if she wasn't mad at the time she may well have ended up so. To try and prevent this and to stop unscrupulous well-off families from committing their relatives in order to get hold of their money, it was necessary for two doctors to certify that a person was of unsound mind. However, in the case of pauper lunatics, those looked after out of the poor rates, only one doctor was needed to sign the certificate of insanity.

The Oxford English Dictionary defines an asylum as *"a sanctuary or inviolable place of refuge and protection from which people can not be forcibly removed"*. The advantage of an asylum to the genuinely mentally ill was that they were removed from the stresses of the outside world and from the derision of their peers. They may not have received any treatment in an asylum, but at least they had the chance to recover in more peaceful surroundings.

The most famous, or notorious, asylum was Bethlem (more commonly known as Bedlam). Founded in 1247 as The Priory of St Mary of Bethlehem it had become a hospice by 1329 and in 1403 there is the first reference to insane men being cared for.

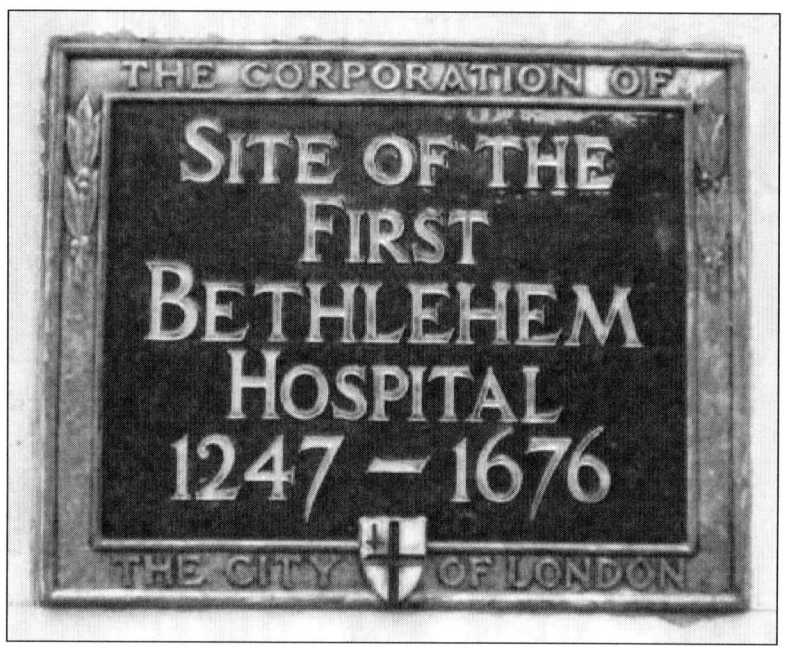

The plaque in Liverpool Street that marks the
site of the first Bethlehem Hospital. (Author)

In 1676 it moved to new premises at Moorfields and became the first custom-built hospital for the insane in Britain. In the early days visitors were allowed free access which led to some people posing as visitors in order to ridicule or tease the inmates. The citizens of London would make excursions on Sundays just to stare at them through the iron gates. Fortunately the practice of allowing free access was discontinued in 1770. A new Bethlem hospital was opened in 1815 and the four storey building housed 200 patients. At the rear of the building was the State Criminal Lunatic Asylum run by the Home Office which survived until 1864 when it was replaced by Broadmoor. The central portion of the Bethlem building still exists and now houses the Imperial War Museum.

To deal with the growing problem of mental illness and the overcrowding in workhouses, a number of Acts of Parliament were passed. In 1808 the County Asylums Act gave permission for the Justices of each County to build asylums, paid for out of local rates. The uptake of this was, not surprisingly, very low so the 1845 Lunacy Act actually compelled the Counties to build asylums and it also established the Lunacy Commission, a government department that would supervise the treatment of all lunatics throughout England and Wales.

As early as 1827 the Middlesex Visiting Justices of Asylums began to look for a site where a pauper lunatic asylum could be built. Two sites were offered to them, one at Gullers Hedge Farm, Hendon and one at Friern Barnet. The site at Friern Barnet was of 45 acres and was opposite the Parish Church of St James the Great, in Friern Barnet Lane (then called Friern Lane). In a letter to the justices[3] Henry Phillips, surveyor and engineer acting on behalf of the land owner Thomas Bensley, described the site thus:

> "…the land is in a most healthy and airy situation at something more than 200 feet above high water in the Thames presenting a very Grand Site for a Mansion or Public Building – it is most abundantly supplied with Water and there is a Conduit on the very summit level supplied by a never failing Spring of the Purest quality for all purposes and which will consequently supply any part of the Estate without the expense and labour of any Engine whatever.
>
> There is likewise an abundance of Gravel in the Estate which will be of much use in making the Airing Grounds, Yards and Walks and will save a great Expense, being on the spot; and as I presume a very considerable part of the land will be cultivated as Gardens its being Tithe free will be a great advantage.
>
> The situation is easy of access from all parts of the town and county, being on the original North Road over Muswell Hill to Whetstone, half a Mile from Colney Hatch, Three quarters of a Mile from the Great North Road at Finchley and within the same distance of the New Road now making at Finchley into the Regents Park, from which Place this land is distant 7 miles and a quarter."

The site at Friern Barnet was visited on Wednesday 20 February 1828 but was rejected in favour of one at Hanwell in the west of Middlesex. A year later 44 acres at Hanwell were purchased from the Earl of Jersey and plans were drawn up by William Alderson for a neo-classical building at whose centre was an octagonal tower from which two wings ran off. The builder was William Cubitt who finished the work in 1831 at a cost of £64,000. Hanwell opened for patients on Monday 16 May 1831 under Dr William Charles Ellis, Resident Medical Director and Treasurer.

By 1851 the population of Middlesex was around 2,100,000. The western part was larger, with 1,400,000 and 945 of these were classified as pauper lunatics. However in the east there was a higher ratio - 1200 pauper lunatics out of a population of 700,000. In addition there were 210 county lunatics and 20 criminal lunatics[4]. Hanwell only had room for 800 patients[5], so the need for a second, larger, asylum in the eastern half of the county was obvious. Thus was the groundwork laid for the building of a Second Middlesex County Pauper Lunatic Asylum.

CHAPTER TWO

Choosing the site at Colney Hatch

On Wednesday 27 January 1847 the Middlesex Justices appointed a committee of 21 to select a suitable site for the new asylum and to negotiate its purchase. Among the criteria were that it should have good transport links, not only to facilitate construction but also to ease the transfer of patients from Hanwell and other parts of Middlesex. It should also be in the countryside and have a southerly aspect.

An advertisement was published in the *Daily News*, *The Times*, *Morning Herald* and *Morning Chronicle*[1]:

Freehold Land Wanted
Middlesex

Wanted about 100 acres of Freehold Land in an airy and healthy situation and well supplied with Water in the Eastern part of the County of Middlesex whereon to build an Asylum for the reception of Pauper Lunatics. A Chalky, Gravelly or Rocky subsoil and easily accessible by Public Conveyance will be preferred.

Proposals are to be sent, sealed up addressed to "The Committee of Justices appointed to provide a Lunatic Asylum for the County of Middlesex" under cover to me at the Session House, Clerkenwell Green before Wednesday the 24th day of February 1847.

Charles Wright
Clerk to the Committee

Replies were received offering land at Colney Hatch; Bagshot in Surrey; Frith Manor Farm, Mill Hill; a piece of land at Winchmore Hill; and "200 or 300 acres at Hornsey in the centre of which stands Hornsey Wood and Hornsey."

A meeting of the committee was held on Wednesday 17 March 1847 at the Hornsey House Tavern at which several sites were considered. After due consideration, the plot selected by the committee was at Colney Hatch and was described thus[2]:

> "...this land is situated at Colney Hatch, between Finchley Common and Edmonton; it consists partly of a wood called Hollick Wood and partly of arable land having a gentle slope to the south with a small running stream at the southern boundary; it is about 7¼ miles from the place where the Hicks Hall formerly stood, 6½ miles from King's Cross by the Great Northern Railway, now in the course of construction and 6 miles as the crow flies from Shoreditch Church. The Great Northern Railway will pass through a corner of Hollick Wood in a deep cutting where it is expected that there will be a station. It is accessible also by high road from the Green Lanes, Tottenham, Hackney etc on the east and by other roads from Muswell Hill, Finchley, Barnet and the Great North Road on the west. Public conveyances to all parts of London leave the foot of Muswell Hill every hour, several coaches pass along the Great North Road and one coach along the Green Lanes. The soil is gravely and it has been stated by Mr Clark, well borer, of Tottenham that good water can be obtained at 250 feet from the surface which will rise to within 150 feet thereof.
>
> Hollick Wood and land contiguous at Colney Hatch; also a farm near thereto in the occupation of Lowels and the other of Clark. The land which Sir William

Curtis is willing to sell consists of 118 acres, 3 roods, 35 poles and land which consists of 8 acres, 1 rood, 30 poles and has been purchased by the Great Northern Railway for temporary purposes. Price of the 118 acres, 3 roods, 35 poles is £150 per acre."

The land was bought for £17,845 6s. 3d. and formed part of the Halliwick estate which had an interesting history. The old road from London to the north had run along Colney Hatch Lane and Friern Barnet Lane and thence through Whetstone and Barnet and had been in existence since at least 1005. Colney Hatch was the name given to a group of about a dozen cottages at the junction with the lane to Betstyle, a hamlet to the east. Halliwick estate, later called Hollickwood, was the main estate in the area and had a manor house, a farm and associated buildings and ran along the east side of Colney Hatch Lane and on the south side of the lane to Betstyle. A south facing slope with a stream at the bottom would have been attractive to early settlers, but it would have been mostly grazing land as the soil was too heavy to be ploughed with the medieval plough. Later on hay and grass were produced which was sent by cart to London in exchange for the manure produced by the thousands of horses there. There is evidence that the estate was already in existence in the early 13th century as King Henry III confirmed Henry de Audley as owner of the estate in 1226, but John de Halliwick disputed this in 1234. The estate was then bought by William de Morton who was a friend of Henry III. Morton lived in Buckinghamshire and may well have wanted a house closer to London to be near the Court.

During most of the 1600s the estate belonged to the Trott family and in 1747 it went to Margaret Nicholl who married James Bridges, Duke of Chandos, who already owned land at Whetstone. 110 acres were sold in 1801 to William Curtis and a further 83 acres to George Knights Smith in 1848. The manor house was described in 1795 as having been "long separated from the estate."

Sir William Curtis (1752-1829) was born in Wapping. His father and grandfather had both been biscuit manufacturers and they expanded into the Greenland fisheries and eventually formed a bank, which was very lucrative. Curtis was elected MP for the City of London in 1790 and became Lord Mayor in 1795-96. He was a supporter of Pitt and the Tories and was made a baronet for "steady voting" in 1802. In spite of being a pitifully bad speaker and very badly educated, he was an important member of the Government because of his City connections. He is said to have invented the phrase "the three Rs". He was mocked for his opulent yacht where he often entertained King George IV, who would also stay at Curtis's house in Ramsgate. He accompanied the King to Scotland where the King presented him with his portrait in a kilt by Sir Thomas Lawrence and inscribed "GB R to his faithful and loyal friend Sir William Curtis." It was said of him that no man of his time was ever subjected to so much ridicule but, despite this, on his death he left a fortune of £300,000 to his son, also Sir William. On his death in 1847 his widow Mary Anne sold 8 acres of the estate to the Great Northern Railway (GNR) and 119 acres to the Middlesex Justices for the site for the asylum.

To finance the building of the asylum bonds were issued and among the investors were a group of men, Michael Gibbs, Deave Barnwell, Charles Perkins and Thomas Moore who bought seven bonds to the value of £110,500. Another group, John Chetwynd Talbot, Charles Thomas Holcombe and Ralph Charles Price, bought £40,000 worth. George Crawshay, the new owner of the Halliwick Estate, invested £10,000.[3]

In 1870 an additional 16 acres of freehold land was purchased from George Knights Smith for the sum of £4,000 and together with land bought from the GNR, the total area amounted to 165 acres.

> **COUNTY OF MIDDLESEX – WANTED**, to borrow, on the security of the County Rates for Middlesex, for the purposes of the Act 8 and 9 Vict, c126, relating to pauper lunatic asylums, the SUM of £35,000 to be advanced on the 6th day of September next. The interest will be paid half-yearly, and the 1-30th part of the principal will be repaid at the end of each year, until the whole shall be discharged. Persons desirous of lending the money are requested to send in sealed tenders, (under cover to me, at the Section House, Clerkenwell,) endorsed "Tender for Loan for the Colney-hatch Lunatic Asylum," addressed to the Chairman of the Committee of Visitors of the Colney-hatch Lunatic Asylum, stating the lowest rate of interest at which they will advance the same before the 28th day of August inst.
>
> JOHN H SKAIFE, Clerk to the Visitors, Section House, Clerkenwell, August 10, 1850.

The GNR were in the course of constructing their new line from Maiden Lane, just north of King's Cross, to Peterborough and the Middlesex Justices approached them and proposed that they build a station at Betstyle; this they agreed to and in return the new asylum would provide the GNR with both gas and water for the station. The railway line would later be extended from the new terminus at King's Cross to York and thence to Edinburgh and which today forms the East Coast Main Line.

So, after a twenty-four year wait, and on a different site, Friern Barnet finally got a lunatic asylum, with a railway station as an added bonus. The building of the asylum would, however, have a dramatic effect on the population of the area which in 1851 stood at a mere 974; ten years later it had risen to 3344 and by 1901 it was a fully developed suburb with 11,566.[4]

CHAPTER THREE

Design

As well as having good transport links, and sited in the countryside, the main requirement that the Commissioners in Lunacy insisted upon was that the new asylum should be no more than two storeys in height. With this restriction and the requirement that the asylum would need to house 1000 patients, it was inevitable that the building would have to be a very wide one.

In 1847 the Middlesex Justices invited architects to submit designs which had to be presented by 1 October. Thirty nine submissions were received, although three of the architects were disqualified as they had privately shown their plans to some of the Magistrates before sending them in; this was, apparently, not an unknown occurrence as it had happened before when the Army & Navy Club was being designed.[1] The estimated costs ranged from £40,000 to £150,000 and after scrutiny the number of submissions was reduced to twelve and then to three. The first prize of £300 was awarded to Samuel William Daukes, the second prize (£200) to Messrs Harris and Godwin and the third prize (£100) to Messrs Allom and Crosse.[2] Although the justices had promised to hold a public exhibition of the plans, this never actually happened and the design by Daukes was chosen without any public consultation. When Daukes was asked what his fee would be he shrewdly said that he would leave that to the Justices to decide. The figure of £3000 was proposed, which he agreed to and he went on to prepare the detailed architectural plans.

In Victorian times two types of architecture were particularly fashionable – Gothic and Italianate, and Daukes had designed buildings in both styles, including a number of churches, a railway station, a registry office at Thornbury, near Bristol and, more relevantly, the Smallpox and Vaccination Hospital on Highgate Hill, which still stands today and now forms part of Whittington Hospital. For Colney Hatch he chose the Italianate style built in brick with stone groins, strings, cornices and window and door dressings and he ingeniously took advantage of the fact that the site sloped gradually from north to south, so that the wings at the rear of the building were actually three stories high. Two tall square towers in each wing were in the style of those at Osborne House on the Isle of Wight which had been designed by Thomas Cubitt and was Queen Victoria's favourite retreat. The exterior bricks of the asylum were made from the local clay and the addition of iron and magnesium produced a pleasant honey colour. The building was finished off with roofs made from Welsh slate which contrasted nicely.

In common with many Victorian buildings, the front, which faced Friern Barnet Road (later to be renamed Asylum Road for a short time) and was the public face of the asylum, was considerably more ornate than the back, which was hidden from public view in order to provide privacy for the inmates.

As with other buildings of the period, there was no damp course and it was not discovered until later that the foundations were only two feet deep, whereas they should have been four feet. Whether this was a change to the plans to reduce the cost of the building or whether it was sharp practice by the builder is not clear.

The building was 670 feet 6 inches deep and had an overall length of 1881 feet 6 inches with a corridor running the length of the building at the front, northern, side – the longest in Europe at the time. To put the size into perspective, it was nearly six times the width of Buckingham Palace.

The central portion of the building contained the chapel (81 feet by 58 feet 6 inches), capable of holding 600 people. The Chapel had galleries on three sides and plain glass windows. In the 1870s the galleries were removed and stained glass windows were installed, along with a lectern and mural texts on the walls. The original organ was hand operated and lasted until 1904 when it was replaced by a modern organ built by Messrs Cartwright.

Leading off the Chapel were various offices. On the right were the dispensary, clerks' offices and attendants' rooms and on the left the waiting room, committee room, and an apartment measuring 30 feet by 20 feet. To the rear of the chapel was the large Assembly Hall (112 feet long) which was used initially for the use of patients during wet weather when they could not use the airing courts to the rear of the building. Later this was used as a dining hall, but eventually the patients would eat in their wards, with the food being transported from the large kitchen. The Board Room was 30 feet by 20 feet and had walls covered with modern Venetian stucco, coloured and polished to represent borders of Carrara marble, and panels of Scienna[3]

Two wings ran off the chapel – the western side, which was the female wing, and the eastern side which was solely for male patients. There were 32 wards in total, fourteen on the male side and eighteen on the female side. Each ward consisted of about 30 to 40 single rooms 9 feet by 6 feet 6 inches on the northern side opening out onto a 4-5 bed dormitory and a day room which was also used for dining. There was also a lavatory, a bathroom, two attendants' rooms, a store room, scullery and two water closets. There was no through access on the first floor – the wards were separated by doors which were kept locked at all times and could only be unlocked by a member of staff.

Walls throughout were unplastered and were whitewashed. An interesting touch was that the corner of every wall throughout the building was rounded, so as to prevent the patients from hurting themselves. The floors were either plain brick, Yorkshire flagstones or, in some areas, black asphalt (then called "patented metallic lava floors") which it was claimed were impervious to water but nevertheless ended up smelling of urine. As can be imagined, the floors were cold in winter and their dark appearance must have made for an extremely gloomy feel. Eventually these floors would be replaced by wooden ones, but it would take some forty years for this to happen. In those areas where there were open coal fires they were provided with heavy lockable fire guards.

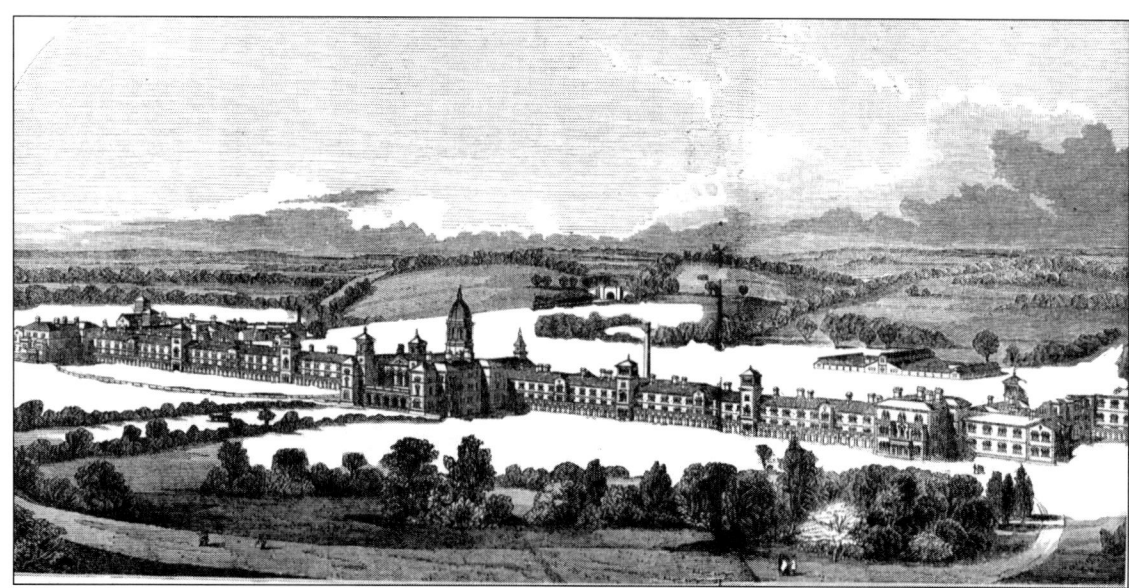

(Barnet Local Studies)

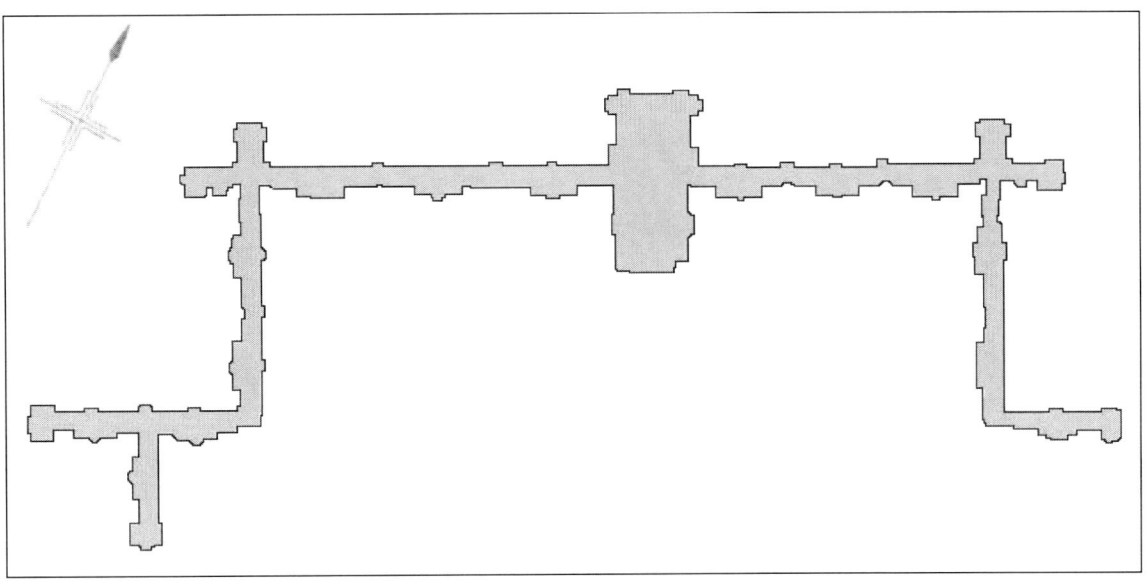

The asylum as originally built. See page 111 for the additions that were made later and page 168 for the original plan

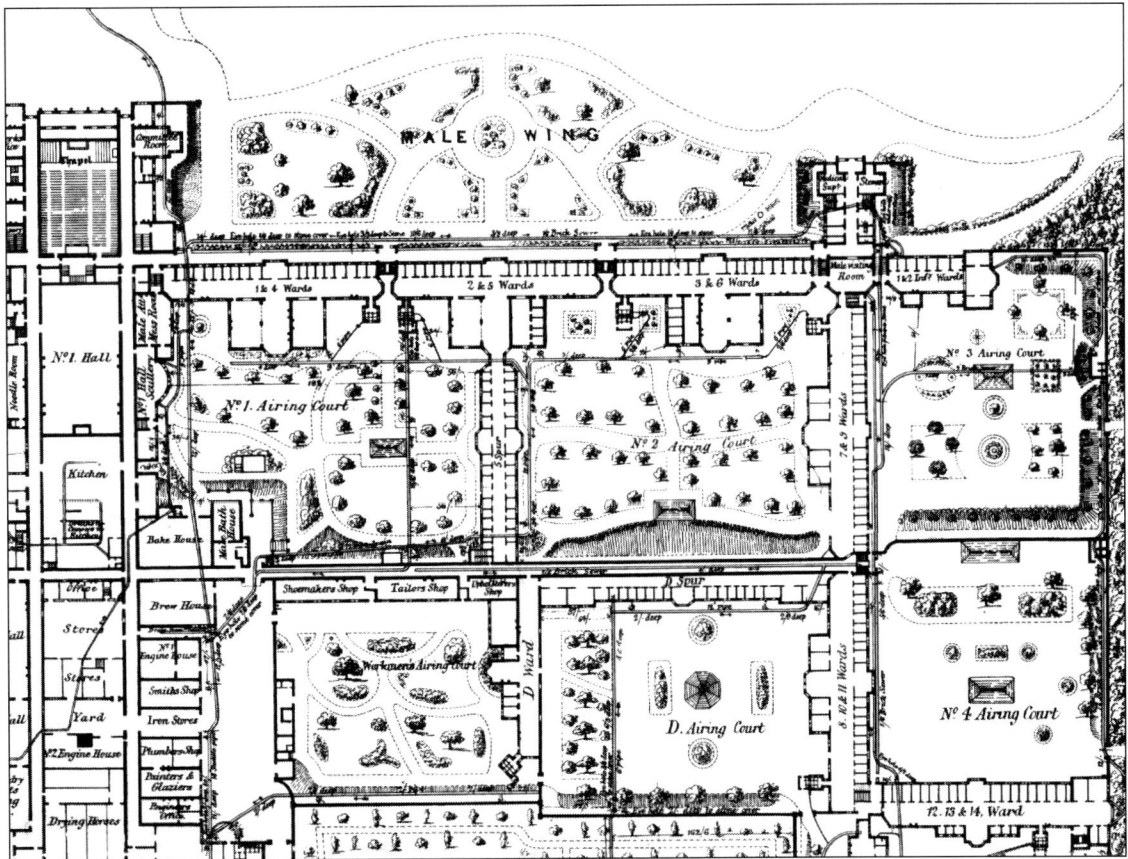

The east wing, showing the different designs of the airing courts. The ornamental gardens to the front of the building were later removed. (Barnet Local Studies)

A distinctive feature of the building was the use of fireproof honeycombed terracotta ceilings, particularly in the long corridor. The windows had iron frames and were of the casement type and for security, those on the wards were designed to only open a few inches at the top. Between the wards there were sheets of opaque glass. Some of the windows would eventually be replaced by sash windows which admitted more light and air.

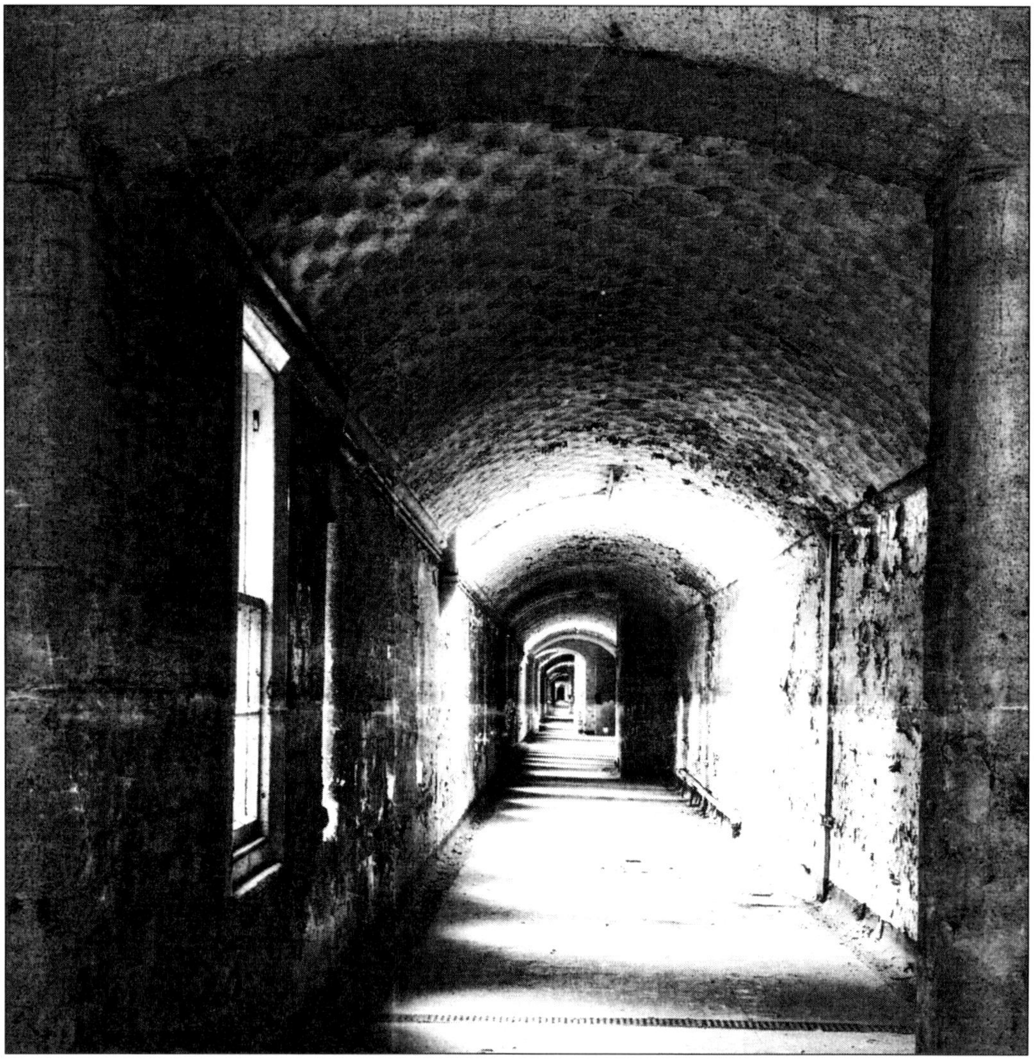

The corridor with its honeycombed ceiling. (FB&DLHS Archive)

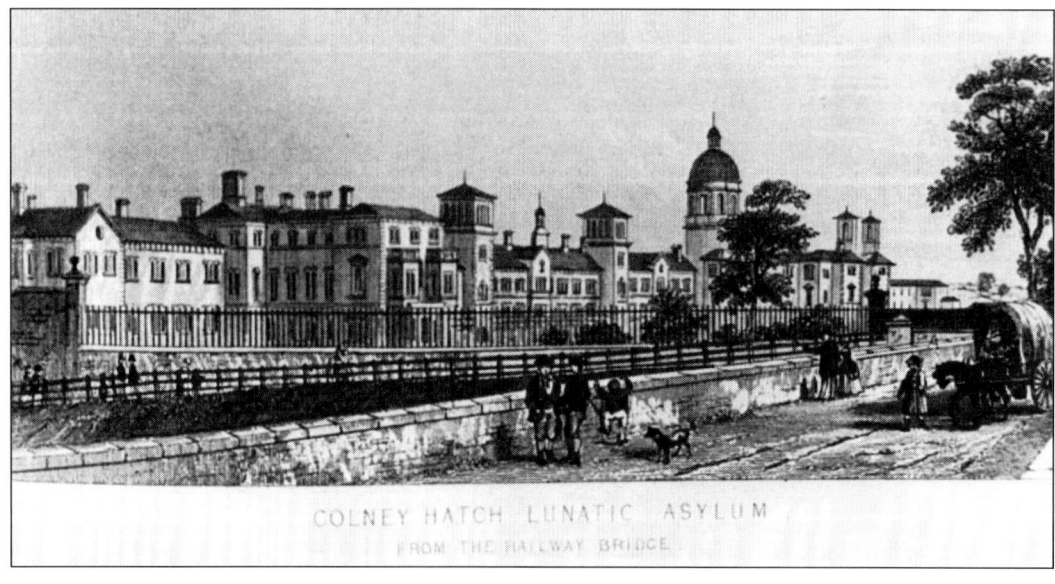

When the asylum was first built there was only a low wall and fence fronting on Friern Barnet Road. (Barnet Local Studies)

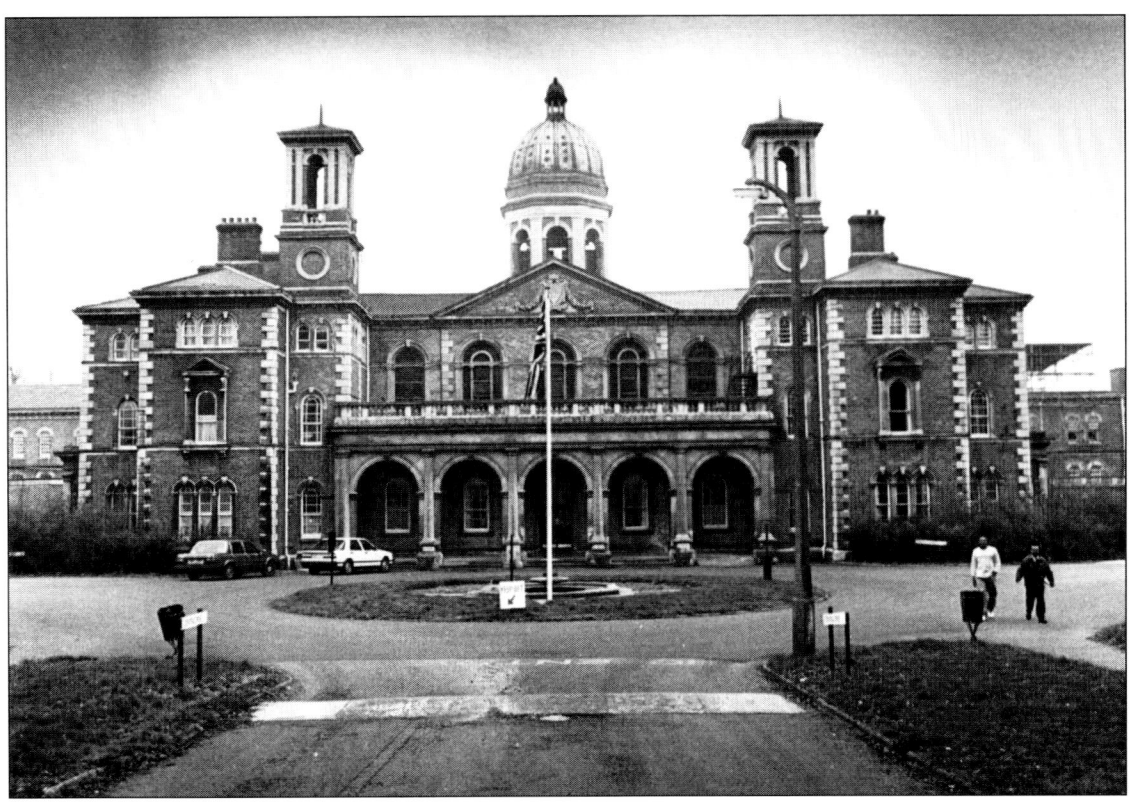

The main building. (Mark Wickwar)

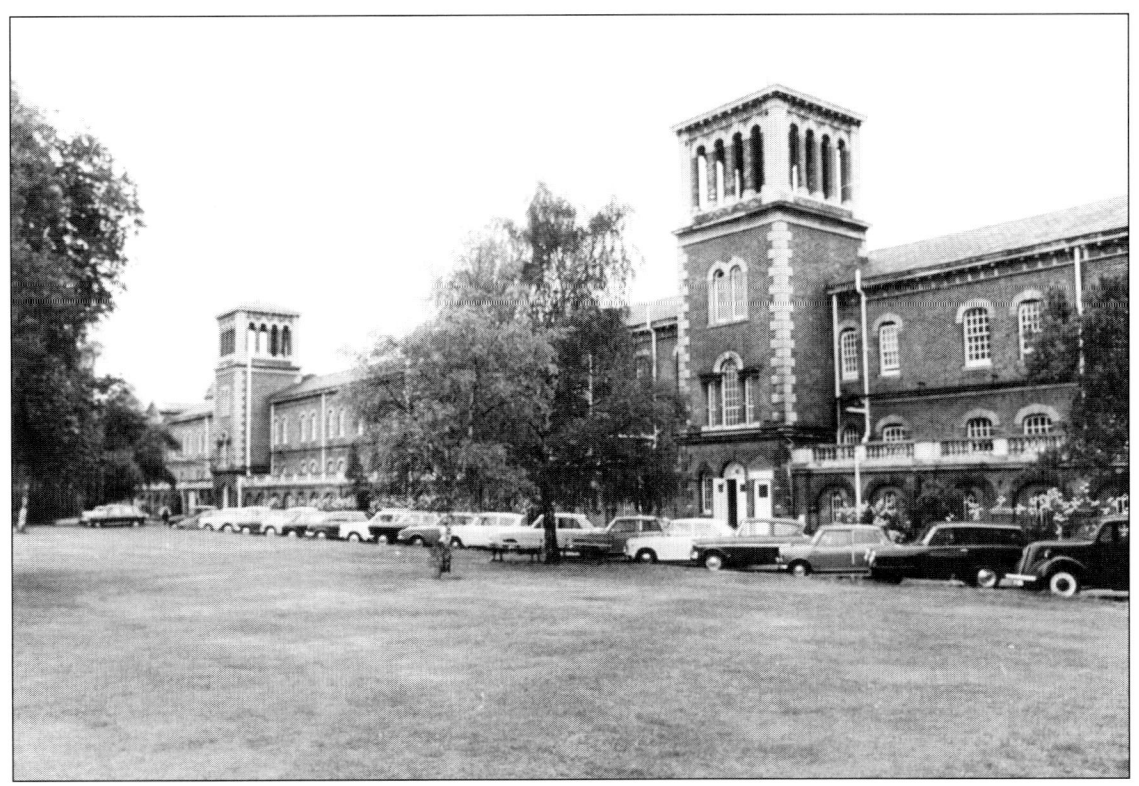

The east wing. (Barnet Local Studies)

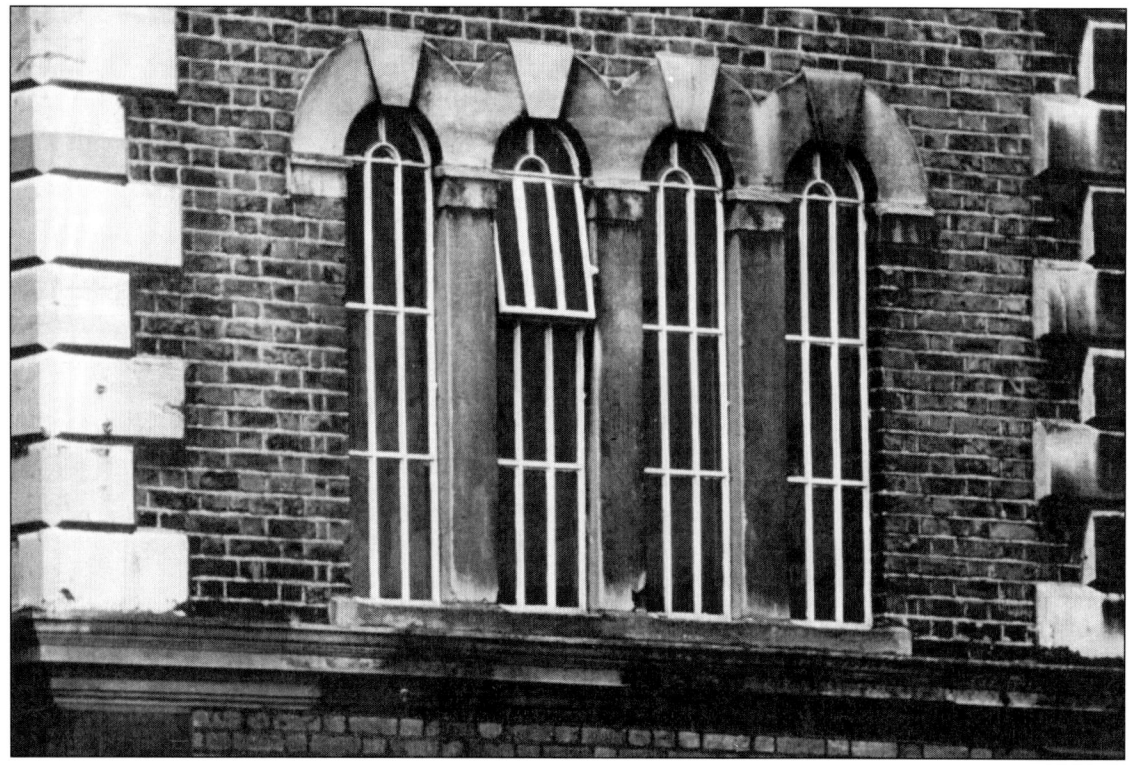

Some of the original windows offered little light or ventilation and were later replaced.
(by kind permission of The Royal Society of Medicine)

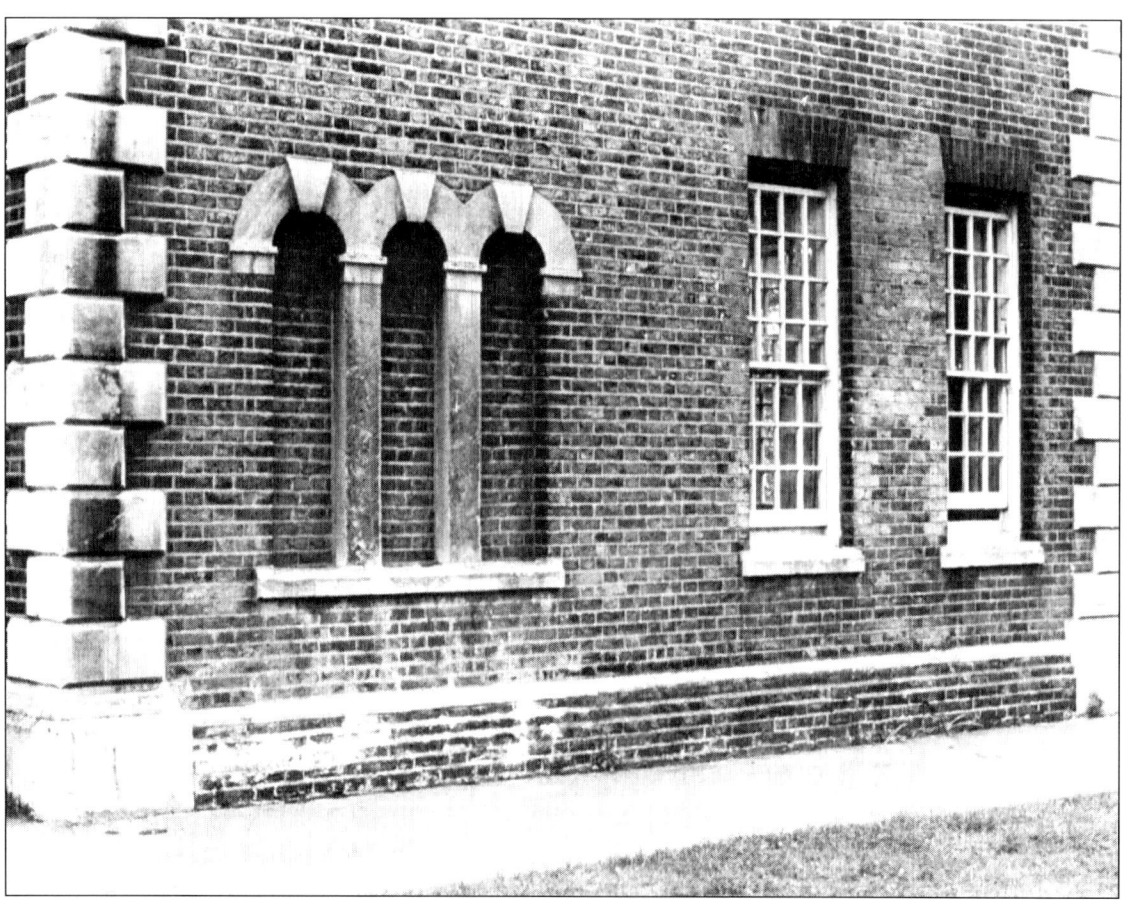

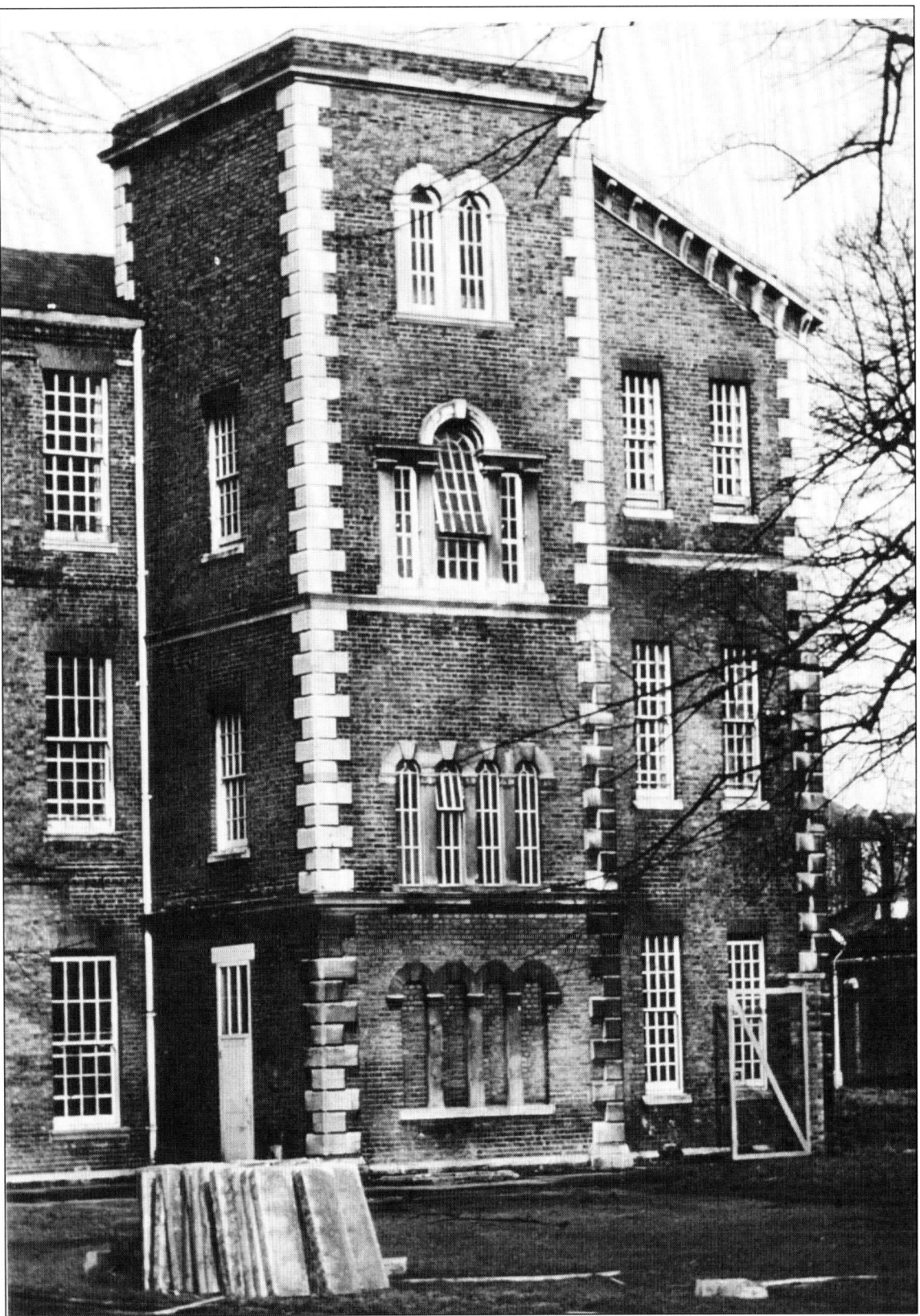

The side wings at the rear were of three storeys. (Barnet Local Studies)

To the rear of the building were a series of what were known as airing courts where the patients could exercise away from public gaze. There were fourteen of these which were laid out as gardens and pathways and each one was of a different design.

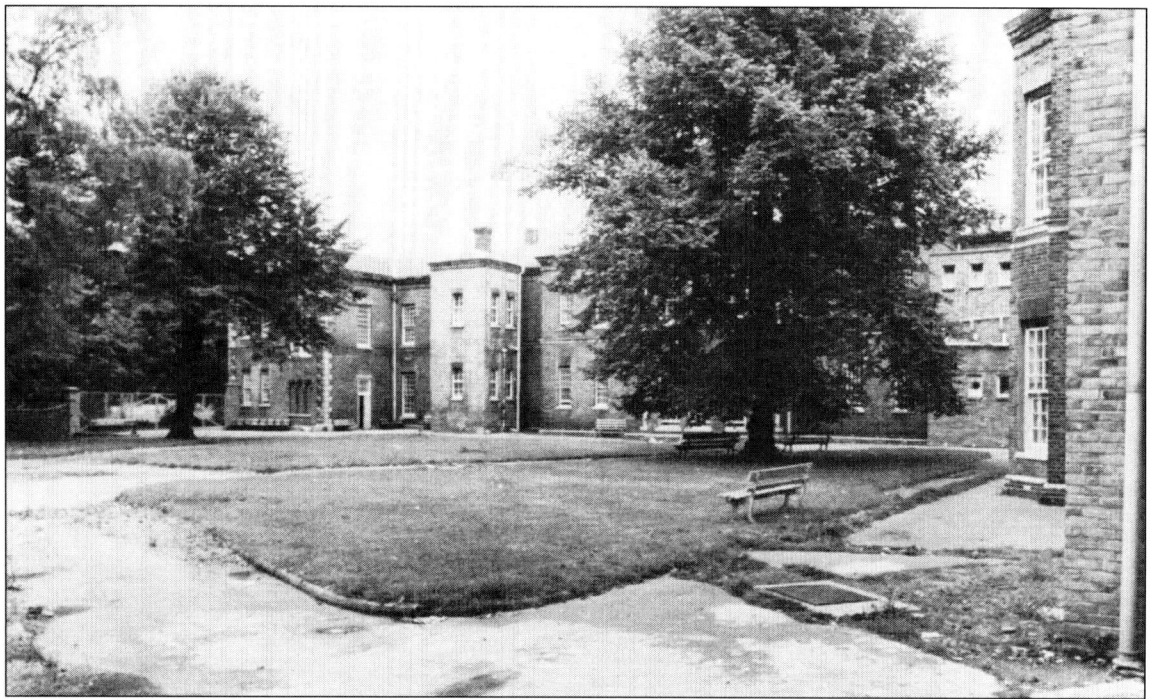

The airing courts offered patients a chance to exercise in pleasant surroundings.
(by kind permission of the Royal Society of Medicine)

In September 1851 the Committee of Visitors of Hanwell Asylum, headed by John Conolly, issued a critical report on the padded cells at Colney Hatch:

> "The padded rooms at Colney Hatch instead of being constructed in the manner which long experience at Hanwell has shewn to be almost free from objection of any kind, are so devised as to comprehend most every imaginable inconvenience – their aspect is gloomy; they are offensive; and they are unsafe. The material with which the padding is covered (caotchouc) is of a black colour and has a most disagreeable smell, whilst the padding of each of the four walls is in one compartment so as not to permit partial removal for the purpose of repair when required, but making it in such case necessary to take down the whole padding of one wall rendering the room useless for several days. There are no Inspection plates in the doors of any of the rooms at Colney Hatch by means of which at Hanwell the Officers and attendants can from time to time so easily ascertain the condition of secluded patients without occasioning them the least disturbance. The substitute for such a plate in the doors of the padded rooms at Colney Hatch is a large opening in the uppermost door furnished with a wooden door that must be entirely unclosed to obtain a view of the patient. As soon as this is opened the head and hands will generally be put through it and will scarcely be got back again without risk."

In rebuttal, a report by W Charles Hood MD at Colney Hatch said:

> "The dimensions of padded rooms are 8ft 6ins long by 6ft 3ins wide and 14ft high with a window 1ft 3in wide by 5 ft 6 ins high. The rooms do not differ from the ordinary sleeping rooms on the ground floor except as respects the padding and wire guard before the window. The covering is dark brown not black. Made from India rubber or Gutta Percha "the smell when first finished is not agreeable, as few things are, but every opportunity is taken during the absence of the patient to allow a current of air to pass through." The door is 1 foot square which enables us

to talk to the patient and to offer him a little refreshment, a piece of tobacco or even some snuff often producing a very beneficial effect."

It may or may not be a coincidence, but Dr Hood resigned in 1852 to join Bethlem as Resident Medical Superintendent.

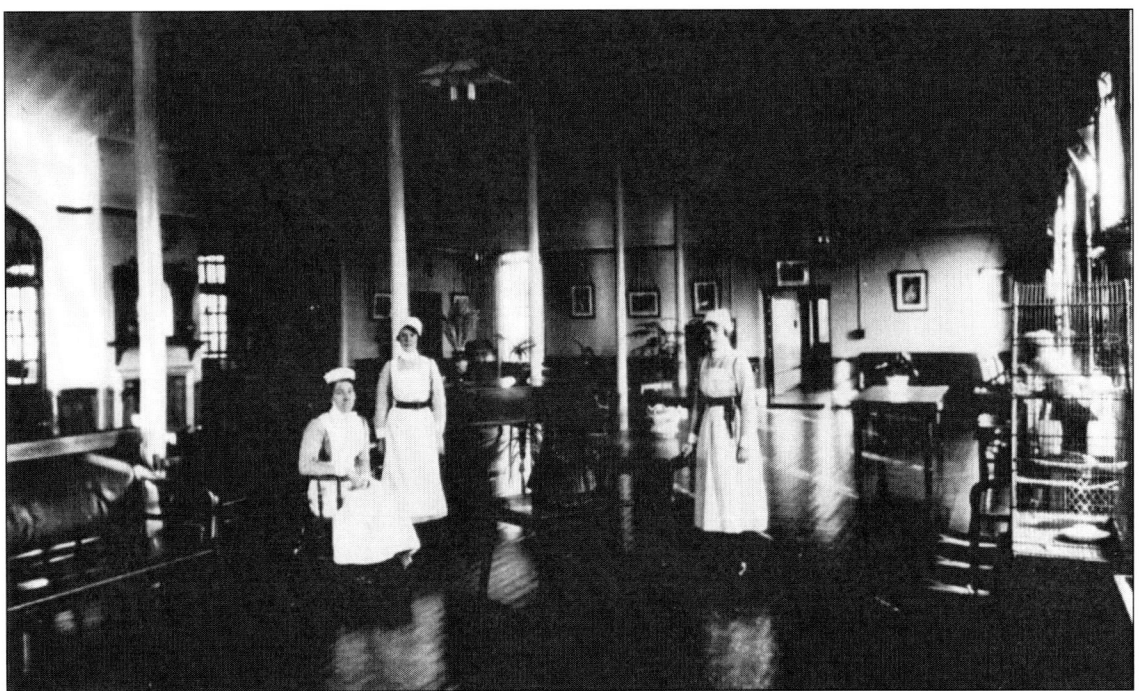

Highly polished floors, framed pictures and a bird in a cage in the reception area (Barnet Local Studies)

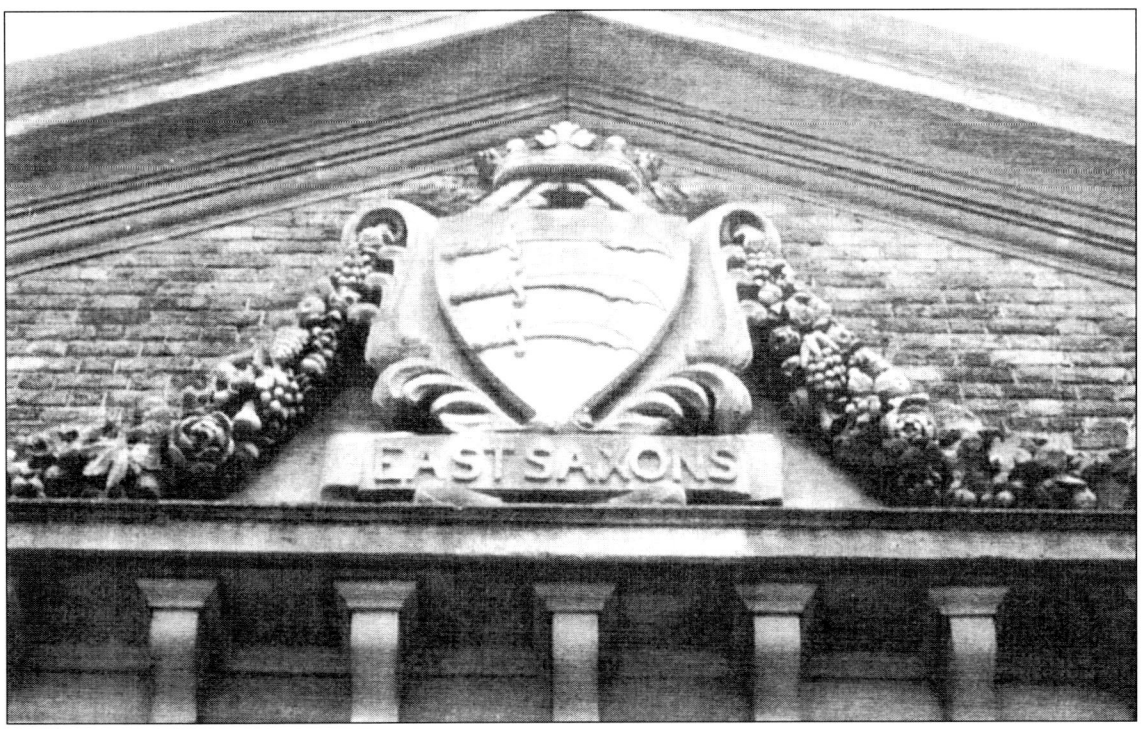

A reference to the fact that Middlesex was once part of the East Saxon kingdom. (Author)

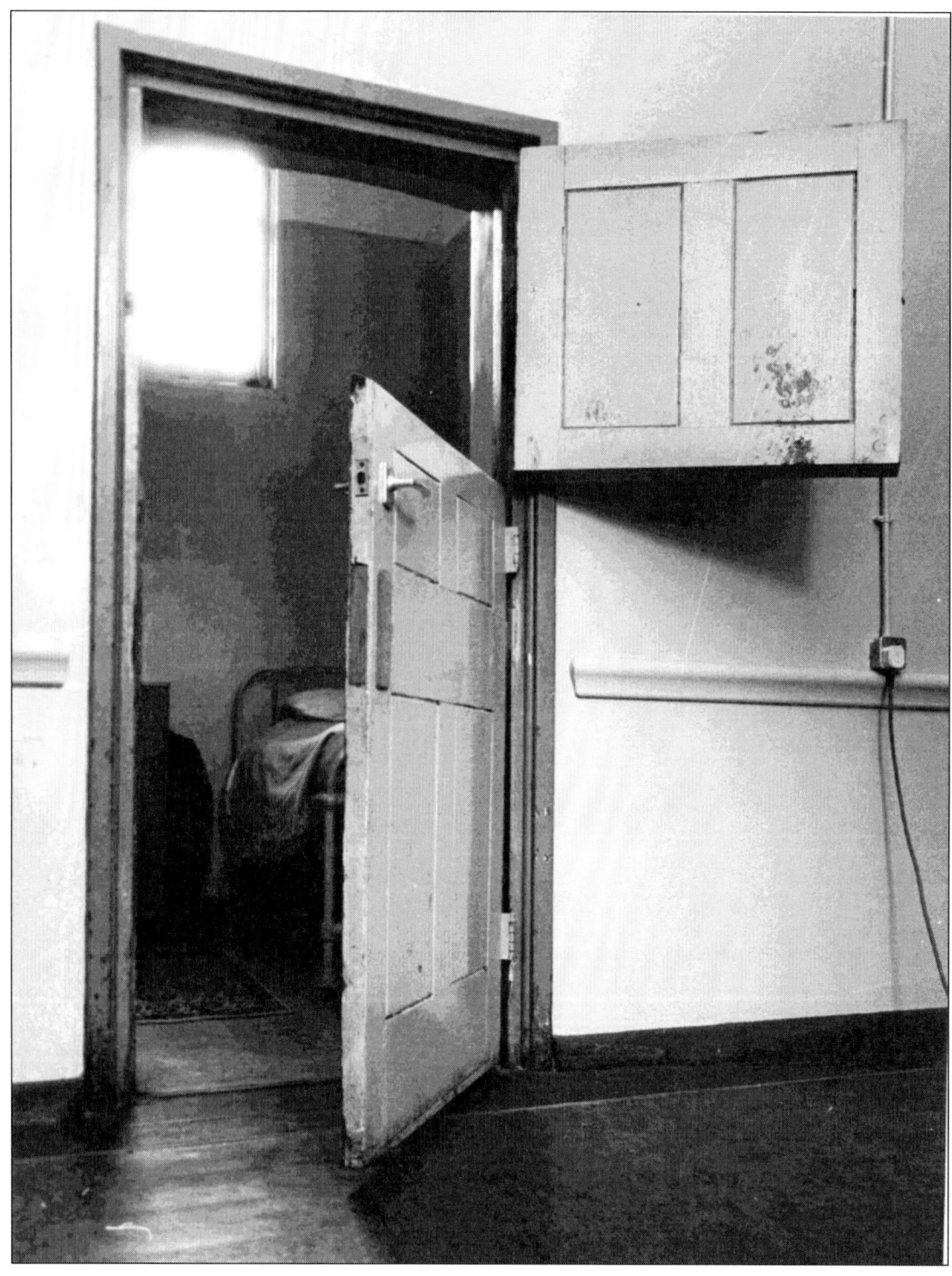

The individual bedrooms were very small. (Barnet Local Studies)

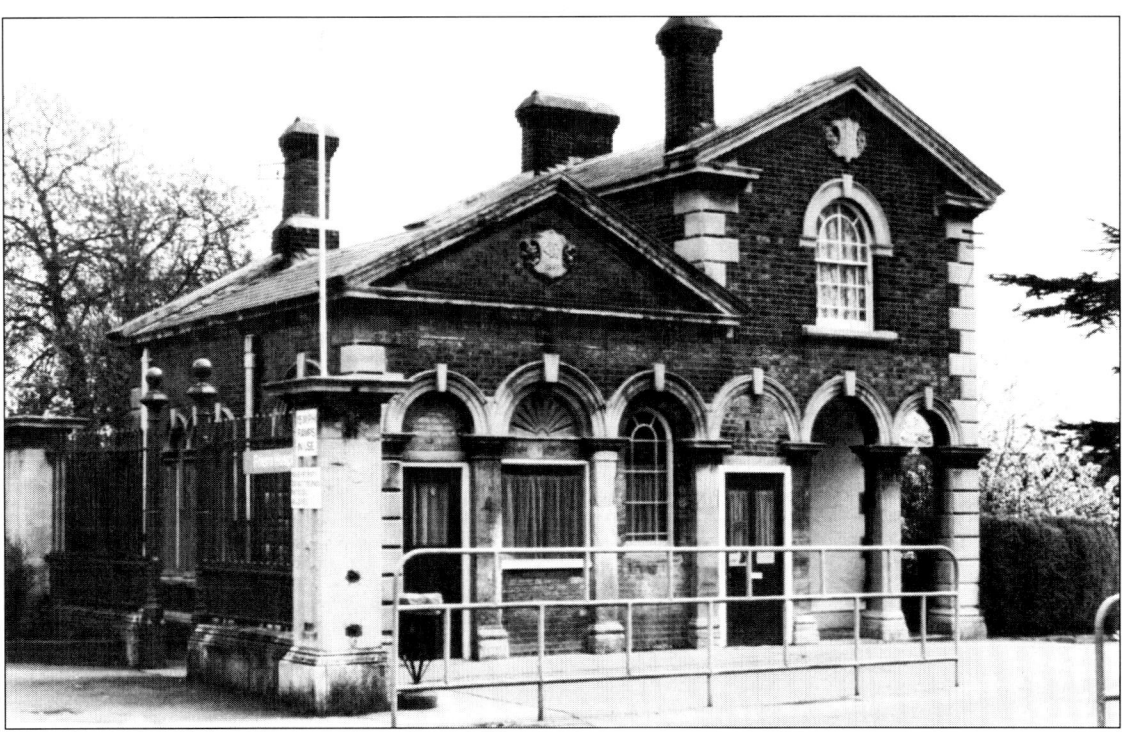

The North Lodge to the left of the main entrance was added in 1888. (John Donovan)

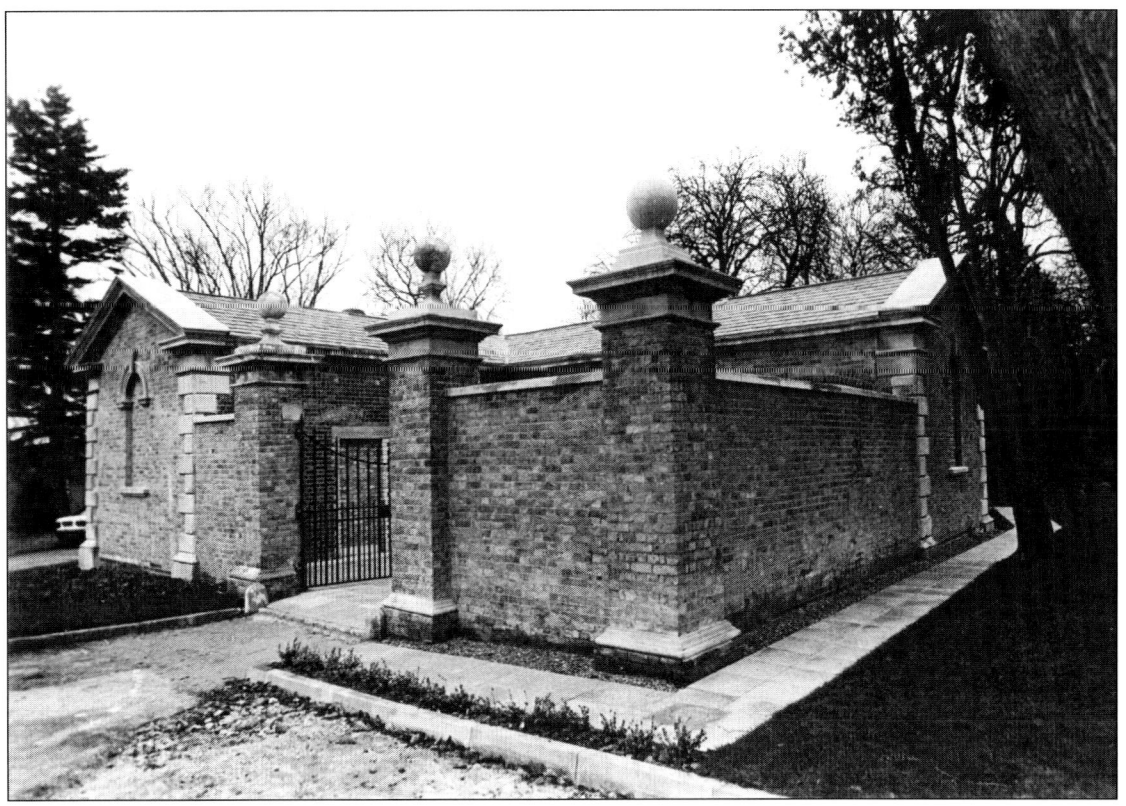

The mortuary was located just inside the main gates and to the west. This was formerly the stables, built for the horses of the visiting Committee of Justices. (Mark Wickwar)

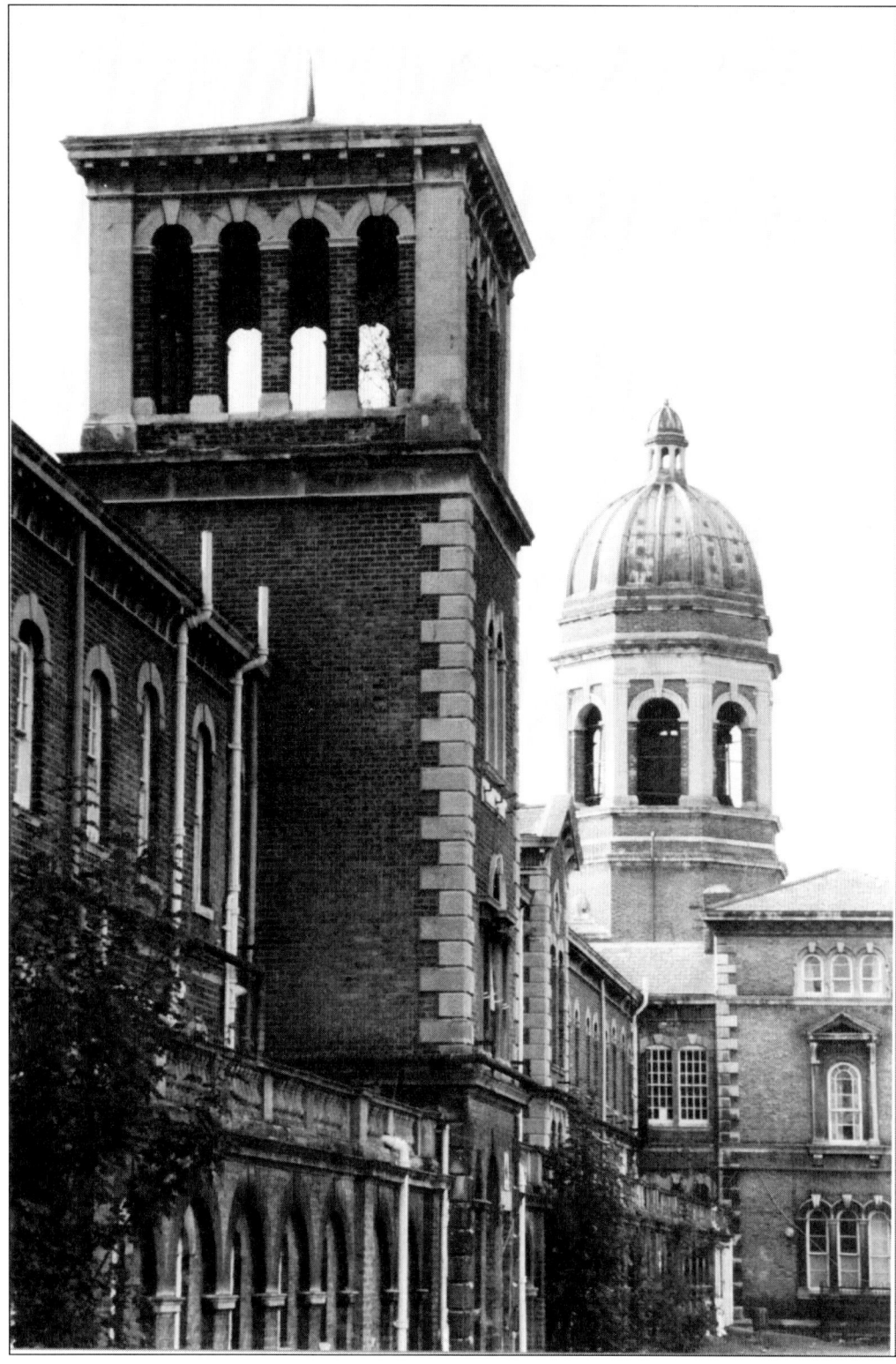

The dome on the main building viewed from the east. The long corridor can be seen running in front of the building. (Mark Wickwar)

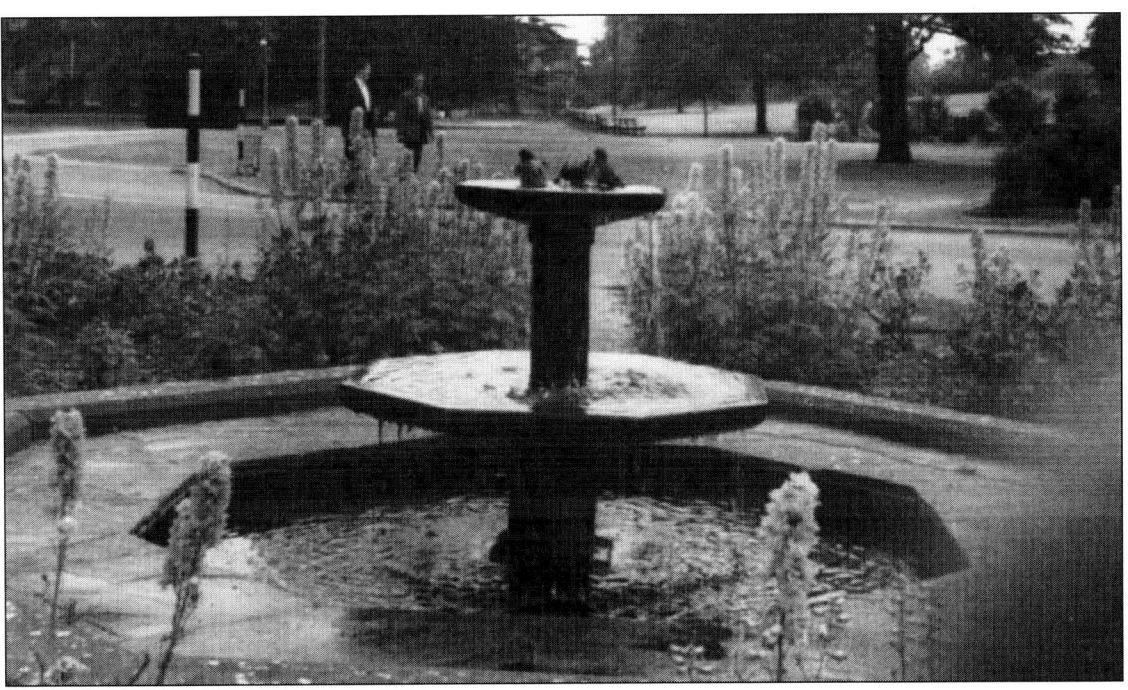

The grounds of the Asylum were designed by William Brodrick Thomas who later went on to design the gardens at Sandringham, in Norfolk and at Buckingham Palace.
(John Rampley Collection)

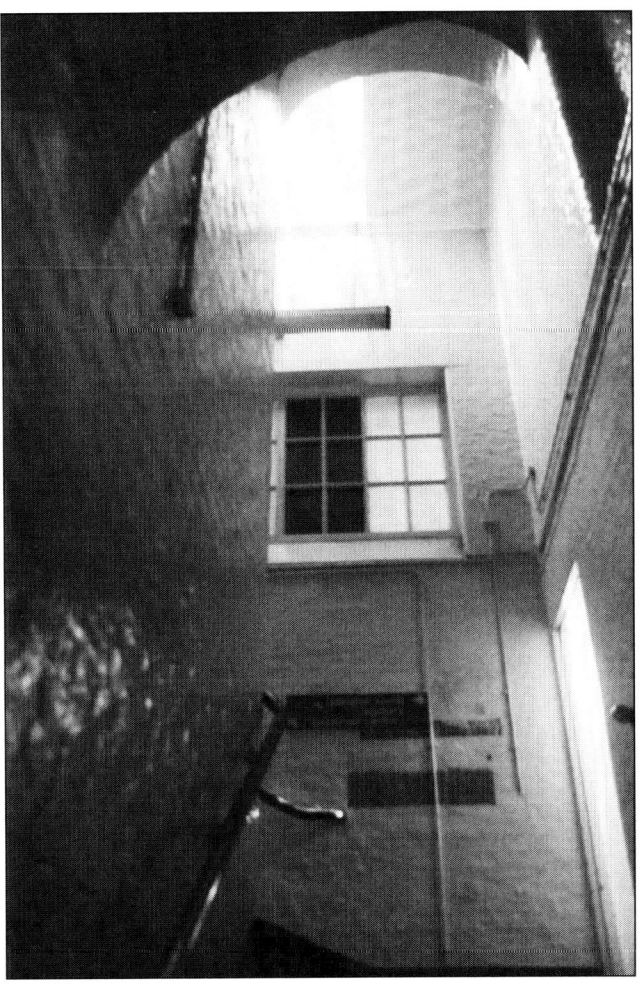

Even the stairwells had honeycomb ceilings. (Percy Reboul)

CHAPTER FOUR

Building the Asylum

Daukes had submitted the names of eleven contractors which he considered would be suitable and the Justices chose George Myers whose tender of £165,000 was £61,000 lower than the nearest rival. In the event, economies were made to the design and the eventual build cost was just in excess of £138,000. Myers went on to build asylums at Bracebridge, near Lincoln and the Essex County asylum at Brentwood so doubtless his experience at Colney Hatch stood him in good stead. The work was financed by various large insurance companies who were able to borrow money on the security of the Middlesex County rate.

The Clerk of Works was Mr C J Shoppee who set about getting estimates for materials and labour. On 27 June 1847 a land agent, John Attfield, was appointed to survey the site and his report was presented in January 1848. Work started immediately and a large number of trees were cut down and the site had been cleared and levelled off by October 1848. Building commenced in March 1849 and an interesting feature of the work was that some of the clay that had been removed during the preparation of the site was used to make bricks, in fact 10 million were made and were being delivered at the rate of 500,000 a week. At the peak, over 1,200 workers were employed and they were housed in huts built on the site.

On Tuesday 8 May 1849 Prince Albert, the Prince Consort arrived at Colney Hatch to perform the ceremonial laying of the foundation stone. The minutes of the Committee recorded that the stone would be placed in the entrance lobby immediately opposite the door, "that a silver trowel would be provided and that refreshments should be provided for the Prince and his suite, the Lord Lieutenant of the County, the Commissioners in Lunacy, and the members of the Committee ONLY, and that no refreshments should be provided for the Committee of the Justices of the County or their friends generally who may wish to attend the ceremony, but that they be informed that there is an inn (the Orange Tree) in the Village where visitors can find accommodation."

The Prince's cortege was met in the village of Colney Hatch by the Foreman of the Works on horse back who escorted it to the site and after passing the outer barrier the cortege passed between the workmen engaged in the building who were drawn up in line on either side of the road.

On reaching the inner barrier the Prince alighted and was received by the Committee of the visiting Justices and the Lord Lieutenant of the County, the Marquis of Salisbury at the head of the Justices of the County of Middlesex. The procession then formed and moved to the Prince's platform where the ornamental Foundation Stone was suspended in front of the Ladies platform. The Chairman of the Committee of Visiting Justices (Benjamin Rotch, Esq) then addressed His Royal Highness, stating the object which the County has in view in erecting "this Additional Asylum."

Daukes then exhibited the elevation of the building and pointed out to His Royal Highness on the General Plan the exact spot where the foundation stone was to be laid, and which would remain a visible and imposing feature in the entrance lobby of the building when it was completed.

The Chairman of the Sessions, Henry Pownall Esq., then presented the current coins of the reign enclosed in a glass receptacle to Prince Albert who deposited them in a cavity under the stone. He declared that the asylum would be "the pride and boast of our metropolitan county" and promised that "no hand or foot would be bound here; rather may the conductors of this asylum surpass the happiest results which have followed the labours of their brethren at Hanwell."

The Assistant Judge, Mr Sergeant Adams, presented specimens of standard weights and measures, in a glass receptacle, to His Royal Highness for deposit in a second cavity beneath the stone. The Rev J Thompson, Vicar of Friern Barnet, then invoked a blessing on the work. The Chairman of the Committee of the Visiting Justices, Benjamin Rotch, then presented the silver trowel to His Royal Highness who spread mortar and the foundation stone was gradually lowered into position. He then malleted the foundation stone, and tried its level both vertically and horizontally and then declared the stone to be laid.

After the ceremony the procession formed up as before and went to the office of the Clerk of the Works to see the various plans of the building. Because the room was only a

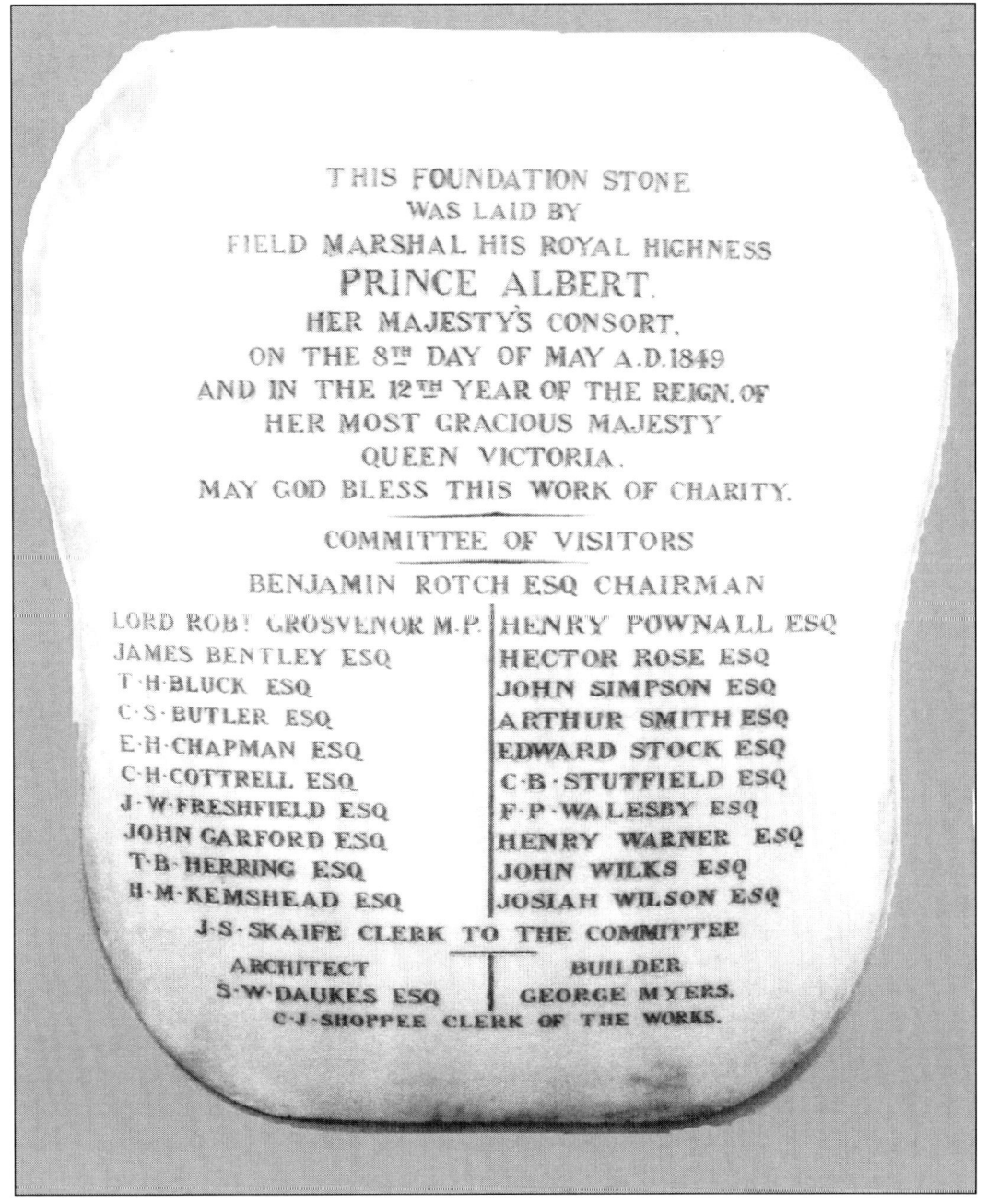

The Foundation Stone. The lettering is in gold. (Rachael Macdonald)

small one, only the Prince and his suite, the Lord Lieutenant of the County, the Lord Mayor and Sheriff, the Commissioners in Lunacy and members of the Committee were admitted.

The Prince's cortege then departed as it had arrived, between the workmen drawn up in line on either side of the road. The remaining visitors were then conducted around the site to see for themselves the progress being made, which was described as "extensive."

The ceremony and the stone cost £34 16s. 0d, the trowel £15 15s. 0d, and the "ample refreshments" provided by Messrs Staples, were paid for by a subscription of 10 shillings per head of the Committee of Justices.

Work on the building progressed and in a letter of 11 July 1849[1] the Committee reported:

> "Your Committee have great satisfaction in stating that from the rapid progress of the works, owing to the spirited exertions of the Contractor, they have every reason to believe that the Asylum will be completed by the time specified viz the 31st of July 1850.
>
> The Architect has reported that the two wings of the resident Surgeons are ready for the first floor and will be level for the roof within the next fortnight. The centre buildings, comprising the Chapel, Assembly room, Kitchen, Scullery, Bake House and stores will be ready for the roof this week and the whole of the long ranges of workshops, the Engine House, Wash Houses and Laundries together with the School Rooms, Pantries, Larders etc are actually at this time covered in, while the other works are progressing so rapidly that it becomes most important for the Clothing and House Linen to be got ready with the least possible delay."

In fact, the work ran a little late and the keys were not handed over until Friday 1 November 1850. The official opening of the railway line between Maiden Lane and Peterborough had taken place on Wednesday 7 August 1850 but it had been operational before then and had enabled bulk supplies of timber, cement, slates, glass, iron window frames as well as food and coal and oil to be delivered to the site, which was doubtless one of the reasons why a building of this size (it had in total 987 rooms of varying sizes plus six miles of corridors) was completed in such a short space of time.

A siding at Colney Hatch & Southgate station ran along the outer wall of the asylum and a turntable was installed which enabled one truck at a time to be passed through a doorway in the wall on to another turntable on the site from where the truck would be pulled by a horse down a short line which led to the gas works which were then being constructed in the asylum grounds.

The business of fitting out the building continued until Tuesday 1 July 1851 when the Chapel was dedicated and the cemetery consecrated by the Bishop of London, Dr Bloomfield. On Thursday 17 July 1851 the first patients, eleven men and five women, arrived and within six months 100 patients were in residence. They were soon followed by patients from the following private asylums in the eastern part of Middlesex[2]:

Barnet Union	Edmonton Union
Hadley	Edmonton
South Mimms	Enfield
Friern Barnet	Hornsey
	Tottenham

East London Union
The Liberty of Glasshouse Yard

Hackney Union
Hackney
Stoke Newingtom

Holborn Union
St Andrew Union
St George Bloomsbury
St Sepulchre
The Liberty of Saffron Hill Hatton
Garden & Ely Rents

Poplar Union
Bromley
Poplar
Bow

Stepney Union
Hamlet of Mile End Old Town
The Parishes of Limehouse, Ratcliff, Shadwell
Wapping, Christchurch

Whitechapel Union
The Precinct of St Katherine
The Hamlet of Mile End New Town
The Liberty of Newton Folgate
East Smithfield
The Parishes of Whitechapel, St George the East,
Clerkenwell, Shoreditch, St Luke Islington,
Bethnal Green, St Pancras

These were followed by those patients from Hanwell who were deemed suitable for relocation.

On 23 July 1851 it was reported that 212 windows in the building were defective and steps were taken to correct the problems, but the justices considered that:

> "when completed the building will be found well-adapted to the purposes for which the County has so liberally contributed…..that of providing an Asylum and a Hospital, a place of recreation, of occupation and cure, to many demented and helpless individuals for whose well-being such expenses are necessary."

1851 was also the year of the Great Exhibition of the Works of Industry of All Nations, a brainchild of Prince Albert, which was held in the Crystal Palace in Hyde Park from May to October and attracted over 6 million visitors. Visitors to the exhibition from home and abroad were encouraged to visit the new asylum by train and a *Guide Through Colney Hatch Lunatic Asylum* was issued for their benefit.

Although the asylum might have been considered suitable at the time of building, by today's standards it was extremely austere. There was, of course, no electricity; heating was by coal fires; there was no gas supply in the kitchens and no blinds or curtains in the wards. The wards and corridors had no lighting at all until 1866 when gas lighting was introduced. Gas cookers were only introduced in 1859 and a washing machine in the laundry was installed only in 1860 – prior to that the 12,000 pieces of laundry a week were all done by hand. Patients were often bathed in the wards in pails and it was not unusual for as many as four patients to share the same water.[3]

The layout of both Hanwell and Colney Hatch asylums – large buildings in a country

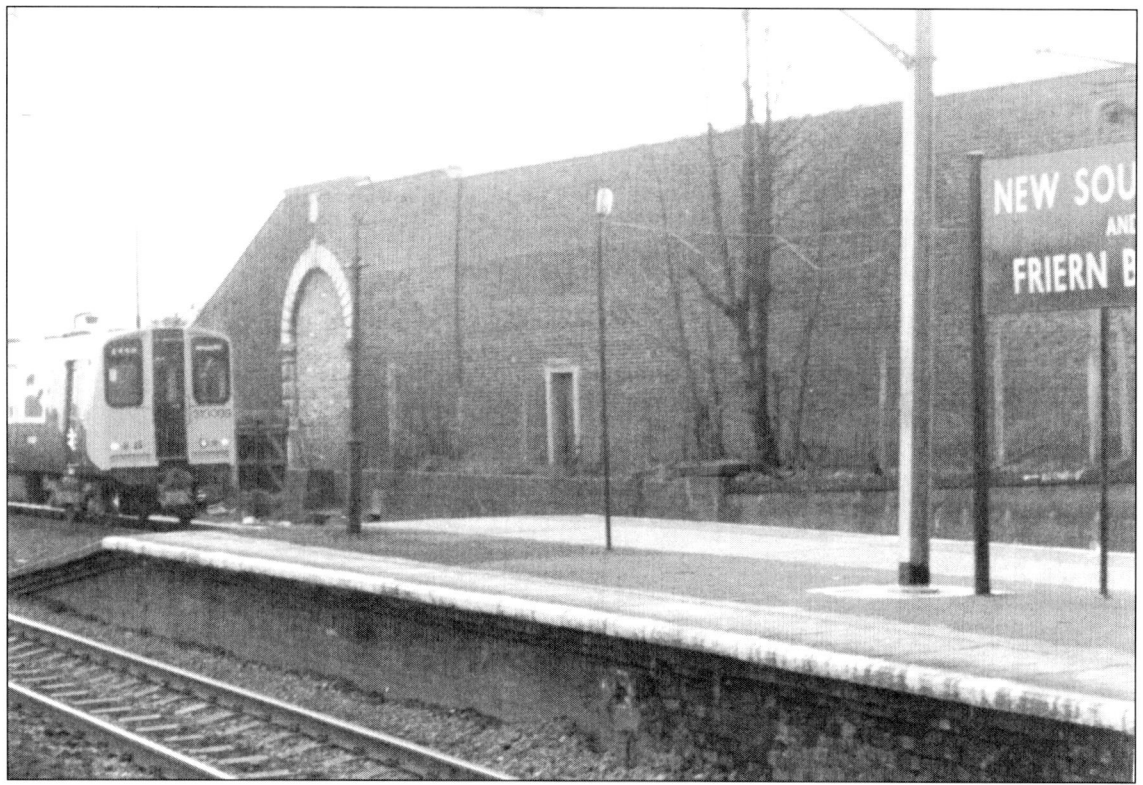

Wagons would be shunted through the gateway to the asylum on the left. (Colin Barratt)

setting - was replicated elsewhere in London where nine more were built before the First World War. A third Middlesex County Asylum was built at Banstead and a fourth at Claybury. Prince Albert laid the foundation stone to one other asylum, the Royal Earlswood Asylum for Idiots in Redhill (unbelievably, that was the official title).

When all the bills had been added up, the cost of buying the land and building and equipping the Colney Hatch asylum amounted to £290,092, equivalent to around £28,314,000 in today's money[4]. This made it the most expensive asylum ever built.

Cost of purchasing land	19,786
Cost of building	139,982
Furniture, fittings & initial salaries	130,324
	£290,092

CHAPTER FIVE

Problems with Sewage

It is not entirely clear whether Daukes underestimated the ramifications of having to deal with the sewage that would be created by over 1000 patients at the hospital or whether there were insufficient funds available. It is more than likely that the latter was the case. Some 100,000 gallons of sewage were generated each day, most of which was distributed over 120 acres of the farm and gardens, but a considerable amount found its way into Bounds Green Brook which ran from west to east along the bottom of the hill to the south of the asylum and thence into Pymmes Brook which continued eastwards to Edmonton.

As early as February 1852 Daukes reported to the Committee[1]:

> "There can be no effectual remedy to the contamination of the water in the brook arising from drainage from the Asylum. Filtering the sewage may be adopted and it would produce large quantities of manure required for the cultivation of the estate. The present manure tank might be adapted. As this tank is remote from the parts of the estate requiring the manure, I would suggest three cesspools be formed in the main drain to receive the sewage of the wings and the centre building. And by erecting a liquid manure pump over each, manure might be drawn up before it reaches the tank and reduce the quantity before it reaches the brook."

On 3 March 1852 Daukes was asked to submit a detailed plan for the work but criticisms began to be voiced by residents in the neighbouring areas. In September of the same year a complaint was received from the Edmonton Board that "Sewage impregnates the brook and the water passes several miles through the Parish." This was followed a month later by a letter from the Tottenham Board that "such a method of disposal is contrary to the Law." The Committee wrote back saying they had already taken steps to prevent the flow of water and sewage. However, the problem continued for several more years and complaints were frequently aired in the local press. It is worth quoting some of these in full, as it gives us examples of the verbose Victorian style of letter writing. In February 1860 the *North Middlesex and Southgate Messenger* carried the following letter:

> "Sir, As the press is the only source through which the Public can complain with any hope that such complaint will be of any avail, allow me through the columns of your valuable provincial to direct your attention, and also that of the authorities, to the great danger and positive nuisance to the Public of the Brook at Colney Hatch, one glance at which must be sufficient to convince you of the truth of my assertion.
>
> In the last three months it has been overflown and impassable eleven times; perhaps the authorities will say there is no danger; have they not put up a post with directions, whether passable or not? Sir, you or any sane person must see the great absurdity of trusting the lives of our fellow creatures to such a foolish and *contemptible thing?* Is it not well known that many of our carters cannot read at all – is the warning of any use to them? - would it be of any use to a blind man? And, sir, who can read it of a dark night, when the greatest danger may be anticipated? For three months it has been all but impassable for females, through the mud which the floods have left on the road and paths. Happy that they can manage to wade Tottenham's disgraceful muddy walks, and arrive safely on Edmonton's comparatively clean paths; there needs no post to mark the boundaries of the dirty parish.

By giving this insertion too will oblige. Your obedient servant,
Bound's Green, Jan 18th 1860. R P A"

This sparked further complaints from aggrieved local residents. The August 1861 issue of the *North Middlesex and Southgate Messenger* carried the following letter:

"The Brook at Colney Hatch.

The Inhabitants of Colney Hatch Park are universally complaining, and we conceive not without good cause, of the noxious state of the Brook, which divides the parishes of Edmonton and Tottenham in close proximity to Lower Park Road. About four of five years since, a public meeting was held at the Cherry Tree Inn, Southgate, to take the matter into consideration, the principal movers being the landowners in the neighbourhood, through whose premises the tainted stream flows, and which they complained of so polluted , that even the cattle refused to drink it. After some discussion, it was resolved, that the Visiting Magistrates of the Colney Hatch Lunatic Asylum should be communicated with, requesting them to remedy the evil complained of, inasmuch as it was patent the cause was produced from the sewage of the establishment being drained into it – the water previous to the erection of the same being to a great extent perfectly pure; if we recollect right however, the only satisfaction the applicants received in reply , was to the effect, that it rested with the parishes to rectify, and a repudiation of any liability on the part of the magistrates. Now it must be admitted, such a doctrine is not only very unjust , but it is by no means compatible with common sense – here is an establishment of great magnitude, containing a multitude of inhabitants, built for the reception of patients for the *whole* of the parishes in the county, and which as a matter of course, requires an outlet for its drainage, and that of a considerable extent, and admitting that this brook is the only available channel for the purpose; it is evident, that to throw the onus of correcting the nuisance committed by the sanction of the county authorities, on one or two particular parishes, is altogether unfair and at variance with common justice, seeing that the expense of such work would not only be enormous for them to incur, but would heavily increase their rate for a long period to come, for a matter not of their own creating, and which they were not consulted upon prior to its existence.

The only course which appears open for the residents in the locality to adopt, is to draw up a memorial and obtain the signatures of the influential inhabitants of both parishes, and forward the same to the Magistrates of the County, requesting them to take the necessary steps for its correction, and that the expense be defrayed out of the County rate, so that each parish in the County may bear its proportionate share of the said expense as the only equitable way of meeting it, on the ground that it has been produced solely by the erection of the Asylum in which every parish of the County has an interest equally as much as Edmonton and Tottenham, and urging, that if proof be needed of the cat that to this cause the nuisance owes its origin, to direct attention to the condition of the stream previous to its entering the precincts of the County property. We cannot think the Magistrates would be so unreasonable as to refuse to attend such an application, but in the event of so doing, it then may be advisable to call upon them to show why they should not be compelled to remedy an evil, for which they alone are responsible and which is of such a character, that if it emanated from any private undertaking, they in their official capacity would immediately exercise the authority vested in them to cause its cessation."

Things had not got any better by November 1861 when the *Messenger* ran an editorial article on the problem:

> "When gentlemen avail themselves of the convenience of railway travelling, and locate themselves within a short distance of the metropolis, the natural inference is that the advantage and benefit to be derived from a pure atmosphere, is one of the principal inducements which leads them often to put up with considerable inconvenience, attendant upon their journeys to and from London. Under these circumstances, we think the inhabitants of Colney Hatch Park have good grounds for complaint, seeing that, previous to the erection of the Lunatic Asylum, the Pymme's Brook was absolutely pure, whereas now it has become a positive abomination and has been a continual matter of complaint.
>
> Recently, a memorial was presented to the Edmonton Local Board of Health, the result of which has been, that a second has been sent to the Tottenham Local Board of Health, and which remains at present for consideration. That it is necessary something should be done to correct the nuisance is certain, for a personal examination, we found in the brook – on the side nearest the railway, where the stream crosses the road leading from Bound's Green to Betstile - that there is a deep deposit, composed entirely of night soil and soap-suds, and that upon being disturbed, the surface of the water becomes in a state of fermentation. To strengthen this assertion, we have been informed by persons who have been employed to clean out the brook lower down towards Broomfield Farm, that our statements are correct, and that insects are bred in the deposit, in marvellous quantities; while the matter is to cause a tormenting irritation on the skin, and other annoyances, which only those who have experienced can describe.
>
> We know not what view the Tottenham Board of Health may take of this subject, but we are inclined to believe that the members of that board, and also those of the Edmonton Board, will not readily lend themselves to fasten a heavy yoke upon the ratepayers of the respective parishes, in the shape of a private improvement rate, seeing that, inasmuch as the Asylum has been erected for the convenience of the whole of the parishes in the county, and it is plainly apparent to any one who chooses to examine the locality, that the nuisance complained of emanates from that establishment, the only equitable plan to be adopted would be, that the remedy be applied, and paid for out of the County-rate, so that each parish may bear a share of the expense.
>
> We shall abstain from any further comments until the decisions of the Local Boards become known, when perhaps we may be in a position to enlighten our readers upon a subject which is of such vital importance to the sanitary condition of the neighbourhood.

The asylum clearly did not relish the thought of having to spend considerable sums of money to alleviate the problems once and for all. In 1869 John Skaife, Clerk to the Visitors, wrote to the Tottenham Local Board that after looking through various Acts of Parliament he had come to the conclusion that the cost of construction should probably fall on the County (Middlesex), but he was not entirely sure of this.[2]

It was suggested that a bridge should be built to replace the "miserable little footplank" across the stream. The road on either side was described as "deplorable" and in a two to three week period in 1869 valuable horses had been injured and "several persons had fallen into the slimy liquid".[2]

On 16 July 1870 the *Barnet Press* reported:

> "The Committee of visitors in their annual report, state that the subject of the disposal of the sewage has engaged much of their attention. The plans for the construction of separate systems of drainage, for the erection of earth closets, and for sewage irrigation, which were approved by the Court, were forwarded to the Commissioners of Lunacy, in order that they might report upon them to the Home Office, and after a protracted correspondence, the Commissioners declined to recommend the plans for earth closets for approval; and those for a separate system of drainage and irrigation were approved by the Secretary of State for the Home Department. The Committee lost no time in carrying the plans into execution, and the separation of the rain water from the sewage by distinct drains was effected. The works connected with the preparation of the land for irrigation with the sewage have been completed, but the Committee are at present unable to say whether this will enable them to comply with the terms of the injunction. They have been repeatedly assured by practical engineers that the system of irrigation which has now been adopted will entirely and permanently purify the sewage, and they hope that these predictions may be verified, but they do not feel at all certain that the proposed scheme will be free from danger and difficulties, and they believe it is very probable that the system of earth closets may still become a necessity."

Although complaints were continuing to be received, the Asylum was fighting back. On 29 October 1870 the *Barnet Press* reported:

> "It having been stated that the plans for disposing of the sewage from Colney Hatch Asylum by irrigation had failed, and that Pymme's Brook was still fouled by sewage from the asylum, Mr Skaife, clerk to the Visiting Justices, has written to the Edmonton Local Board, stating that (with reference to the alleged recent fouling of Pymme's Brook by the Asylum) there was no truth in this charge; that no sewage had gone into the Brook for many months; and that the state of the stream has been improved by the effluent water from the Asylum. The sewage from the private houses was no doubt the cause of the fouling complained of – Mr Sheppard assured the Board that the Committee of the Asylum were most anxious to prevent any impure water going into the Brook – the Surveyor said there had been an improvement since he reported a fortnight ago – He was instructed to watch and report again if necessary."

A sad personal tragedy was reported in *Tottenham & Edmonton Weekly Herald, Southgate Messenger, North Middlesex & West Essex Advertiser* on 8 Oct 1875:

> "On Saturday Dr Hardwicke, Coroner, held an inquest at Colney Hatch upon the body of George Reeves, aged 46, who fell a distance of about 70 feet while filling the earth closet coppers at the Lunatic Asylum with mould. The accident occurred on the Thursday of the previous week and the injured man lingered for seven days afterwards. The jury returned a verdict of Accidental Death"

The problem with sewage was finally resolved when Friern Barnet Local Board opened a sewage works at Cromwell Road in 1898 to serve the whole district. The effluent from the hospital was thereafter safely treated and no further complaints were received.

Whilst it is easy in hindsight to criticise the asylum for its seemingly unneighbourly behaviour, it should be remembered that sanitary conditions in London at this time were

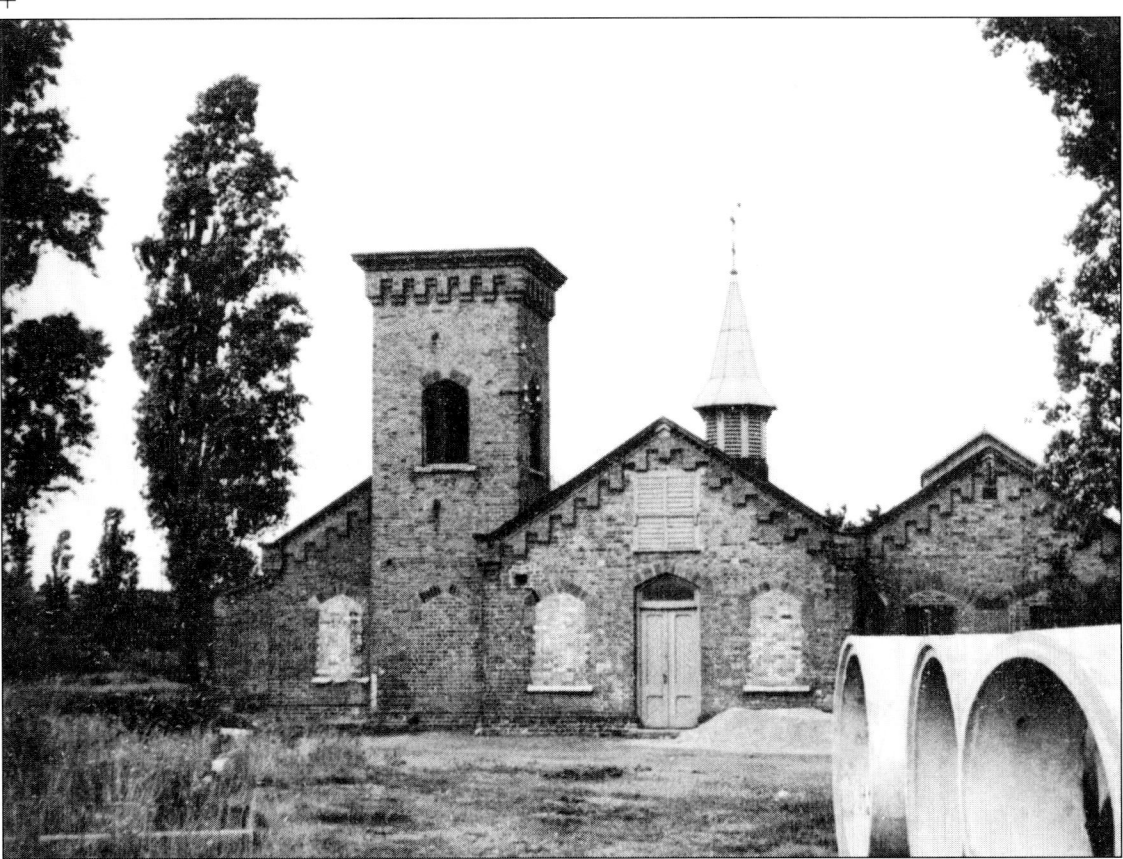

The Friern Barnet UDC Sewage Treatment Works at Cromwell Road.
This photo was taken shortly after it closed in 1962. (John Donovan)

generally awful; most of London's sewage was dumped directly into the Thames which became polluted and malodorous. Diseases such as typhoid and cholera were rife and it was not until it was realised that contaminated water was the cause that a remedy was looked for. In 1856 a new body, the Metropolitan Board of Works, was formed and it commissioned Sir Joseph Bazalgette to come up with a solution. A massive programme of works saw the creation of new sewers leading down to the Thames which emptied into larger sewers that ran parallel to the river. These in turn emptied into large settlement tanks at Dagenham and the liquid effluent was then piped into the Thames each day just after high water, which prevented it being carried upstream. After this London became a much healthier place.

CHAPTER SIX

Gas and Water

The asylum generated its own gas from coal which was transported by rail to Colney Hatch station and thence into the asylum. Trains would run into a siding running alongside the outer wall of the asylum and the trucks would be uncoupled and would be put one by one onto a turntable and then moved through a doorway in the wall, through a boiler house and onto another turntable that linked with rails which led down to the gas works at the south east corner of the grounds where there were two 30 foot gasholders and one of 50 feet.

Under an agreement between the Justices and the GNR on 27 March 1850 the asylum actually supplied both gas and water to Colney Hatch station. On 7 April 1852 the Station Master had reason to complain about the gas supply[1]:

> "On Saturday last the porter asked the gasman on duty to turn the gas on. After waiting a considerable time he went back and asked again and was challenged to a fight by the gasman. We must be properly supplied with gas when required. The lights in my office are almost nightly turned off before I leave it. Gas is turned off immediately after the 10 o'clock train."

The supply of gas to the railway was taken over in 1859 by the newly formed Southgate and Colney Hatch Gas Light & Coke Company which had built a gas works on the eastern side of the railway, opposite the asylum. Initially it had two small gas holders and produced about 1.5 million cubic feet of gas and possessed just 3 miles of mains and had only 65 consumers[2]

In February 1861 the *North Middlesex and Southgate Messenger* carried the following:

> "Misfortunes it is said seldom come alone, and in this instance the assertion has held good, for in the first week of the past month one or two accidents happened on this line of railway, but we believe without any peculiarly disastrous results – one of these occurred at the Colney Hatch Asylum, from the fracture of the tire of a wheel attached to a luggage train when passing the station, and although it was midnight when it happened, considerably impeded the traffic for several hours on the following day. The most disastrous affair, however, occurred at about 7pm on January 10th when, as the train was about to leave the station for King's Cross, an explosion of gas took place, to the imminent risk of the passengers, fortunately as far as the train and those attached to it were concerned, the guard only was slightly injured, and the window of an unoccupied compartment of a first class carriage demolished. Upon examination however of the premises, a very different state of affairs presented themselves, the roof of the gentlemen's waiting room, in which several persons had been sitting prior to the arrival of the train, had entirely disappeared, while the room was found in a state of indescribable confusion; the furniture therein having been destroyed and lying in the midst of bricks, rafters and rubbish; the porters room which adjoined, had also been severely shook and rendered unsafe, while the partition wall on the side dividing the waiting room from the Station master's apartments, was rent open nearly from end to end, and as we understand, so violent was the shock, that it instantly deposited the occupant on the opposite side of the room, in a most unceremonious manner It fortunately happened that a gas fitter who had been at work during the day for the Southgate and Colney Hatch Gas Company, had taken his seat in the train at the time the explosion occurred, and having immediately alighted, he took the measures to cut off the communication in the main – but nevertheless the gas with

which the main and the room was charged become ignited, and considerable exertions had to be used to subdue the fire. Recent examination has led to suppose that the action of frost must have had some effect upon the iron, for the main was found split in one or two places where the escape had occurred, and that almost immediately under the platform – probably assisted by the vibration of the trains passing to and fro.

It is perhaps necessary to state that the Railway Station is supplied with gas from the works of the Colney Hatch Asylum; rumour ever busy, immediately having been asserted that the accident was connected with the Southgate and Colney Hatch Gas Works: at the same we take the opportunity of observing, that notwithstanding the severity of the weather, and consequently the increased amount of labour which has been entailed, these works were never in a more efficient state, and this must be solely attributed to the characteristic watchfulness, combined with order and regularity, which has been exercised by the individual in charge."

In August 1861 the same paper reported that the Asylum had helped out yet again:

"On Thursday July 18th, a fire, which might have been terminated in a serious manner, broke out on the line of the Great Northern Railway. Along the embankment on the London side of the Colney Hatch Station, and parallel with the Southgate and Colney Hatch Gas Works, a quantity of railway sleepers have been stacked for some few months past. On the morning named, between 9 and 10 o'clock, it was discovered that one or more of these stacks had been ignited (as supposed by a spark from an engine) and from the inflammable character of the timber, being imbued with tar, it quickly extended from stack to stack, to the number of seven, and covered a space of upwards of twenty yards in length, and four or five in breadth, the whole of which were at one time blazing away together. The fire engine from the asylum was quickly brought to the spot, and run along the line of the railway, the hose being put to the tank of the Gas Works, but as the machine refused to work in that quarter, it was found requisite to run it down the embankment into the yard of the Southgate and Colney Hatch Gas works, and after sundry oilings &c, was ultimately brought to play with good effect. In the interim an engine was brought from London, per railway, and obtained a supply of fluid from the tank in which the refuse of the Colney Hatch Asylum is deposited. By one o'clock all danger had ceased, but as the wind was blowing the whole time from the west quarter, the charcoal, ashes, smoke and sparks were all carried on to the buildings of the Gas Company, the gas holder being sufficiently heated as to rarify the gas, and cause it to rise some inches out of the tank.

Upon examination, after the danger had ceased, the Board room and dwelling house of the man in charge, together with the adjoining premises, showed that the ashes had penetrated to the most remote corners. In order to prevent a recurrence we think that the salvage which has been re-stacked, together with the portion not injured should be at once removed, as it is not impossible for it to again take fire, and perhaps with more disastrous results than on the present occasion."

In 1927 a recommendation was made by the Commissioners that electricity should be installed in the hospital and this was eventually completed in 1935 at a cost of £22,500. The hospital continued to produce its own gas for cooking and heating until 1933 after which it got its supply from the Southgate and District Gas Company which had taken over from the previous gas company. The gasworks was then demolished.

As part of the initial investigations to see if the Colney Hatch site was suitable, a trial bore hole was made in 1848 to verify that water was available. The company responsible for the exploration reported that the geology consisted of 12 feet of yellowish brown clay; then 98 feet of blue clay; the next 1 foot 6 inches was stone, then 30 feet of hard coloured clay; and then 23 feet of pebbles and sand charged with water to the chalk, making a total to the surface of 188 feet 6 inches. They estimated that 200,000 gallons a day could be drawn from any well bored and that the water "is of most excellent quality and rises to within 109 feet of the surface."[3]

Water was drawn up by steam driven pumps in an engine house situated to the north west of the site at such a height above the level of the asylum building that the flow of water was assisted by gravity. The water was first stored under the engine house in a 9 feet deep reservoir where it was settled before being transferred to the main asylum building on the west side, the female wing, via a 4 inch main which then increased to 5 inches on the eastern side. To the south of the building water was supplied to the farm by a 2½ inch main and to the carpenters' yard by a 2 inch main and then down to the gas works by a 1 inch main and was transferred by pipe to the east wing. After some years, tanks were installed in the dome of the main building to increase the supply.

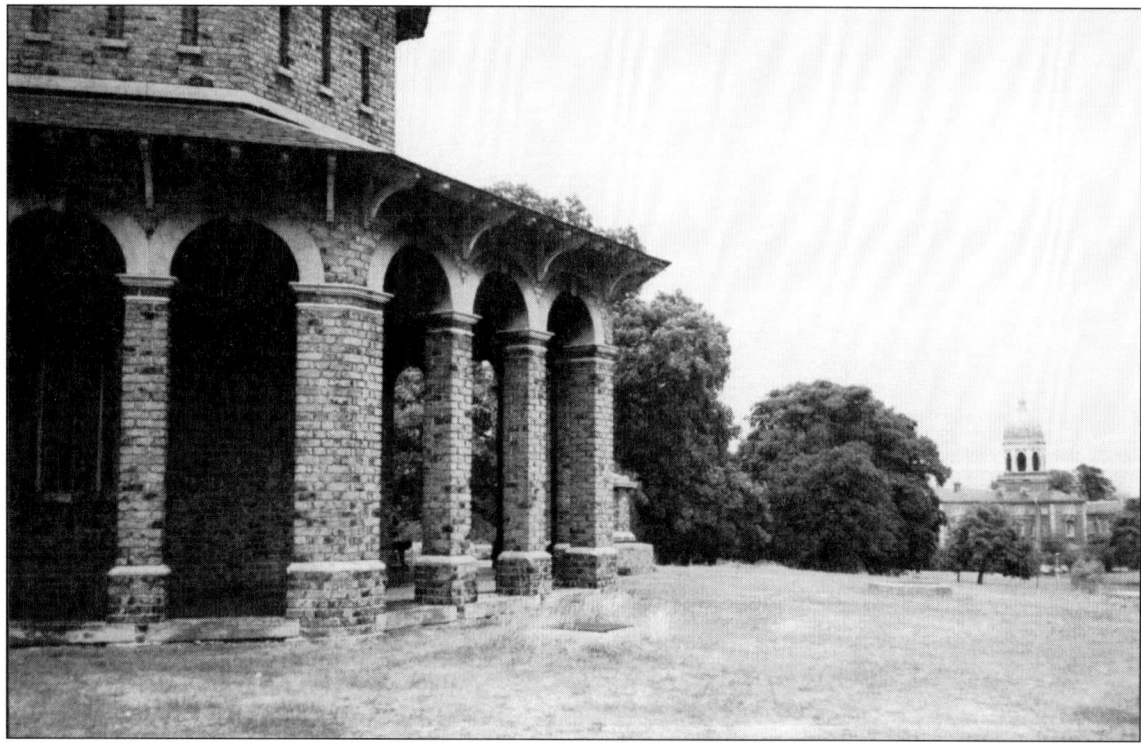

The pump house was higher than the main building, the dome of which can be seen on the right. (Barnet Local Studies)

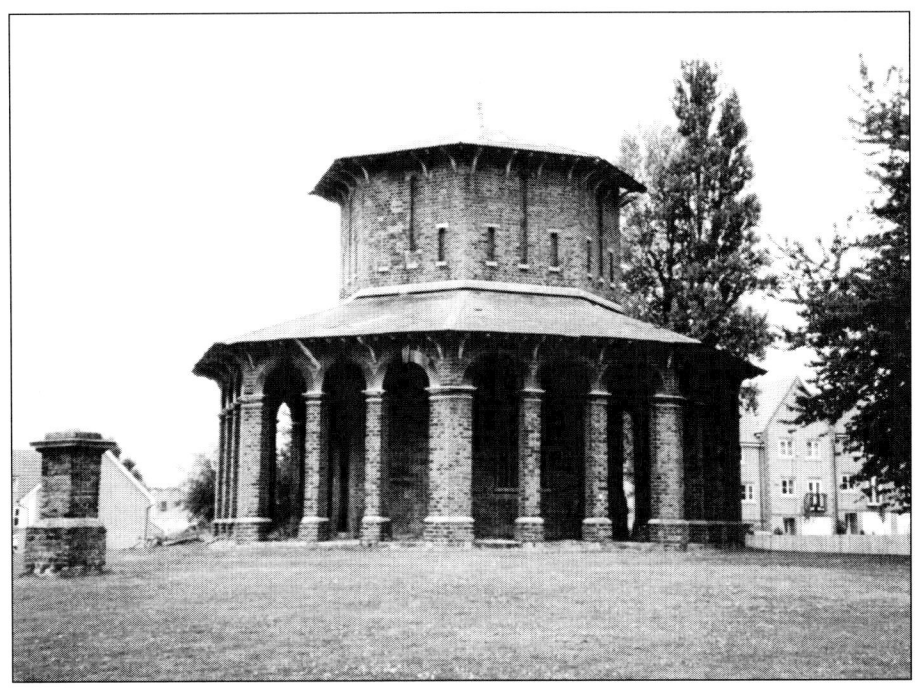

The pump house was an elegantly designed building. (Author)

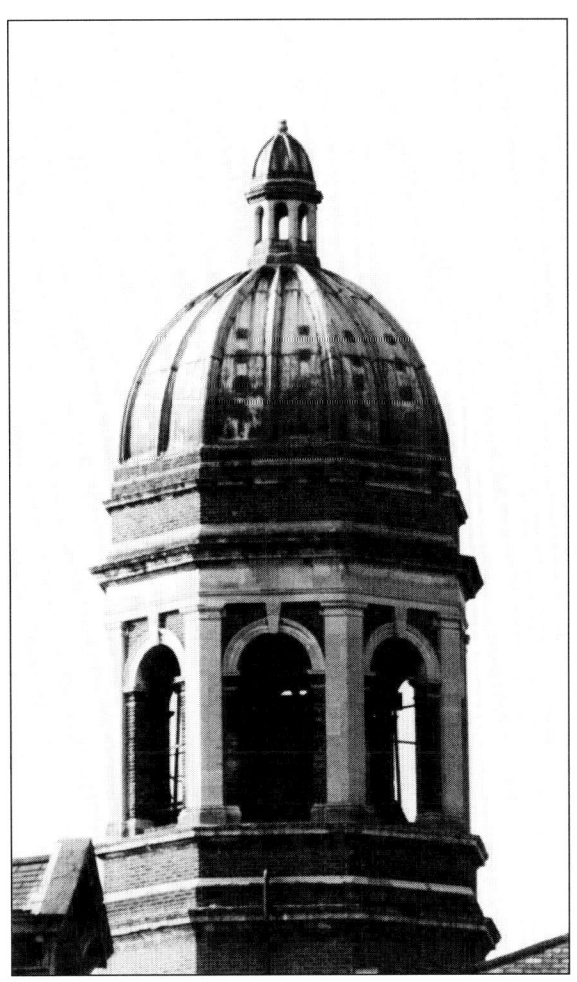

Water tanks were installed in the dome
after the fire of 1903. (Mark Wickwar)

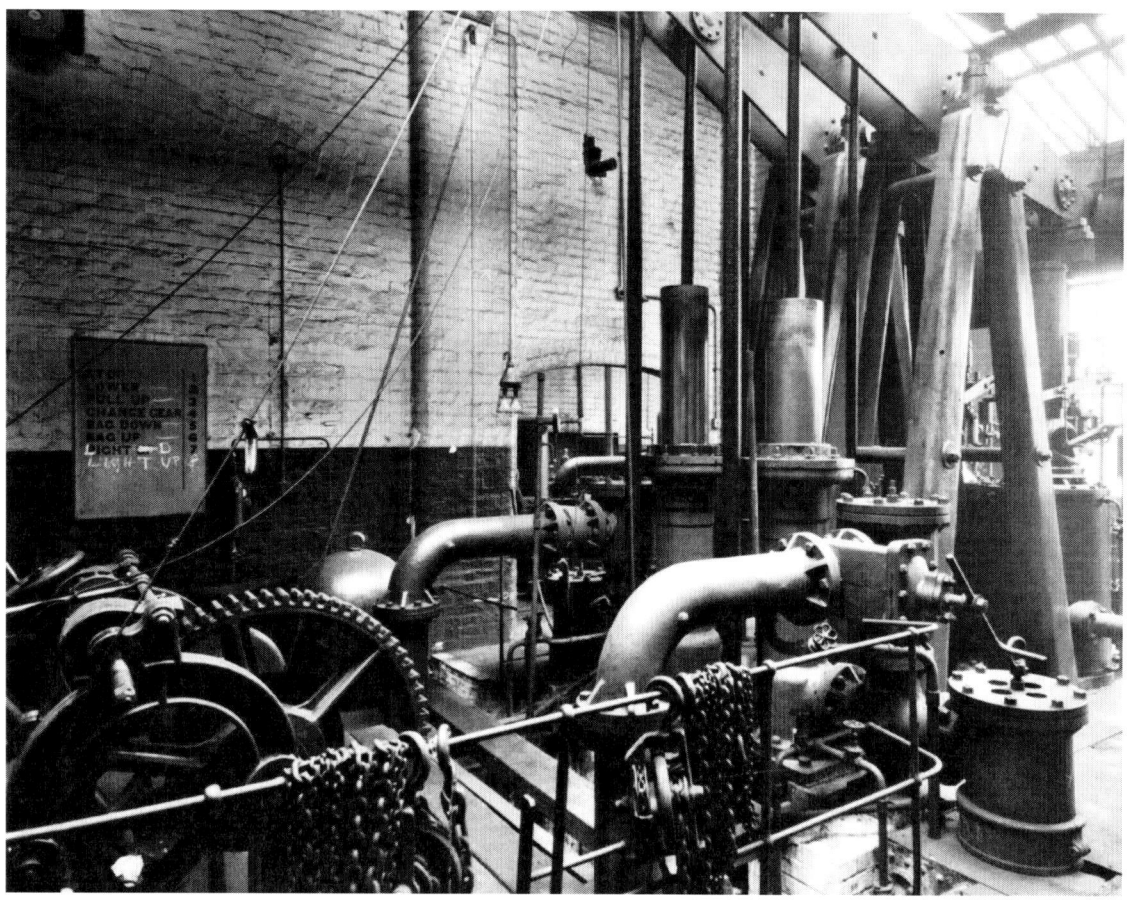

Well machinery photographed in 1938. (City of London. London Metropolitan Archives)

CHAPTER SEVEN

The Early Days

When it first opened the asylum had accommodation for 1036 patients, 428 males and 564 females plus 44 in the infirmaries and by the end of 1852 it had grown to 1244 patients, 515 male and 729 female, and they were being looked after by 18 officers, including two Resident Medical Officers and 72 male servants and 74 female servants. Together with administrative posts the staff totalled 164 and the annual wage bill amounted to £5,458 12s. 0d.

On 28 July 1851 the first death was recorded at the asylum when Catherine Doudan, alias Regan, a pauper, died of congestion of the brain and lungs during a fit of epilepsy[1]. There were more than 45 more deaths recorded within the first six months of opening. The first baby to be born to inmates was an ungiven-name boy to Jane and James Browning, of no known occupation, on 9 April 1852.

The asylum was administered by a committee of Visiting Justices known as the Committee of Visitors who spent a week every year thoroughly inspecting the asylum. They produced annual reports every January; these were very detailed and ran to over 200 pages. The introduction to the 1876 report gives an idea how comprehensive their work was:

> "We have, on the days above referred to (26-30 June 1876) made our annual statutory visit to this asylum, for inspection, inquiry and report. We have, as usual, seen every patient in residence, identifying each person with a name on the register, conversing with many (especially the convalescent), listening to all complaints brought forward, and looking into the patients' general treatment and accommodation. In the discharge of these duties we have, accompanied by the medical staff, visited each ward in both divisions, the offices, chapel and workshops."

Not surprisingly, these reports often led to disagreements between the Commissioners and the asylum's management committee. Whilst the annual reports were extremely comprehensive, they only gave a snapshot of conditions and could not take into account the daily problems involved in running such a huge enterprise.

A number of high profile cases of people being wrongly committed to lunatic asylums led in 1858 to pressure from the public at large and from newspapers and organisations such as the Alleged Lunatics' Friend Society for a public inquiry to investigate. Wilkie Collins' capitalised on this disquiet with his popular novel *The Woman in White,* initially published in serial form in 1859, which centred round a woman who had been wrongfully incarcerated in an asylum.

At that time, of course, knowledge of the causes of so-called lunacy was very slim and doctors put forward various reasons for it. In 1852 a Henry Hollan suggested that it was all based on dreams[2]:

> "If it were an object to obtain a description of insanity, which might apply to the greater number of cases of such disorder, I believe this would be found in the conditions which most associate it with dreaming; viz, the loss, partial or complete, of the power to distinguish between unreal images created within the sensorium and the actual perceptions drawn from the external senses, thereby giving to the former the semblance and influence of realities – and secondly, the alteration or suspension of that faculty of mind by which we arrange and associate the perceptions and thoughts successively coming before us"

As well as the enlargements of the asylum, a number of changes were made to the interior as time progressed. When it was built there was no interior decoration and almost all of the wards had no curtains. In 1857 curtains and blinds were installed in the galleries, recesses and Day Rooms and work started on painting the wards blue and white. This may seem an odd choice of colour – yellow would have been more cheerful – but it was widely considered at the time that flies were repelled by the colour blue and many kitchens in country houses were painted in this colour. In 1860 gas cooking ranges were introduced and the open fireplaces in the kitchens were done away with. In the same year the first washing machine was installed in the laundry and work was started on building a high wall around the hospital grounds. In 1865 a two-storey convalescent home and Fever Infirmary for females was opened. With the main building plus residences, offices, farm buildings, airing courts, a laundry and gas and water works, yards and lodges there were 20 acres of buildings on the site and including the burial ground, kitchen garden and other land the total area was 119 acres. The farm covered an additional 10 acres.

In 1873 the cemetery ceased to be used as a burial place and from that date bodies were buried in the Great Northern Cemetery which had been built in 1861 in Brunswick Park Road. A cross was later erected on the site in the grounds of the asylum with this inscription:

> In this Sacred Ground
> Has Been Interred
> The Remains of 2,696 Inmates of this Asylum
> And this Monument
> Has Been Erected
> To Their Memory
> By the Committee of Visitors
> 1883

The area covered by the asylum cemetery was comparatively small and it is possible the bodies would have been buried in an upright position to save space; this was not an uncommon practice where pauper burials were concerned. A simple calculation shows that burials had been taking place at the rate of over two a week.

The name Colney Hatch originally referred to the tiny hamlet at the junction around Friern Barnet Lane and Colney Hatch Lane, but it was later used to describe the development of houses to the east of the railway line in the 1860s, which was named Colney Hatch Park. Once the name Colney Hatch became synonymous with the asylum, people from outside the area were reluctant to move there. Pressure from local residents forced the authorities to change the name and they opted for New Southgate, although it had no connection with the nearby "old" Southgate[3].

The railway station had opened in 1850 as Colney Hatch and Southgate. In 1855 it changed to Southgate and Colney Hatch and in 1876 it then became New Southgate and Colney Hatch. The name Colney Hatch was dropped altogether in 1923 when it was renamed New Southgate and Friern Barnet.

In 1852 the asylum received a letter from Robert Morris, Rector of Friern Barnet, explaining that the parish was undergoing considerable alterations as a result of the opening of the railway and the building of the asylum and there was therefore an increase in the size of his congregations, particularly as families of the attendants at the asylum were coming to church. His appeal for funds to help cope with this was, not surprisingly, turned down by the Asylum Committee[4] but it did highlight the effect that the asylum was having on the area.

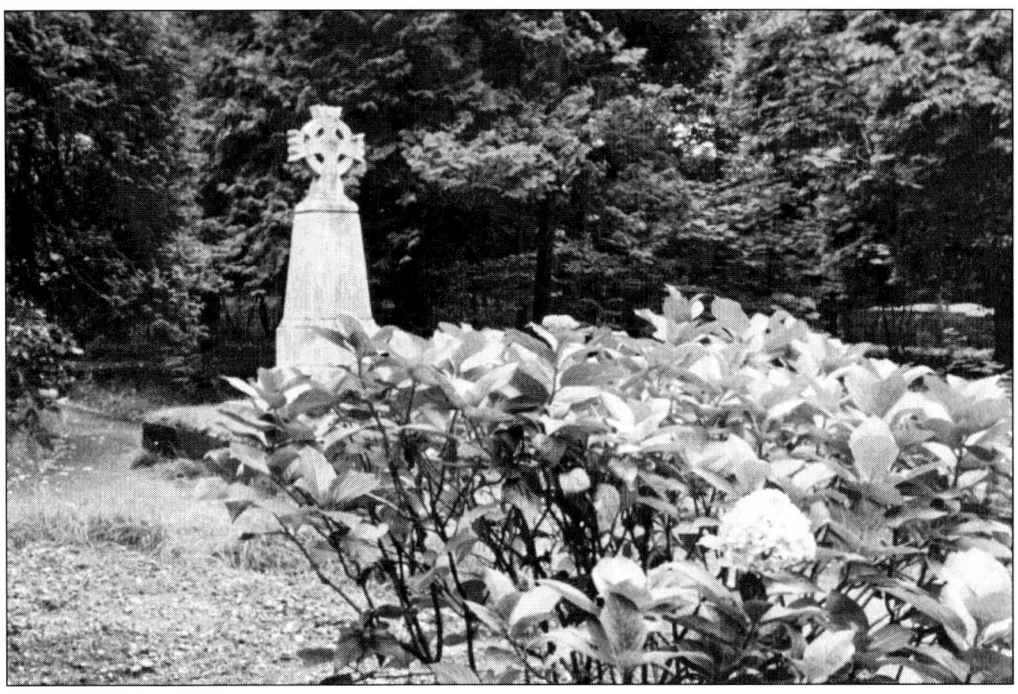

The cross (above) was later removed and replaced with a simple marker.
(by kind permission of the Royal Society of Medicine)

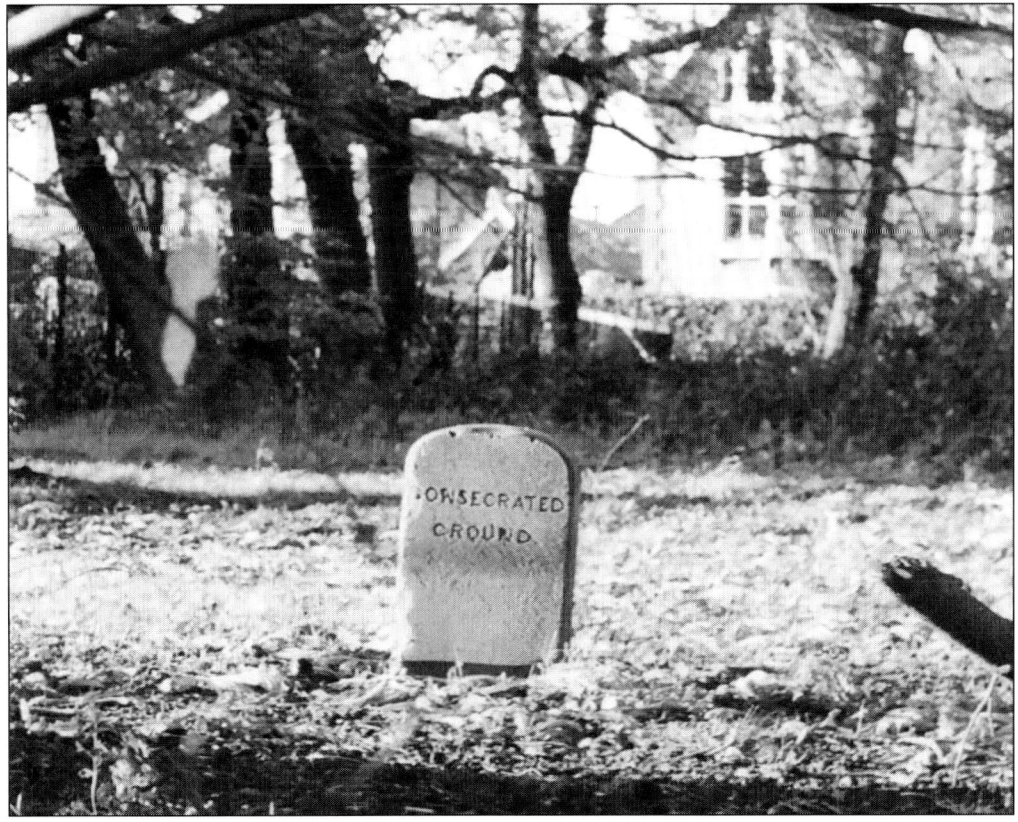

The marker. (Colin Barratt)

CHAPTER EIGHT

Housekeeping

The Victorians kept meticulous records from which we can get a glimpse of just how big an operation the running of an asylum the size of Friern was.

The accounts for 11 August 1852[1], when there were 1236 patients in residence, give an idea of the kind of expenditure involved in running the asylum:

	£	s	d
W Carr - Cheesemongery	282	8	6
Capper & Gray - Grocery	84	19	10
Layton Hulbert & Co - Tea	168	1	2
Charnely & Abraham – Wines & c	164	4	6
Reid & Co – Beer	36	2	6
Paton & Charles – Soap	7	0	0
William Clark – Grocery	180	18	4
Pinchin & Johnson – Oilman's Stores	86	6	5
Thomas Wood & Co – Coals	264	12	0
H & J White – Tobacco & Snuff	64	15	7
R Russell – Coffins	24	14	6
J Lyne – Brushes & Brooms	18	2	9
G Reynell – Advertising	54	12	5
J & A Bradley – China & Glass	14	6	11
E Jones & Sons – Drapery	142	3	6
G & M Pooley – Hay & Straw	44	4	6
Henry Young	15	12	0
Bruce Johnson – Livestock	89	16	0
J Butt – Harness &c	13	4	9
J Davis – Potatoes, Hay &c	202	17	5
W Patten	69	17	7
J A Granley – Bricks	32	16	0
	£2075	**18**	**8**

The provisions consumed in 1858, when the asylum had grown to 1295 with 145 staff, were as follows[2]

Bacon	5,241 *lbs*
Beef and mutton	198,285 *lbs*
Pork	10,816 *lbs*
Beer	69,742 *gallons*
Bread	430,241 *lbs*
Butter	18,443 *lbs*
Cheese	36,577 *lbs*
Cocoa	13,290 *lbs*
Eggs	5,680
Flour	431,843 *lbs*
Milk	19,587 *gallons*
Hops	367 *lbs*
Potatoes	245,286 *lbs*
Sugar	21,640 *lbs*
Tea	5,284 *lbs*
Treacle	27,332 *lbs*

Sick patients consumed the following:

Wine	91,320 *oz*
Brandy	10,392 *oz*
Gin	10,392 *oz*
Porter and Ale	34,400 *pints*
Fish	15,330
Biscuits	12,775
Eggs	16,618

The dietary requirements of the large number of Jewish patients were provided for by the purchase of kosher food supplied by suitable outside companies.

By 1950 the kitchens were supplying 64,000 meals to patients and 9400 to staff every week[7], an average of some 10,000 a day. With a very limited budget it is not surprising that there were complaints about the quality of the food, as this letter from January 1890[6] shows:

> "Patients (Females): The fresh beef on Sundays and Fridays is almost invariably hard and generally wanting in flavour. The patients very aptly term it "old cow" On Thursdays the Canadian pork is much disliked and a large proportion of patients will not eat it. The fish and rice dinner is very tasteless and at the best is not satisfying. I would suggest that potatoes be served instead of rice also that bread and cheese be allowed after a fish dinner. Head Attendants and Nurses: Baked mutton makes a good dinner but when it is served 5 or 6 days a week (as I am told it is) is apt to pall and disagree. Very many of the nurses suffer from indigestion, due in part, I believe to the monotony of the diet. The quantity is sufficient. Assistant Medical Officers: The improvement in eggs and cheese is much needed. Except for some six weeks in the year the eggs are always foreign and very musty and are rarely eatable. Even half the quantity on new laid eggs would be much appreciated. The cheese that is served is the same as that for the patients."

For the first seventy years the patients' daily meals were:

Breakfast	*Dinner*	*Supper*
6oz bread	7oz uncooked meat	6oz bread
1 pint cocoa	4oz dumplings	2oz cheese
½ pint beer	12oz vegetables	½ pint beer
	10oz pie (Saturdays)	
	14oz stew (Thursdays)	
	1 pint soup (Mondays)	

One pint of cocoa comprised ½ pint cocoa, 1oz treacle, and ¼ pint milk.

Soup for 900 patients comprised 112lbs of leg and shin of beef, 60lbs of peas, 50 lbs of rice, 20 lbs Scotch barley, 40 lbs onions, salt, pepper and herbs

Stew for 900 patients comprised 112lbs of meat, 560 lbs of potatoes, 120 lbs onions, salt and pepper

Until 1921 the meals were always served in the same way[8] - patients ate at long forms and bare tables with no table cloths. At breakfast, a basin was used for porridge and then for tea or coffee; bread and butter was placed on the tables for those who could sit up, or on the bed clothes, or on chairs by the bed for those unable to get up.

Dinner was served in a basin or a tin pannikin, with pudding on the saucer. Meat was served already cut up and was eaten with a spoon – knives and forks were not provided until after 1921. From this date drinking glasses were provided and bread was cut up into thin slices rather than large chunks, and butter and jam was placed on small plates and spread with a knife provided for the purpose.

The farm occupied the southern part of the site and helped to make the asylum virtually self sufficient in milk, meat, vegetables and eggs. In 1851 there was a cow-house for 23 cows, calf pens, dairies, piggeries, stabling loose-boxes, cattle and cart sheds, a slaughter house and a cowman's residence.[3] The farm was enlarged in 1859 to include additional space for cows, which would then number 36. It was calculated that in 1854 the cost of keeping a cow was roughly the same as for a patient. The livestock would sometimes have been obtained from local farmers as Committee minutes in 1923[4] showed:

> Purchased from Mr Morley of Gallants Farm 2 freshly calved cows at £44.10 each and average daily yield of milk was 18 quarts each.

Pigs, and 200 sheep, were also kept on the farm and the crops included wheat, potatoes, clover, mangold wurzells (for cattle feed), cabbages, onions and rye In the years when surpluses were produced, these were sold to other asylums and helped to produce a profit in most years.

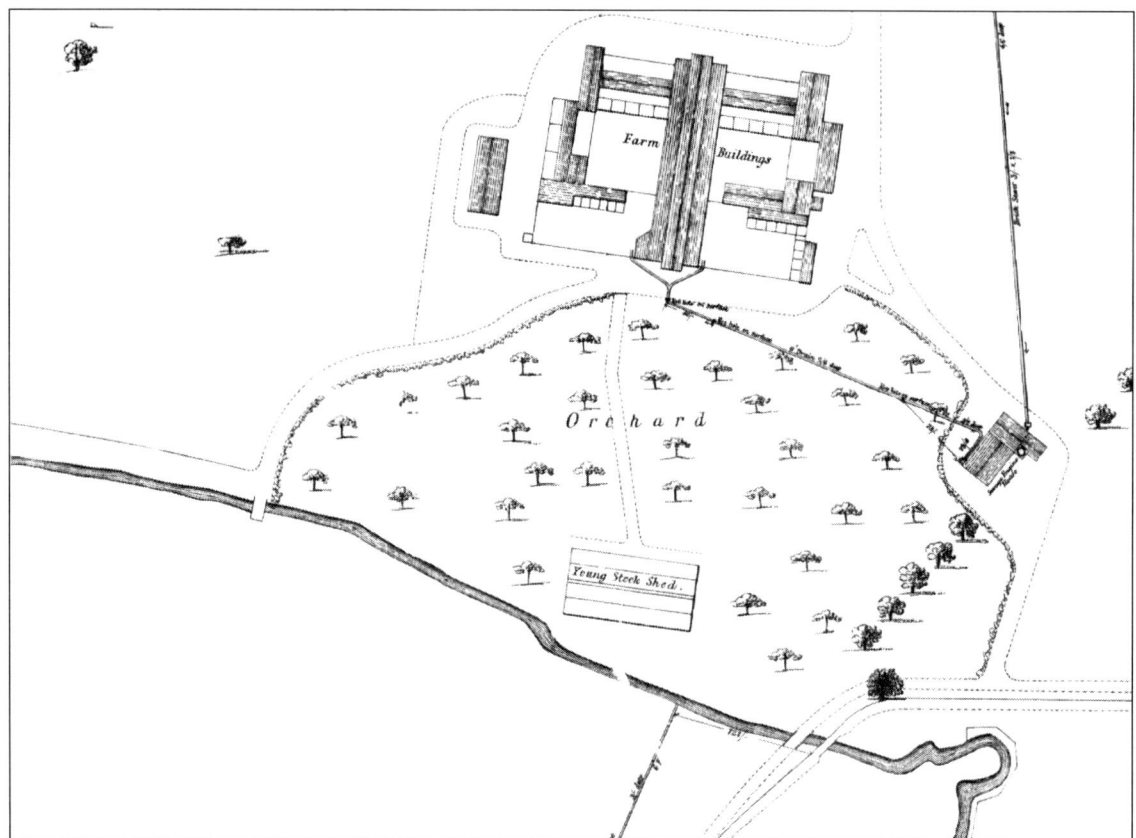

The farm buildings were situated on the southern end of the site.
Bounds Green Brook runs west to east along the bottom, just below the orchard.
(Barnet Local Studies)

A bacon curing plant was installed in 1912 and a milk cooling shed was also built. The asylum was also supplied with fruit from the orchard which was situated to the south of the farm buildings and adjacent to Bounds Green Brook.

A report in June 1918[5] reported;

> Inmates of the asylum are entirely kept in vegetables except 4 months potato supply and large quantities of meat, fruit, milk, rabbits etc are supplied. This farm is an example of what can be done on the heavy clay lands of Middlesex when properly tilled. Many nooks and corners, formerly lawns etc have been made full use of by planting sunflowers, artichokes etc. Sports grounds are temporarily abandoned as such and used for food production.

It seems surprising today but patients were issued with two pints of beer a day at dinner and was much appreciated. Initially this had been supplied by a firm of wine merchants but from 1852 the Asylum had its own brewery which lasted until 1890 when the LCC had taken over the running of the asylum and decided to replace this with milk which was served with lunch. The Commissioners in Lunacy, however, were opposed to the withdrawal of beer as they felt that while some patients were intemperate, the majority would only benefit from it, particularly those who worked in the laundry or on the farm.[9]

In the early days the male patients were dressed in corduroy suits except for when attending Church or any function when they were expected to wear their best suits or boots. Very few patients had been issued with underclothes and socks were seldom darned, except by the few patients who knew how to darn their own. After 1921 patients were gradually issued with tweed suits and they were expected to wear these, together with boots, when attending church or special functions

Nearly all the male patients wore beards, which was the fashion anyway, and their hair was closely cropped. Later, shaving kits were issued to those patients who could be trusted.

CHAPTER NINE

Patients

The 1852 Annual Report gave the breakdown for patients admitted that year, from which it can be seen that the majority were from the working class:

ADMISSIONS 1852

Occupation	No.	%	Occupation	No.	%
Labourers	30	8.60%	Horse jockey	1	0.29%
Servants	15	4.30%	Accountant	1	0.29%
Boot & shoe makers	14	4.01%	Parliamentary agent	1	0.29%
Painters & glaziers	12	3.44%	Surgeon	1	0.29%
Tailors	12	3.44%	Medical student	1	0.29%
Carpenters	10	2.87%	Commercial traveller	1	0.29%
Merchants clerks	10	2.87%	Goldbeater	1	0.29%
Porters	10	2.87%	Looking-glass silverer	1	0.29%
Soldiers & pensioners	9	2.58%	Stonemason	1	0.29%
Hawkers	8	2.29%	Gas fitter	1	0.29%
Law writers & clerks	7	2.01%	Type founder	1	0.29%
Nurserymen & gardeners	7	2.01%	Bookbinder	1	0.29%
Mariners	7	2.01%	Brush maker	1	0.29%
Bricklayers	6	1.72%	Sealing wax maker	1	0.29%
Silk weavers	6	1.72%	Chairmaker	1	0.29%
Bakers	5	1.43%	Copper scourer	1	0.29%
Cabmen & conductors	5	1.43%	French polisher	1	0.29%
Booksellers & stationers	4	1.15%	Tin plate worker	1	0.29%
Cabinet makers	4	1.15%	Mother of pearl worker	1	0.29%
Compositors & printers	4	1.15%	Uhl cutter	1	0.29%
Stablemen	4	1.15%	Hairdresser	1	0.29%
Drapers & haberdashers	3	0.86%	Stamper	1	0.29%
Artists	3	0.86%	Engine driver	1	0.29%
Hotel keepers & publicans	3	0.86%	Brass finisher	1	0.29%
Watchmakers	3	0.86%	Brass maker	1	0.29%
Corn-chandlers	3	0.86%	Dyer	1	0.29%
Coachmakers	3	0.86%	Turner	1	0.29%
Coopers	3	0.86%	Pavior	1	0.29%
Engravers	3	0.86%	Musician	1	0.29%
Coal porters	3	0.86%	Farrier	1	0.29%
Chimney sweeps	3	0.86%	Soap boiler	1	0.29%
Sadlers & harness makers	2	0.57%	Comb maker	1	0.29%
Wire workers	2	0.57%	Toll collector	1	0.29%
Shipwrights & boat builders	2	0.57%	Milkman	1	0.29%
Blacksmiths	2	0.57%	Green grocer	1	0.29%
Curriers	2	0.57%	Fancy leather worker	1	0.29%
Wheelwrights	2	0.57%	Fishing tackle maker	1	0.29%
Custom & excise officers	2	0.57%	Stays cottoner	1	0.29%
Cork cutters	2	0.57%	Grave digger	1	0.29%
Costermongers	2	0.57%	Furniture broker	1	0.29%
Pocket-book makers	2	0.57%	Bristle sorter	1	0.29%
Whip makers	2	0.57%	Brickmaker	1	0.29%
Jewellers	2	0.57%	Clock case maker	1	0.29%
Paper hangers	2	0.57%	Glass cutter	1	0.29%
Butchers	2	0.57%	Plasterer	1	0.29%
Fishmongers	2	0.57%	Policeman	1	0.29%
Architects & builders	2	0.57%	Dustman	1	0.29%
Merchants clerks	1	0.29%	Others	47	13.47%
Boot finisher	1	0.29%		349	100.00%

Building Trade	18.93%		Domestic	5.45%
Retail	16.05%		Printing	3.16%
Manufacturing	15.24%		Other	35.13%
Clerical	6.04%			100.00%

It is important to remember that the asylum was originally set up to deal with *pauper* lunatics, who had previously been incarcerated in workhouses. The Committee, in commenting on an Annual Report from the Commissioners in Lunacy which had called for additional comforts for the inmates, said:

> "The Commissioners do not appear sufficiently to bear in mind the fact that the Colney Hatch Asylum is established for Pauper Lunatics only, and that many luxuries and appliances suggested by them are quite unsuited for that class of patients, and could not be provided but at a cost which would be most justly complained of by the Parishes chargeable for their support, and which would, even if granted to the patients during their residence in the Asylum, tend to aggravate the distress of those discharged as recovered, who on their return to their homes and former condition would have to forego those comforts which by long use had become almost necessary."

Nevertheless, the conditions at Colney Hatch were superior to those of lunatic patients in workhouses. Charles Hood, Physician to the Male Department at Colney Hatch described the condition of four patients received from the Clerkenwell Workhouse in 1852.[1]

> ".....they were admitted in an emaciated, dirty, and neglected state. Two of them were tightly restrained by strait-waistcoats, worn under a coat, so as to prevent any use of their arms and hands. One was in a most miserable state of bodily suffering, having extended bed-sores, and a large angry-looking blister on the nape of his neck; this, unprotected by lint or dressing from the irritation caused by a dirty, coarse, patched shirt. The poor fellow at first showed some disinclination to proceed to his ward, but this difficulty arising entirely from fear on his part, and bodily suffering incident upon his sores, was, by a little encouragement, overcome, and within half an hour he was cleanly clad, his sores dressed. And expressions of gratitude escaped him."

The records are littered with reports on patients and their behaviour, but a few examples will give a flavour of what was happening. *The North Middlesex and Southgate Messenger* carried a report in July 1858:

> "On Saturday night, June 19, a patient in the County Lunatic Asylum, Colney Hatch, effected his escape from the establishment by making a hole through the wall of the building, eighteen inches in thickness, by means of a nail or similar instrument. The most singular part of the affair is yet unexplained, as to the manner in which he obtained his clothes – as each patient is locked in his sleeping apartment, and the clothes laid outside the door until the following morning. We hear that he was captured and taken to Marylebone Workhouse, and has since been safely housed in his old quarters, and is now labouring under a fit of mania."

The 3 March 1900 issue of *Barnet Press* carried the following:

> "Dr Danford Thomas, the Middlesex Coroner, held an inquest at the Colney Hatch Asylum on Saturday on Hyman Alberge, aged 41. Henry Rawlings, charge attendant, said that he found Alberge crouching by the door of the dormitory unconscious. Morris Cohen was sitting on the next bed. Alberge had both eyes black and closed. Cohen's hands were swollen and covered with blood. Joseph Goudge, night attendant, visited the room at 5.30 and found all the patients in bed except Cohn and the deceased, both of whom were sitting up. The eleven patients were locked in the room. Dr Seaward, Superintendent of the Asylum, said that Cohen was not of a quarrelsome disposition. Amos Nicholls, an inmate, said that he saw the two men struggling and heard blows. He thought the men were playing. Dr H J Tisard, medical officer, said that the death was due to syncope,

from shock, whilst suffering from a general paralysis. The jury found the verdict "Manslaughter" against Cohen whilst of unsound mind. As a rider, they emphasised the need for visits from the attendants at more frequent intervals than every one and a half to two hours, and suggested the advisability of some means of communication between the attendant and those in the dormitory."

The 29 September 1900 issue of *Barnet Press* carried the following:

"Particulars of some very remarkable incidents at Colney Hatch asylum for lunatics transpired on Saturday. It seems that as far back as February 11th 1871, Mrs McCann, who resides at 21 Sandycombe Road, Richmond, sent her father, Mr Gilbert Macaulay, to Colney Hatch Asylum. Till the beginning of the present month he was well and comfortable. On September 7th Mrs McCann received the following telegram, which had been handed in at New Southgate: "Your father is sinking fast. Seward"

Mrs McCann despatched a wire to the asylum authorities asking for further information and on September 10th she received a second telegram in these words: "Funeral Friday 11 o'clock. Letter follows. Colney Hatch" The second telegram was handed in at New Southgate at 11.17 on September 10th and on receipt of the tidings , which seemed to confirm their worst fears, Mr & Mrs McCann prepared for the funeral and the lady went out to order the mourning garments. She had no sooner returned home than she found a further telegram awaiting her, also dated September 10th and handed in at 12.12. This was as follows: "Please ignore previous telegram. Macaulay in the usual health. Superintendent. Colney Hatch" The letter which followed in due course was dated London County Asylum, Colney Hatch, N. September 10th and was in these terms: "Madam, when your telegram was replied to it concluded that your father, Gilbert Macaulay, was dead; but upon inquiry it was found not to be the case. In the event of his death, notice will at once be sent to you informing you of the day and time of his funeral. Yours faithfully, Robert Sterland, Acting Clerk of the Asylum"

Mr McCann then wrote for an explanation. In reply the subjoined letter was forwarded from Colney Hatch to his wife, dated September 15th, this being over three days after he had written: "Madam, if you call at the asylum tomorrow (Sunday) to visit your father, you will be able to see the medical superintendent on the subject you mention. Yours faithfully, Cecil F Beadles, Acting Medical Superintendent." On the same day (September 15th) a letter was despatched from Colney Hatch, signed "W J Seward" in which the writer regretted to inform Mrs McCann that her father had died at 6.30 that evening. The letter also stated that when Mrs McCann's first telegram was received the clerk at the office supposed he was dead and Mr Seward said he was sorry the mistake should ever have occurred. A printed form enclosed said that the cause of death was senile decay and exhaustion. Mrs McCann also received intimation that the funeral would take place at the Northern Cemetery at New Southgate on Friday at 11am precisely. The form likewise stated that the mourners wishing to see the deceased must be at the asylum at 10 o'clock on the morning of the day named. Mr & Mrs McCann arrived at the asylum a few minutes after ten o'clock. They found the body placed in the coffin and in the hearse and were subsequently unable to see the deceased. The deceased, it is stated, was an artist of no mean merit."

A report on 19 December 1919[2] stated:

"On the 13th at about 6.30pm Thomas Bradley, a patient in 12 ward made a determined attempt to escape from the Hospital under the following circumstances: He lowered himself from the scullery window of Ward 12 (where he was employed as a sculleryman) by means of a rope of his own construction made from patients neckties. Failing to judge the total height he fell into the Airing Court with violence and sustained a severe sprain of the right ankle with other bruises and abrasions. He was however able to scale the Airing Court wall with the assistance of a garden seat, but failed to get over the Boundary Wall. Suffering from severe pain he struggled round the building until he met the Head Night Nurse of the Villa, who immediately informed the Head Night Male Nurse. He was brought back to the Male side about 4am"

There was some criticism of the bathing arrangements as the provision of toilets was inadequate and the normal bathing facilities were considered unacceptable by the Commissioners in Lunacy. The supply of hot water was inadequate and about three men and from three to six women were bathed in the same water.[3] In fact it was not until 1883 that every patient was bathed in fresh water.

Among the many suspects in the notorious Jack the Ripper murders in Whitechapel between 1888 and 1891 were two people who were patients at Colney Hatch Asylum. Aaron Kosminski was a Polish Jew who was transferred to Colney Hatch in 1891 from an asylum in Mile End. He suffered from auditory hallucinations, had a dread of being fed by other people and refused either to wash or bathe. In 1894 Sir Neville Macnaughton, the Assistant Chief Constable, issued a memo in which he named one of the Ripper suspects as "Kosminski" whom he described as having a great hatred of women and having strong homicidal tendencies. The case notes at Colney Hatch indicate that he was not violent, although he did once brandish a chair at an attendant and threatened his sister with a knife. He died in the asylum March 1919.

David Cohen, another Polish Jew, was also a suspect. He was committed in December 1888 and was described as violently antisocial, exhibited destructive tendencies and had to be restrained. He died in October 1889 but it was never clearly established whether Cohen was his real name, as foreign names were often difficult to understand or spell and it may have been a generic name for a Jewish patient, much as "John Doe" is today for an unknown person.

One of the most fascinating patients at Friern was Dorothy Lawrence. Dorothy was born probably in 1888 and, having been abandoned by her mother was adopted by a guardian of the Church of England. She had an ambition to become a journalist, a rare occupation for a woman in the early days of the 20th century. She had a few articles published in *The Times* and at the outbreak of the First World War in 1914 she tried to become a war correspondent. Having been thwarted in this ambition in 1915 she went to France, managed to acquire a uniform and disguised herself as a man. She then managed to work her way into the Front Line and join the Royal Engineers 179 Tunnelling Company where she survived detection for ten days. She was eventually spotted, was detained in a French convent at St Loos and was court martialled. She was returned to England and wrote a book *Sapper Dorothy Lawrence: The Only English Woman Soldier* in 1919. She lived in Canonbury until 1925 when she claimed that she had been raped by her guardian. In what was almost certainly a cover-up she was declared insane and was committed to Colney Hatch Lunatic Asylum where she remained until her death on 29 August 1964.

In November 1854 new rules were posted on a board at the entrance gate and 1000 leaflets were printed for distribution to visitors.[4]

1. The Visiting days are Monday and Thursday in each week

2. After 1st January 1855 no Visitors to Patients will be admitted through the gates on Visiting days before 11 or after 2

3. Not more than two persons together will be allowed to see any one Patient, and no Patient will be allowed to see more than one party of Friends on any day without the special permission of the Medical Superintendent of the Department

4. No children in arms to be brought in

5. No gifts of Money, Food, or any other articles are to be brought to any Patient unless with the special written permission of the Medical Superintendent of the Department, and such gifts are in that case to be delivered to the Officer in Attendance and not to the Patient. And no Visitors are to partake of any Food either themselves or with a Patient during their visit

6. No Gratuities are to be given to the Attendants or Stewards

7. The Friends of Patients are recommended not to prolong their visits to them as long visits are injurious to the Patients

8. Any person committing a breach of any of these Regulations will not again be permitted to visit a Patient in the Asylum

The local Police would often become involved, as Richard Testar recalled:

"In the early 1980s I was a Police Inspector stationed at Golders Green. This was the Divisional Headquarters covering a large area, including New Southgate and Friern Barnet. I ran a team of police officers and worked early shift, evenings and nights. We had quite a heavy involvement with Friern, especially when patients went missing. They were obviously vulnerable and I did my best to deploy as many officers as I could to search the area once we had received a description from the Hospital. Generally it didn't take long to find them, and often it was the result of an emergency call from a member of the public who had seen the person acting irrationally. We would return the patient to the care of the hospital; we had to be aware, however, that not all patients were compliant, and some were enjoying their freedom and resented being detained. Strangely though, many mental patients had a liking for the Police; maybe we gave them a sense of security! I can recall finding missing patients wandering the streets in the middle of the night. Sometimes the hospital staff was not even aware they had escaped until we told them.

Friern Hospital seemed a sinister and unfriendly place at night and that long corridor and the poor lighting added to the sense of spookiness. On more than one occasion I can recall returning a patient to the Hospital at night and to be greeted by the duty orderly, only to realise that the person was not a member of staff at all, but another patient – on one occasion he was even wearing a white coat!

One evening I was called to Friern where a patient had died. I went with a newly trained policewoman, and found that the deceased, a young woman, had been placed in a small side room. It was very hot in the room, and I remember the policewoman asking to be excused as she feared she would faint. As I remember, the deceased had recently returned to the Hospital after some form of home leave,

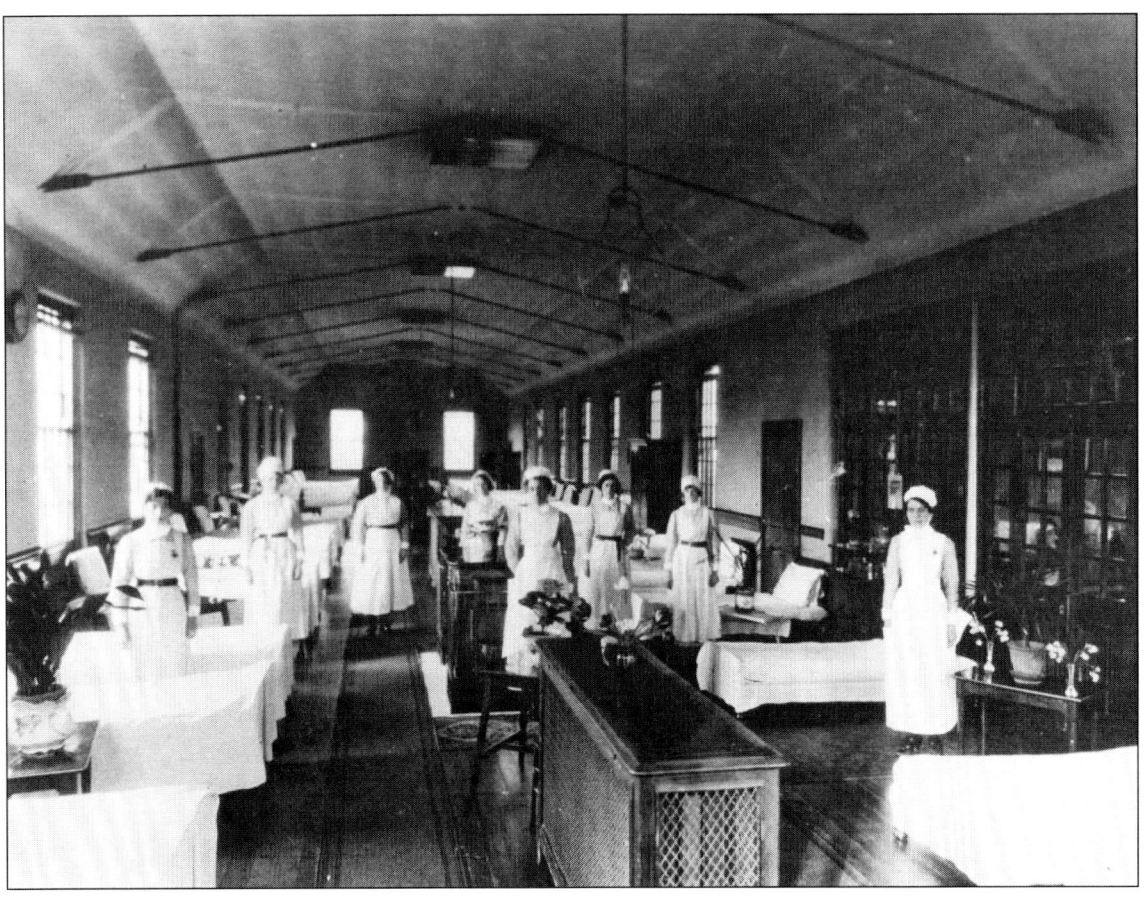
An open ward   (Barnet Local Studies)

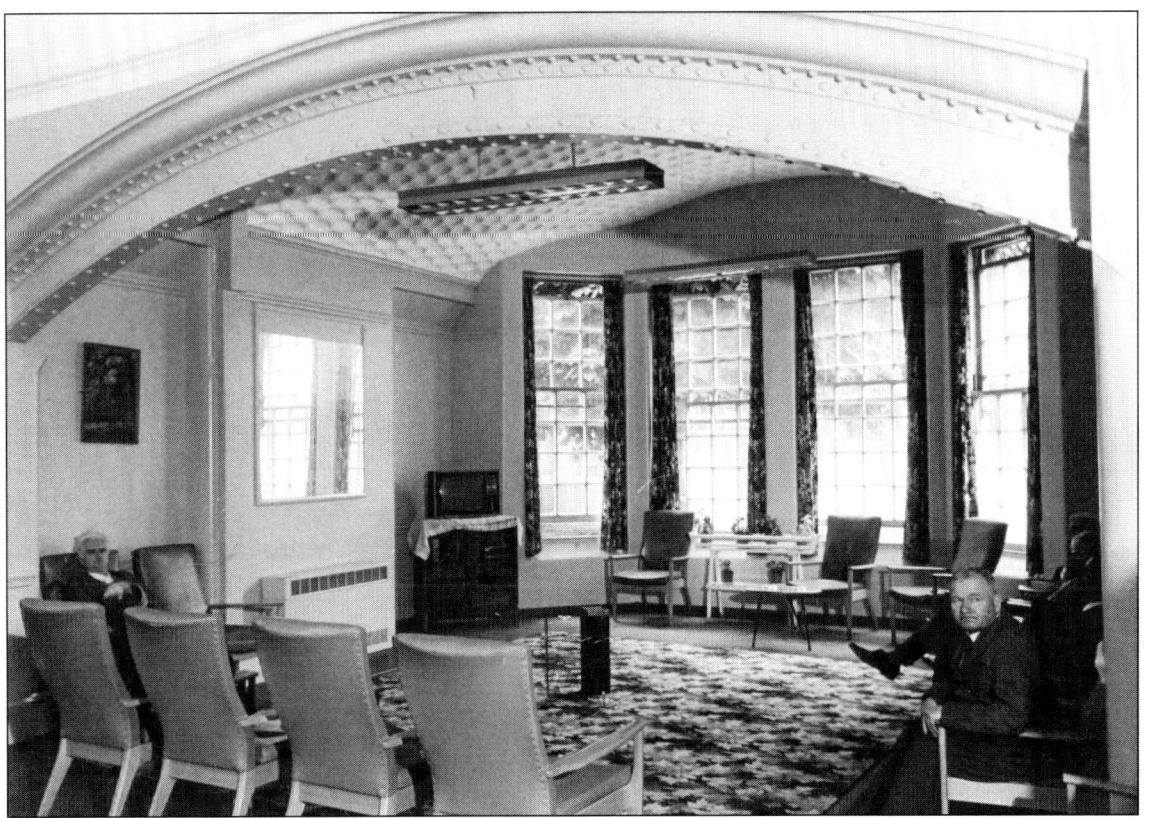
The patients' lounge, with its distinctive honeycomb ceiling, photographed in 1973.
(by kind permission of The Royal Society of Medicine)

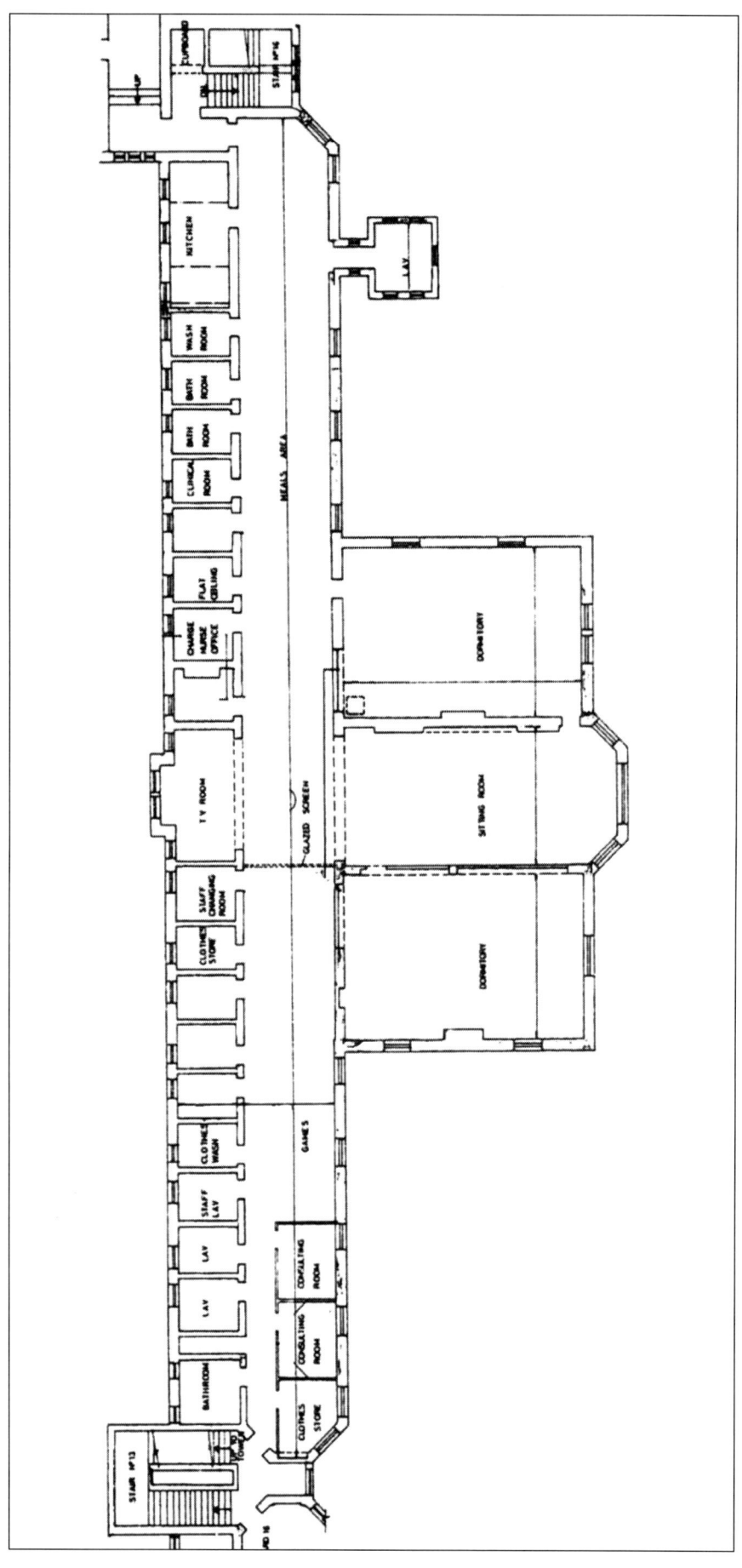

Layout of a first floor ward, Ward 15, in 1982.
(Royal Free Hospital Archives)

and her sudden death naturally aroused the suspicions of the hospital staff, as bruises could be seen on her body. She was examined by a police surgeon who declared that the bruises were not caused by violence, but the normal effect of death where the blood ceases to flow round the body. The local CID was called however, although after investigation, the verdict was "death by natural causes."

I was told there was a padded cell at Friern, although I never saw this, but I clearly remember the padded cell at St Bernard's at Southall. This had a high ceiling, large brown leathery pads fixed to the four walls and door and a gulley running around the floor on all sides so that the patient could go to the toilet. Only the most violent patients were put in the padded cell, when no other restraining measures worked.

Police obviously had the power to detain and return patients to the Hospital when they were under a compulsory order. Police had another power under Section 136 of the Mental Health Act which enabled them to detain any person 'in a public place' who appeared to be mentally unstable, and who needed to be immediately detained 'for their own safety and that of others'. In these cases the person was normally taken to the psychiatric wing at Barnet General Hospital where they were 'deemed' and detained by the Hospital for the purposes of assessing them".

An example of severe mental disturbance was reported in *The Times* of 15 September 1965. A 25 year old female patient at Friern had died of acute peritonitis brought on by her swallowing needles. She had often swallowed metal objects and had undergone several operations. Doctor Subir Bal gave evidence at the inquest:

> "She swallowed a fork when she came to see us. She was a hysterical psychopath. This is an organic disease and she could not help what she was doing. It was a pattern of the disease. Our consultant thinks it was a death wish that made her do these things."

In early 1977 a confidential monitoring report[5] was submitted to the North East Thames Regional Health Authority which was critical of various aspects of patient treatment at Friern. Amongst the allegations was that voluntary patients were illegally locked in wards and were forcibly administered drugs. There was also criticism of the treatment of the elderly:

> "We are at a loss to account for the fact that an institution we so much admire because it is like a teaching hospital among mental patients should in this manner have neglected the interests of the old. Elderly patients are housed sometimes for years in the admission wards and the oldest patient, a lady of 104, lives on a rehabilitation ward. The hospital should consider how to mount a psychogeriatric service."

The report also revealed that Friern had a worse accident record than a hundred years ago with 454 patients having accidents in the previous six months and 53 staff being assaulted – far higher than any other similar hospital in the Region.

The report did, however, have praise for Friern;

> "We have criticised Friern's methods not because the hospital is a bad one as a result of them but because in our belief they prevent it from becoming superlative."

The Regional Health Authority did not publish the report and was critical of it when parts

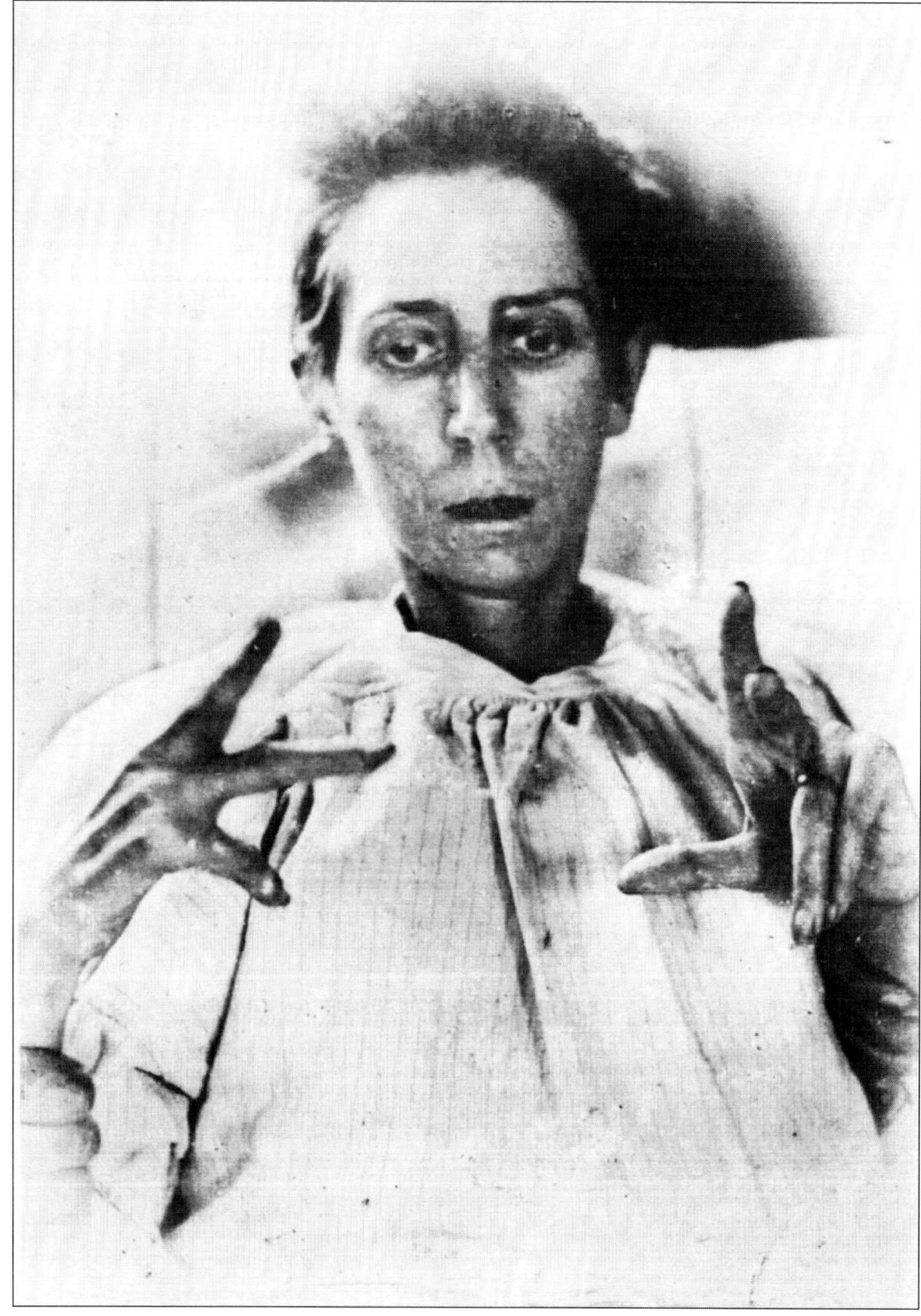

This patient was one of many photographed at Colney Hatch between 1890 and 1910 as part of the study of mental illness. She appears to be suffering from chorea – uncontrollable spasms of the limbs and body.
(Wellcome Library, London)

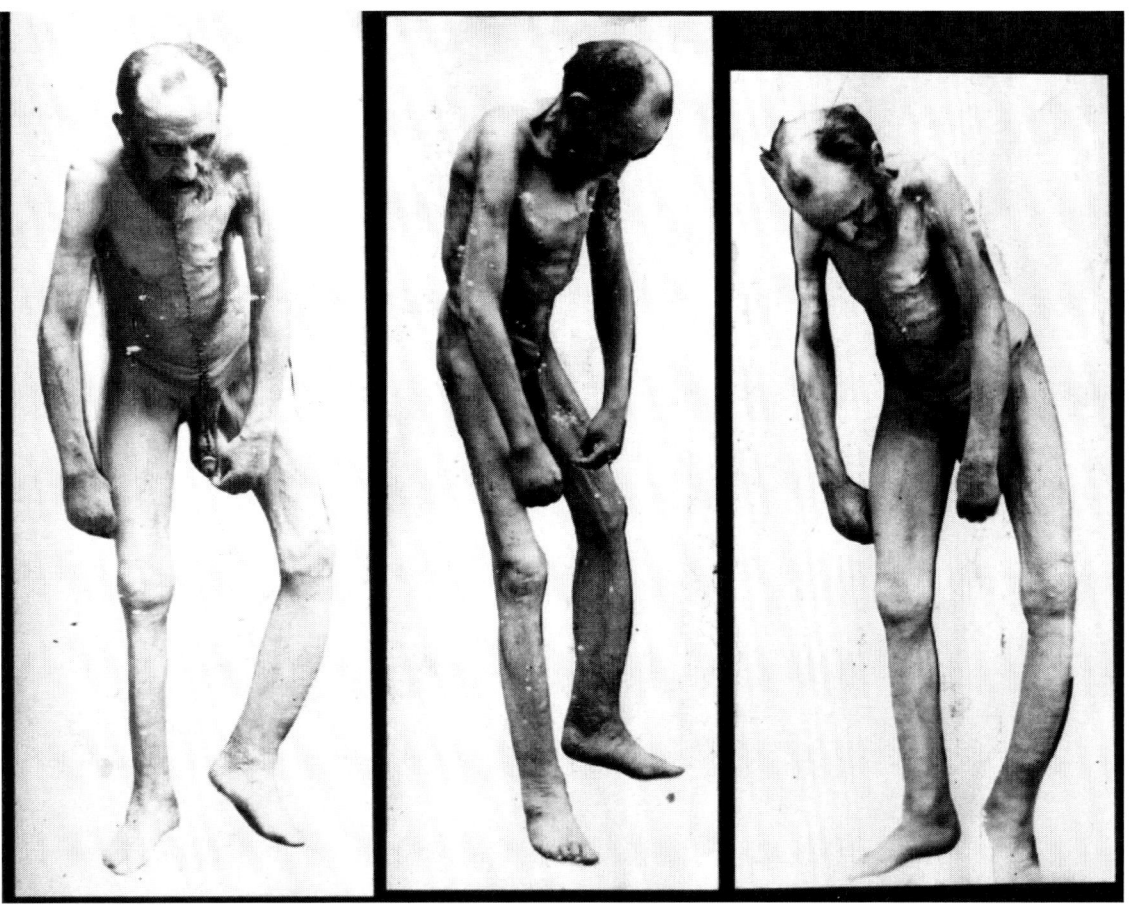

This poor emaciated man has obviously had major surgery at some time,
as can be seen by the stitch marks on his trunk.
(Wellcome Library, London)

of it were leaked to the press:[6]

"Our situation is analogous with situations which arise in every other hospital. If someone starts wandering off the ward they have to be stopped. If a patient confronts you in a very violent state, you have to take action there and then without considering the precise legal situation."

A report in 1970[7] gave an idea of the problems that were peculiar to Friern:

"The suggested bed ratio of 0.5 beds per 1000 population was totally inadequate for the area served by Friern Hospital. The area contained a higher percentage of psychiatric illness than most and contributing to this is the higher proportion of schizophrenic patients in urban areas, the itinerant population, large numbers of single person households, with high rates of suicide and attempted suicide, the many old people living alone, the urban problem of drug addiction, the use of many premises in the catchment area for rooming houses for the psychiatrically ill who gravitate towards the area, the large number of railway termini, the police stations, prisons and rooming houses. To equate the bed requirements of this type of area with rural, suburban, or even other types of urban areas, would be most unwise. It is suggested that a bed ratio of 1.0 per 1000 population would be imperative. It is considered that any less provision would result in an intolerable burden on the community. In addition insufficient beds will encourage the bad medical practice of too cursory assessment, incomplete treatment, and precipitate discharge."

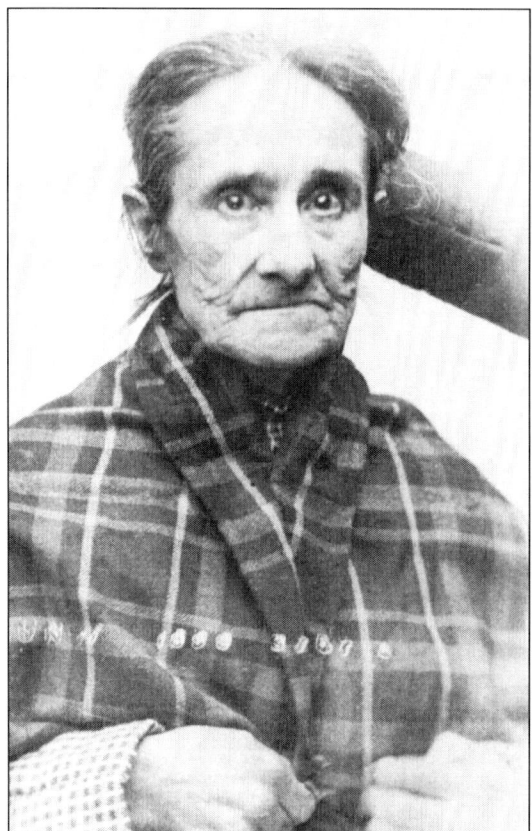 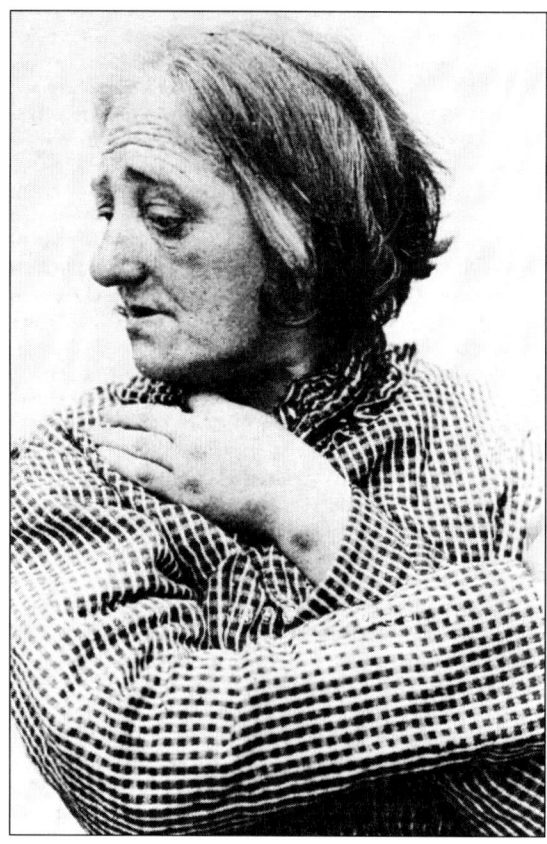

These patients, photographed in 1899, were described as suffering from melanhcolia. Today they would be diagnosed with Parkinsonism
(by kind permission of The Royal Society of Medicine)

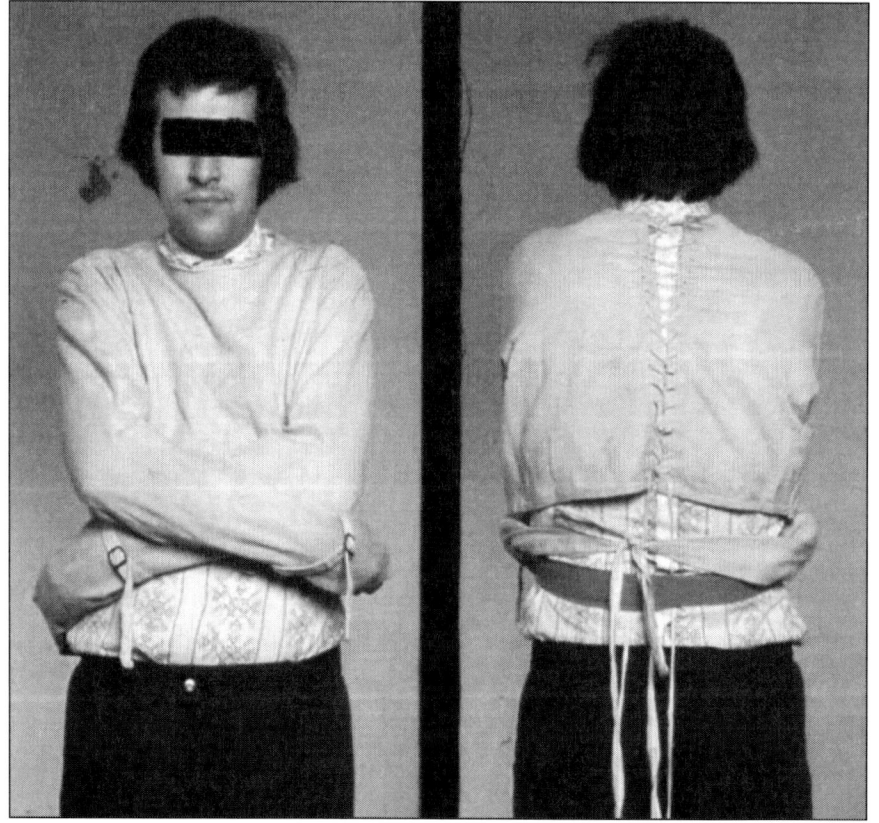

Where violent patients needed restraint, a strait jacket would be used
(courtesy of Royal London Hospital Archives)

One constant feature of the patient population at Colney Hatch Asylum, and later on at Friern Hospital, was the ratio of females to males, which averaged 1.41:1, as the records show:

Year:	1851	1858	1911	1917	1927	1934	1942	1965
Males	179	521	947	994	1005	1120	976	899
Females	331	774	1520	1613	1546	1499	1075	1037

The propensity for females to suffer more from mental illness than males was recognised right from the beginning in the design of the asylum, with eighteen female wards and fourteen male wards, but it is interesting that even in post-Victorian times there were more women patients than men; this may have been a reflection on the population of the catchment area which was mainly working class and where women were subject to more economic and social pressures than men.

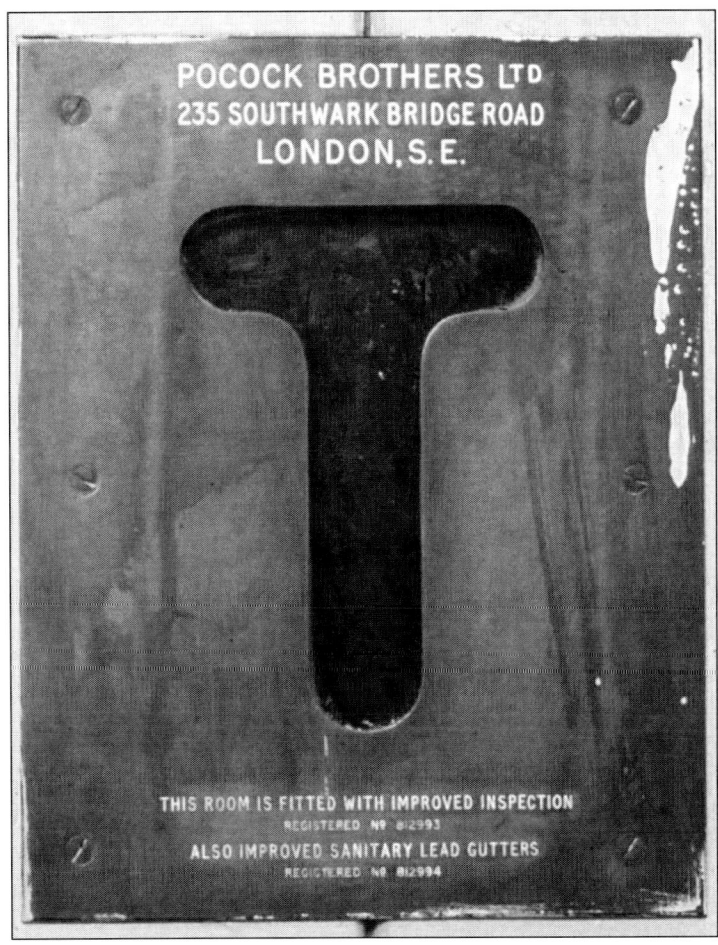

A peep hole to a padded cell
(courtesy of Royal London Hospital Archives)

CHAPTER TEN

Treatment

The building of large publicly-funded lunatic asylums coincided with the introduction of more humane ways of treatment. The pioneer in the field was Robert Gardiner Hill who was house surgeon at Lincoln Lunatic Asylum between 1835 and 1840. Hill introduced the non-restraint system which he described as "the total abolition of instrumental restraint in the treatment of the insane that, in a properly constructed building, with a sufficient number of suitable attendants restraint is never necessary, never justifiable and always injurious." The success of his methods was proven at Lincoln where "patients acquired habits of self control, which is one great step towards cure; the proportion of recoveries increased; comfort and good order prevailed in the place of noise and uproar, and not one fatal accident occurred." In 1857, after analysing the results of his work at Lincoln, he wrote *A Concise History of the Entire Abolition of Mechanical Restraint in the Treatment of the Insane*.

Hill's example was carried on by Dr John Conolly who had been appointed as resident physician at Hanwell in 1839. His success at Hanwell, which was a much larger asylum than Lincoln (800 patients compared with 100), and the success of the non-restraint system led to its gradual adoption throughout the country, including Colney Hatch. An indication of the importance of his work can be seen from a commendation he received when he was presented with a testimonial plate on 31 March 1851[1]:

> "With the name of Dr Conolly is associated the most successful efforts of more enlightened times to substitute kindness and occupation for cruelty and neglect in the treatment of persons labouring under mental disease and it would be difficult to point to any instance in which the distinction of a public testimonial has been more honourably earned."

Although Conolly was feted for his work, he was not above criticism. In 1859 Rosina Bulwer Lytton, wife of Edward Bulwer Lytton, an MP and novelist, accused her husband of murdering their daughter, of adultery, brutality and refusal to grant her and adequate allowance. Bulwer-Lytton had her abducted and certified insane by Conolly and L Forbes Winslow, another celebrated doctor, and committed to the Wyke House Lunatic asylum in Brentford. There followed a huge scandal and both Conolly and Winslow were forced to reconsider their decision and Rosina was subsequently released. She went on to become a prolific author.[2]

Even with today's advances in medical science, the causes of mental illness are not fully understood, and there are a number of theories ranging from genetic disorders, disease or injury and stress to viruses and deterioration of the brain. The asylum kept detailed records of all the patients, including the reasons for their admission. These were categorised as either moral or physical, moral being seen as the event that triggered the person's decline whereas physical was the result of illness. The lack of expertise at the time did not enable doctors to offer more specific reasons for their illness.

The following examples from the first year the asylum was open give some insight into life at the time. The high rate of intemperance was reflective of the problems that drink posed; there was no minimum age for drinking and until 1839 there were no restrictions on opening hours in pubs, so drunkenness was rife and its effect on families, particularly the womenfolk, was often disastrous.

Not surprisingly, the "loss of property" was a significant cause - these were *pauper* lunatics.

CAUSE OF ADMISSION
1851-1852
MALES

Moral

			overall
Sudden shocks, frights	29	32.58%	12.66%
Reverse of fortune, loss of property	12	13.48%	5.24%
Domestic grief	7	7.87%	3.06%
Loss of situation, dread of poverty	7	7.87%	3.06%
Unfaithfulness	6	6.74%	2.62%
Want of employment	6	6.74%	2.62%
Loss of wife or children	3	3.37%	1.31%
Disappointed affection	3	3.37%	1.31%
Erroneous views on religion	3	3.37%	1.31%
Jealousy	3	3.37%	1.31%
Pride	3	3.37%	1.31%
Unhappiness at home	1	1.12%	0.44%
Non-success in business	1	1.12%	0.44%
Responsibility and over-anxiety	1	1.12%	0.44%
Sudden loss of several cows	1	1.12%	0.44%
Suicide of a brother	1	1.12%	0.44%
Regret for a theft	1	1.12%	0.44%
Over-excitement at Great Exhibition	1	1.12%	0.44%
	89	100.00%	

Physical

			overall
Intemperance and debauchery	57	40.71%	24.89%
Congenital deficiency	16	11.43%	6.99%
Injury to head	14	10.00%	6.11%
Epilepsy	14	10.00%	6.11%
Over-study	6	4.29%	2.62%
Paralysis	6	4.29%	2.62%
Masturbation	5	3.57%	2.18%
Fever	4	2.86%	1.75%
Old age	4	2.86%	1.75%
Disease of lungs	3	2.14%	1.31%
Fatigue and over-exertion	3	2.14%	1.31%
Chorea (twitching)	2	1.43%	0.87%
Disease of brain	2	1.43%	0.87%
Bad company	1	0.71%	0.44%
Delirium tremens	1	0.71%	0.44%
Injury to retina	1	0.71%	0.44%
Disease of liver	1	0.71%	0.44%
	140	100.00%	
TOTAL	229		100.00%

One cannot help wondering what happened to the man who suffered "over excitement at the Great Exhibition" – would he have been released after he had calmed down or would he have spent the rest of his life in Colney Hatch? In the 1800s anyone suffering from epilepsy was classified as a lunatic, in fact at Colney Hatch about 25% of men and 20% of women were epileptic. Nowadays, of course, epilepsy is treated as a medical condition. It is a sobering thought that today 1 in 10 of adults may suffer from anxiety or depression and 1 in 50 is likely to experience a severe psychotic illness, such as schizophrenia, in his or her lifetime.[3]

Understandably, the females were most affected by the deaths of children and other relatives. In Victorian times more than half the children died before they reached their fifth birthday and the average life expectancy among the working classes was only 17 years.[4]

CAUSE OF ADMISSION
1864
FEMALES

Moral

			overall
Religion	3	15.00%	5.08%
Death of a child	2	10.00%	3.39%
Diasppointment	2	10.00%	3.39%
Death of a daughter	1	5.00%	1.69%
Death of a son	1	5.00%	1.69%
Death of a father	1	5.00%	1.69%
Death of a niece	1	5.00%	1.69%
Death of relatives	1	5.00%	1.69%
Death of a sister	1	5.00%	1.69%
Death of an employer	1	5.00%	1.69%
Distress of mind	1	5.00%	1.69%
Domestic afflictions	1	5.00%	1.69%
Fright	1	5.00%	1.69%
Ill-treatment by husband	1	5.00%	1.69%
Over study	1	5.00%	1.69%
Poverty and disability to work	1	5.00%	1.69%
	20	100.00%	

Physical

			overall
Epilepsy	20	51.28%	33.90%
Parturition	7	17.95%	11.86%
Intemperance	6	15.38%	10.17%
Irregular menstruation	2	5.13%	3.39%
Fracture of skull when a child	1	2.56%	1.69%
Fright to mother	1	2.56%	1.69%
Having an operation performed	1	2.56%	1.69%
Surpressed menstruation	1	2.56%	1.69%
	39	100.00%	
	59		100.00%

An asylum was precisely that – a place of refuge from the outside world where people could be looked after in safety and without outside pressures. However, it is not difficult to imagine the effect on perfectly sane inmates (with minor afflictions such as epilepsy, drunkenness or depression) of being confined alongside irrational, deranged and violent patients.

There were only two Medical Officers in 1851, Dr W C Hood, in charge of the male department and Dr J G Davey of the female department. Both these men had gone within a year, to be replaced by Dr D F Tyerman who ran the male side for the next ten years and Dr W G Marshall who stayed in charge of the female department until 1890. Dr Tyerman, who was a keen cricketer, encouraged patients to take up the game and he arranged for the land in front of the male wing to be levelled out so that proper matches could take place.

Each doctor had one assistant until 1859 when each was given an extra assistant. The number of doctors remained at this level until 1939 when their number was increased to nine.

The advertisement for Dr Davey's replacement included details of the Victorian heating and lighting arrangements on offer.[5]

> **Middlesex County Lunatic Asylum Colney Hatch.**
>
> Wanted a Resident Medical Officer for the female department of this Asylum. He must be a doctor of medicine; a fellow licentiate of the Royal College of Physicians of London, Edinburgh or Dublin; a member or fellow of the Royal College of Surgeons and a member or licentiate of the Apothecaries Company. The salary will be £200 per annum with Board and an allowance of Coals and Candles. His services will be required in the middle of June next. Candidates are requested to send their testimonials addressed to the Committee of Visitors under cover to me at the Sessions House, Clerkenwell, before the 17th day of May next and to attend the Committee at that place on Thursday 18th of May next at 12 o'clock precisely.
>
>   John S Skaife
>   Clerk to the Visitors
>
> Sessions House
> Clerkenwell
> April 22nd 1852

Since there was virtually no treatment that could be offered to patients, the roles of these doctors was mainly of a supervisory nature and they were responsible for maintaining casebooks and preparing annual reports.

By the twentieth century, when some treatment was becoming available, a sense of the frustration that medical staff felt can be seen in this letter dated 31 July 1947 sent by the Superintendent at Friern to Sir Allen Daly, Medical Officer of Health at County Hall.[6]

> "….one great need has become outstandingly clear that is a full time psychotherapist. The patients whom we see there can be roughly divided into four groups – those for home admission to hospital or voluntary or certified patients is desirable; those for whom little or nothing can really be done; those who can be helped by what has been described as "supportive treatment" i.e. psychotherapy to a limited degree, with or without drugs; and, lastly, those for whom the only real treatment is prolonged or intensive psychotherapy at the hands of a really experienced doctor. It is at present almost impossible to deal with the last group and there appears to be no provision in the Council's service for this type of treatment."

Even as late as 1949 the medical staff only numbered fourteen and, of these, only two were psychiatrists and there was only one psychotherapist.

In early Victorian times at Colney Hatch the only treatment consisted of bleeding and purging, the administration of herbal remedies and hot and cold baths. These latter two remedies were introduced by the Superintendent of the Male Department from 1862 to 1881, Dr Edgar Sheppard, who was a strong believer in hydrotherapy and in particular the Turkish Bath. The Turkish Bath had been used in asylums in Cork, Ireland, and in Haywards Heath and results seemed encouraging.

The London & Provincial Turkish Bath Company was approached by Sheppard in 1864 and asked to quote for the building of a Turkish Bath in the asylum. The plan had originally been for an installation of 1500 square feet but, at £500, it was considered too expensive and a smaller version, of 700 square feet, was installed and opened in 1865 at a cost of £300.

The rooms were heated by radiant water heaters and even though the doorway was covered only by a blanket the temperature reached 190ºF.[7] The early results looked promising:

> "It was a case of melancholia – a young intelligent man he seemed, but had lost a child, and could not be brought to believe in its death, but fancied it had been stolen. Dr Sheppard said it was a very bad case; he could not get any sleep. Had not more than three hours' sleep in four days and nights. Was in the bath nearly an hour, sweated very well, epidermis peeled off in the most extraordinary manner. He was very comfortable all through the bath, and afterwards while cooling, and despite the conversation going on between four or five persons present as to the bath itself, fell off into a sound sleep. Dr Sheppard woke him, and he said he felt very comfortable. He went to bed at eight and slept soundly till six next morning, when he took exercise – a new man. Dr Sheppard says it was a bad case, but now he will be right in about ten days."

In the Annual Report of 1866 the secretary noted that:

> "Several of the Patients themselves, when coming before the Committee for their discharge, have attributed their cure in some measure to its influence."

Initially, and despite the preponderance of female patients at Colney Hatch, it was the male patients who were being treated in Turkish baths:

> "Up to the present time it has not been used for Female Patients in consequence of the Nurses being ignorant of the duties required, but the Committee have authorised the Medical Superintendent of the Female Department to send certain number of Nurses to London for instruction."

By 1866 females were being regularly treated:

> "Previous to her having the baths she suffered from small abscesses of a furuncular character, which she prevented from healing by constantly picking, and she would sit listlessly about the ward, not taking any interest in objects around her. After the third bath her habits became much improved, her health re-established, and she began to employ herself in needlework and general household work, ands is a most useful Patient during the remainder of the time she resides at the Asylum."

Visitors from other asylums came to Friern to inspect the Turkish bath and Sir Robert Armstrong-Jones, who was the Superintendent between 1882 and 1888, took the idea with him when he took up his new position at Claybury Asylum.

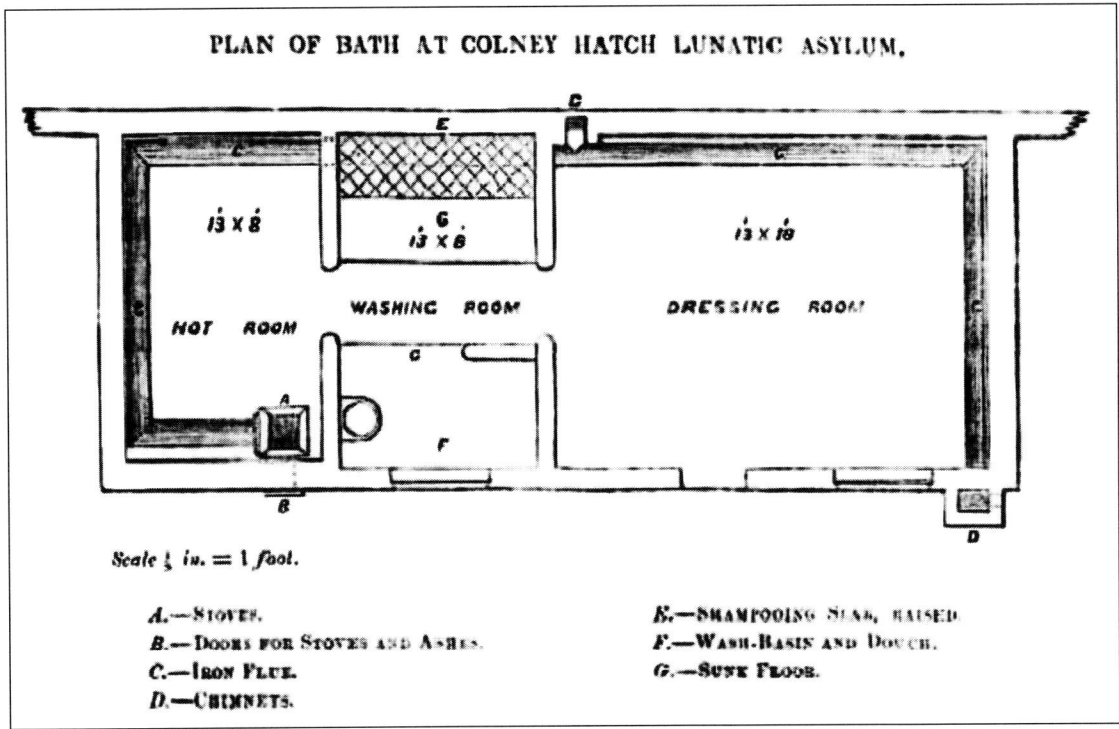

(www.victorianturkishbath.org.)

The large number of patients with epilepsy led Dr Tyerman to start recording the number of fits that they suffered. The figure amounted to 10,000 each year for male patients, and when female patients were investigated the total number was found to be an incredible 82,962[6]. Tyerman theorised that fits were being influenced by changes in the weather and climate and instituted a five year study of the changing weather conditions by means of meteorological apparatus. Not surprisingly, there was found to be no correlation.

Friern was a pioneer in the study of the brain currents of mental patients when in 1937 recordings were taken from schizophrenics with a portable two-channel electro-encephalograph (EEG). A new type of therapy was introduced in 1945 at Friern. Insulin Coma Therapy involved injecting large doses of insulin which burned up all the sugar in the body and induced a coma. It was hoped that the brain, being in a relaxed state, would somehow start to heal itself. In fact, it proved very harmful and in some cases led to death, so it was discontinued in 1948.

In 1949 Lithium, the first psychotropic, or mood-influencing, drug was introduced to manage manic-depression, or bipolar disorder as it is known today. It was highly successful and is still widely used today.

In the early 1950s the first antipsychotic drug, Chlorpromazine, was marketed in the UK by May & Baker Ltd who had invented sulphapyridine (M&B 693) which had saved Winston Churchill's life when he was suffering from bacterial pneumonia. Chlorpromazine was marketed as Largactil and became known as "the liquid cosh" because it reduced patients to a trance-like state. From this point of view it was ideal for hospital staff as it reduced the number of violent outbursts, but its effect on the patients was often to reduce them to listless zombies. One of the side effects of this drug was what was known as "Largactil Tan" whereby patients have sensitivity to sunlight resulting in them getting burned if exposed to it for too long. Largactil also made women produce breast milk. Other anti-psychotic drugs included Stelazine and Haldol. Stelazine (a member of the trifluoperazine family) had several side effects, including a dry mouth, and to counteract this another drug, Kemadrine (procyclidine) would be prescribed but this too had side effects, and so these cocktails of drugs might alleviate the original symptoms but ended up making the patient feel physically unwell.

In 1974 Friern conducted preliminary trials of a new drug, propranolol, amongst schizophrenics. The results were strikingly effective – six patients lost all their symptoms and another five showed definite improvement. Like many drugs, however, it did have quite serious side effects, including possible heart failure and making asthma worse.[8]

Impiramine was another new drug, which was used for the treatment of depression. The tranquiliser Valium (diazepam), which raised serotonin levels and induced a feelgood sense of security and assertiveness and made people feel "better than well."[9] It became widely prescribed, particularly by general practitioners. Such was the effect of these drugs that at the time it was claimed somewhat optimistically that they would eliminate mental illness by 2000.[10] One problem with these minor tranquilisers was that they can be effective for short-term relief of symptoms, but quickly become less effective. Anti-depressant drugs include Anafranil, Gamanil, Parnate and Prozac took longer to take effect but they were ineffective in about a third of cases.[11]

Prefrontal leucotomy involved drilling holes in the skull and severing the frontal lobes from the rest of the brain and the first such procedure was performed at Friern in 1946. Operations were carried out on 30 mostly chronic patients with a bad prognosis. Eight of the patients were subsequently discharged, 13 improved in varying degrees and only nine showed no appreciable change.[12]

Electro-convulsive therapy (ECT) was also carried out. A patient would be injected with a drug to dry the mouth and stop them from swallowing their tongue and they would then normally be anaesthetised (although not always) and then a gag was put in the mouth and electric shocks would be passed through the brain by means of paddles. This is a somewhat controversial treatment as the results can not always be predicted; some psychiatrists claim that it does not damage the brain, whilst others think that it does. The comedian Jo Brand, who early in her career was a Mental Nurse at Bethlehem Hospital, described in her autobiography[13] one of the effects of ECT:

> "When I was a student, we had a woman admitted with the worst case of agitated depression I have ever seen. She cried out constantly, could not sit still, wandered around the ward all day wringing her hands and clutching at her face and clothes, and was so completely overwrought with emotion, desperate and sad, that it was painful to witness. This woman had about five sessions of ECT and the transformation in her was absolutely unbelievable. She became calm, articulate, relaxed, and communicative and her mood was happy and contended. I could not believe what I was seeing. On the other hand, I witnessed many patients who were given ECT, on whom it had no effect whatsoever."

The hospital at Friern was poorly equipped – it did not even have its own X-ray equipment until 1939 and that was brought by St Bartholomews' when they transferred there at the start of the war; it was left at Friern after they departed in 1946 and new equipment did not arrive until 1960. Until 1939 patients needing X-rays were treated at Passmore Edwards Hospital at Bounds Green.

Patients' meetings were part of the treatment and gave people an opportunity to express

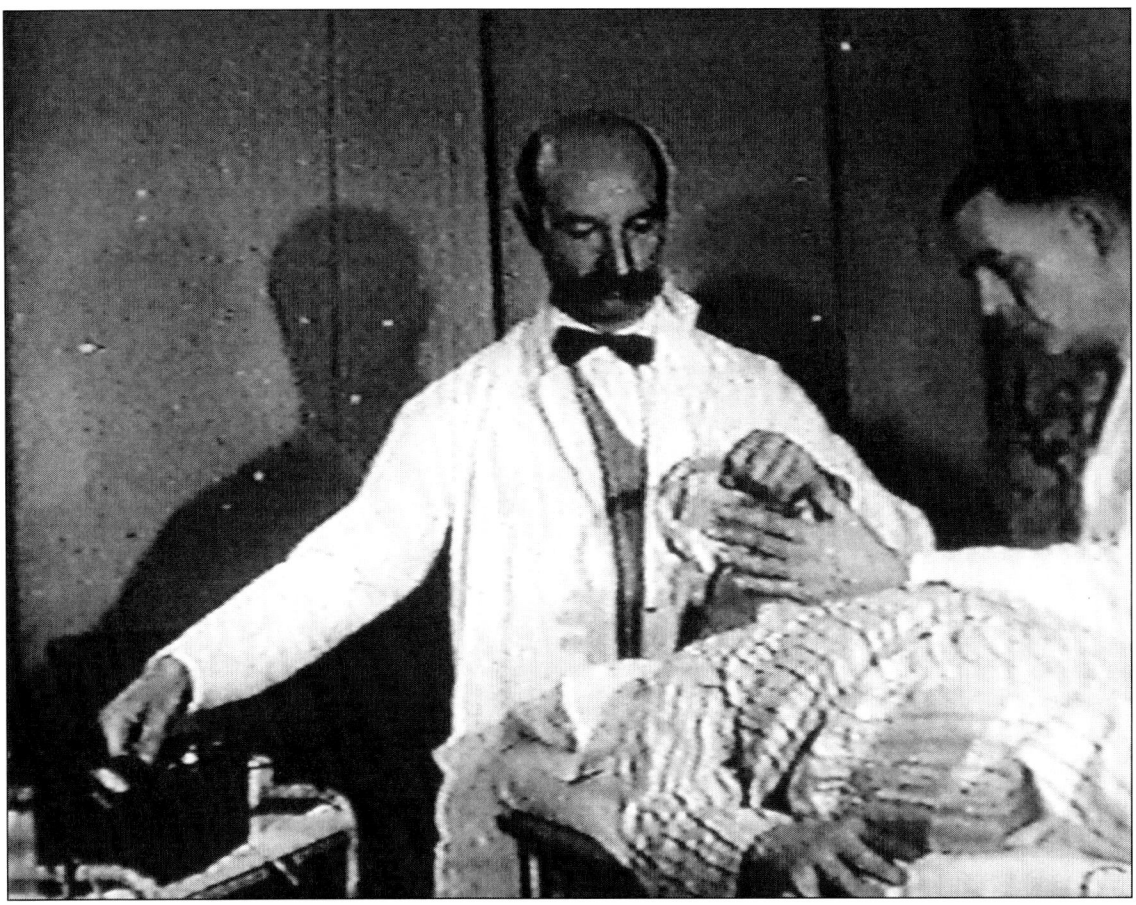

A patient undergoing electro convulsive therapy at Friern in 1950.
(Time Marches on at Friern)

their criticisms or comments to the staff. Group therapy sessions were sometimes useful although these could degenerate into chaos if disturbed patients were present. A former patient, Mary Comyns, confirms the positive benefits:

> "I had spent three separate months during the previous ten years in Claybury Hospital as a patient and the peace and quiet and freedom to roam the woods in my Community Ward, and the discussion groups in which we discovered that our problems and symptoms were general, and not peculiar to ourselves alone, were something I was very grateful for".

An important part of treatment was physiotherapy and Friern had appointed a full time physiotherapist before the Second World War and two were employed during the war when St Bartholomew's was looking after general patients, including wounded service personnel.

Relaxation exercises helped to reduce stress and tension while ultra violet light treatment could alleviate bedsores, a particular problem with elderly or immobile patients. Ultra sound was introduced in the 1970s and was beneficial in treating torn muscles and ligaments. Although there were positive benefits to keeping patients mobile, particularly the elderly, their co-operation was not always forthcoming and they could not be forced into receiving treatment.

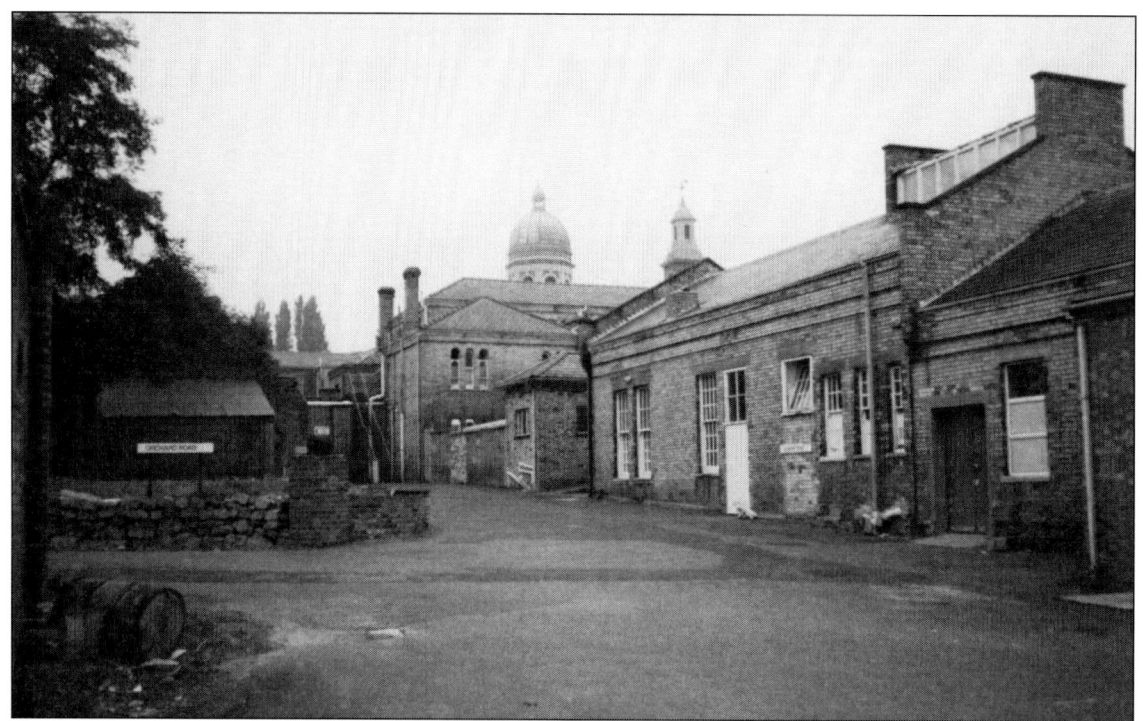

The gymnasium, on the right of the picture. (Barnet Local Studies)

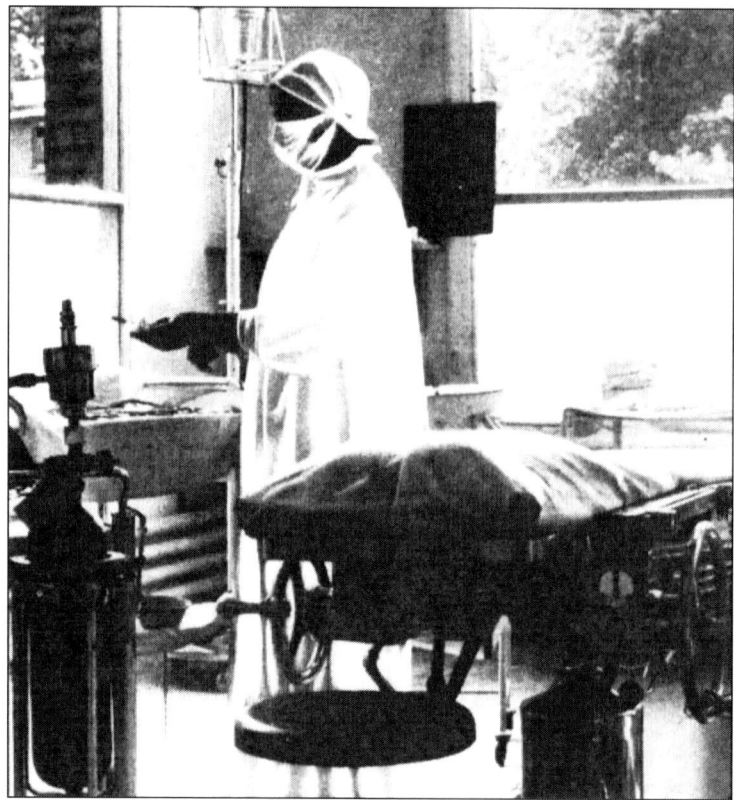

The operating theatre
(FB&DLHS Archive)

CHAPTER ELEVEN

Work and Therapy

From the very beginning it was the intention to make Colney Hatch as self-supporting as possible, hence the inclusion of a farm and orchards, bakehouse and brewery and the creation of independent gas and water supplies. To this end it was desirable that patients would do most of the day-to-day work of the asylum. There was, of course, an ulterior motive to this: patients who were occupied were less likely to be either bored and listless or overly manic.

As we have seen, many of the early patients were from the labouring classes, being either artisans or labourers. Thus carpenters, painters, gardeners, upholsterers, tinsmiths, seamstresses, and basket makers were given jobs commensurate with their experience. Brush making actually made a profit and money was saved when patients who had been painters and decorators were put to work to brighten up the wards.

Articles made in the year to 31 March 1891

TAILORS' SHOP	No	UPHOLSTERERS' SHOP	No
Patients' Trousers	993	Bedside Carpets	592
Patients' Coats	489	Mattresses	232
Patients' Vests	298	Mattings	226
Waterproof Aprons	58	Bed Sackings	215
Attendants' Trousers	34	Blinds	98
Attendants' Vests	33	Sofa Cushions	88
Cloth Capes	15	Chair Cushions	42
Waterproof Leggings	15	Strong Shirts	24
Attendants' Coats	15	Canvas Aprons	18
Attendants' Jackets	11	Strong Rugs	18
		Horse Cloths	6
		Rick Cloth	1
Repairs		*Repairs*	
Patients' Trousers	6,514	Bed Sackings	1,712
Patients' Coats	3,891	Mattresses (re-made)	1,589
Patients' Vests	3,071	Pillows	1,146
Patients' Strong Dresses	273	Chaff Beds	1,072
Attendants' Trousers	167	Blinds	516
Patients' Cloth Capes	83	Canvas Rugs	310
Attendants' Coats	40	Sofa Cushions	208
Attendants' Vests	12	Chair Cushions	177
		Carpets	97
		Mattings	83
SHOEMAKERS' SHOP		Padded Rooms	76
Canvas Boots	19	Kneelers	59
Leather Boots	6	Rubber Covers	12
Cloth Boots	6		
		Hair & Fibre Picked	lbs
Repairs		Horsehair picked (male patients)	24,082
Boots & Shoes soled & welted	5,007	Fibre picked (male patients)	4,665
Boots and Shoes repaired	4,484	Hair picked (female patients)	13,936
Boots & Shoes locked & strapped	1,981		
Attendants' Belts	69		
Leggings	75		

Articles made by Female Patients

Dresses	2,378	Petticoats	628
Aprons	1,868	Flannel Shirts	508
Shirts	1,530	Bed-Gowns	483
Men's Caps	1,381	Uniform Dresses	431
Chemises, Linen	1,177	Drawers	396
Uniform Aprons	780	Stays	376
Uniform Caps	744	Hoods	111
Chemises, Flannel	634	Slops	48

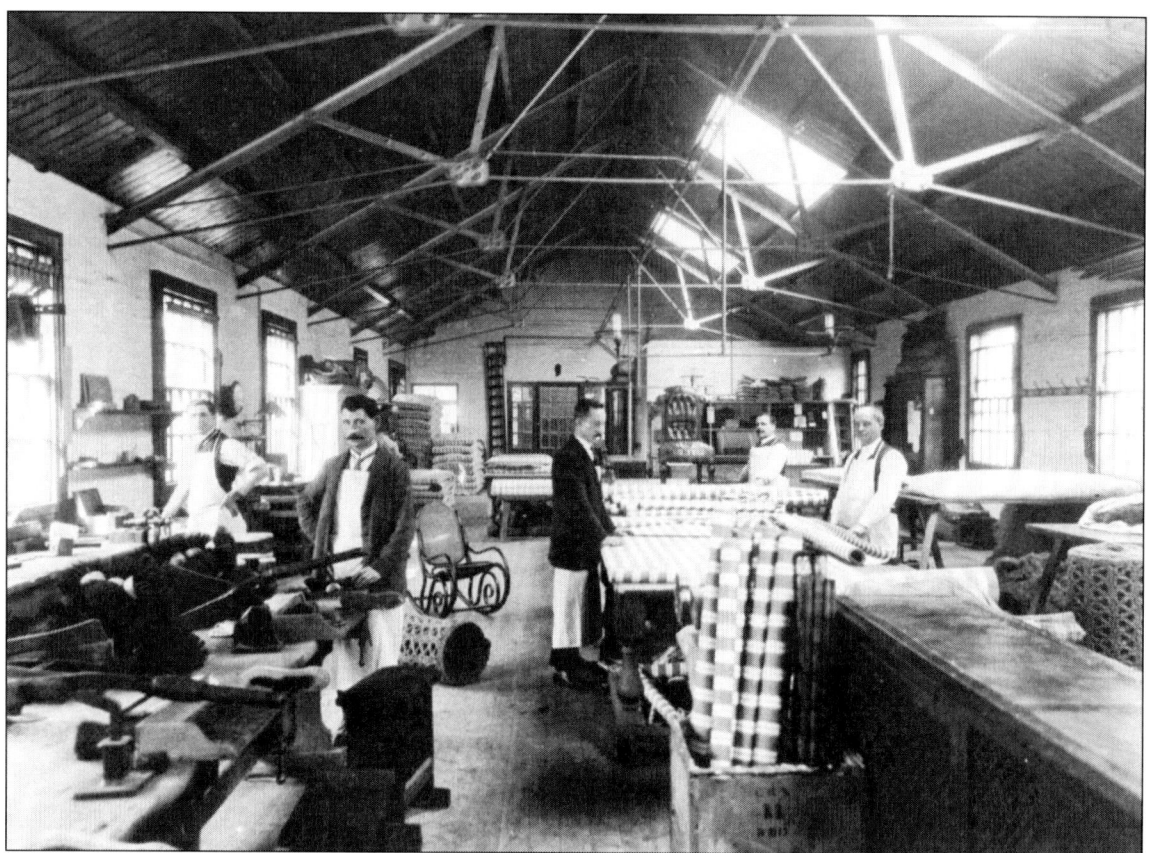
The upholstery workshop. (By kind permission of the Royal Society of Medicine)

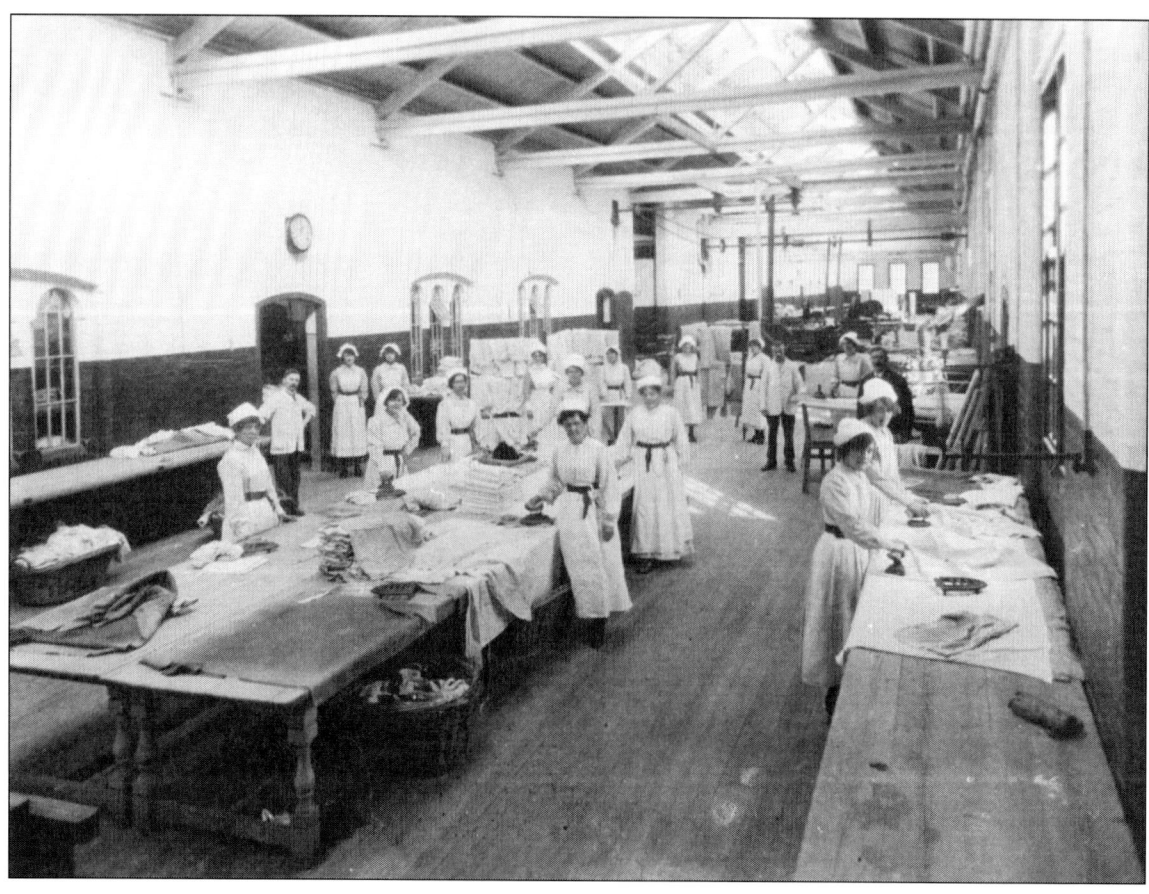
The laundry in the early 1900s. Machines were later introduced
to cope with the increasing demand. (Barnet Local Studies)

Patients helped out in the laundry, in the kitchens and workshops unskilled female patients did domestic work. A particular problem was getting patients to work on the farm. Most of them had lived all their lives in the metropolis where agriculture was unknown and the spade was looked upon as an emblem of poverty rather than an instrument of support. In the early days the Commissioners were critical of the small number of patients who were employed in work (in 1861 it was only 44%) but while patients were encouraged to participate, they could not be forced to. Charles Hood summed it up when he said: "The insane mind might be lead, but it will not be driven." Inducements such as tobacco and snuff were offered instead. Those patients who were too incapacitated to work were taken into the airing courts and exercised for three hours in the morning and three hours in the afternoon or taken for walks in the grounds.

A somewhat dramatic report in *The Sentinel and Finsbury Park to Finchley & Enfield Advertiser* of 16 January 1914 gives us a good idea of the importance to the patients of work:

> "Late at night the big bell at Colney Hatch Asylum rang loudly. The attendant at the gate shivered in his overcoat, gazed through his observation grill at the form of a man, and asked him what he wanted.
>
> Quite cheerfully the man outside said, "I have come back to you, sir. I've come aboard. I am the escaped lunatic."
>
> The man was Woodhouse, the fugitive lunatic, who had enjoyed five days' free leave of absence, eluded all efforts to recapture him and at the end had returned to give himself up at the asylum gates. When Woodhouse was searched a sheaf of newspaper cuttings relating to his escape were found in his pockets.
>
> The friends of Woodhouse are supposed to have declared that he is not insane; and this story of his return will, in the opinion of some go to prove it. For outside the asylum he has to take a slender chance of getting work. In the asylum work is provided for him – on the farm. Outside the asylum, as an ill-paid labourer, he might have no other than his working clothes. In the asylum he has a Sunday suit. He has regular meals too, and a room of his own to sleep in. The best medical care is taken of him and there are times of amusement and play. To "escape" from this looks like lunacy: this must have been borne in the mind of Woodhouse by a brief "outside" experience and so he returned."

In the later part of the twentieth century, therapy replaced work. Once a patient's condition had been stabilised by the use of drugs he or she could participate in the various therapy programmes that were being developed. The introduction of Occupational, Recreational and Social Therapy after the Second World War proved very successful. One of the male Staff Nurses at Friern had a particular musical ability and it was felt that he could fulfil a useful function by devoting his whole time to such matters as organising concerts, teaching patients various musical instruments and organising a choir. The title Music Therapist was not given to him as he held no special qualifications, but his activities increased so that he also became responsible for such things as the use of a 16mm cinema projector in wards for patients who could not come to the cinema, arranging coach outings, and in fact doing much that might come under the heading of "Social Therapy" or "Recreational Therapy" A 'most satisfactory degree of co-operation existed between this therapist and the Remedial Gymnast who organised all patients' sports and athletics.'[1]

During the 1950s it was found that even the most deteriorated patients benefited from courses of Occupational Therapy, together with Recreational Therapy, and physical training. Difficulties were encountered to begin with in raising the enthusiasm of some of the nursing staff whose cooperation was essential in the success of the treatment, but these problems were eventually largely overcome.

An Industrial Therapy unit was set up and was equipped with machines for woodworking and metalworking. Patients were encouraged to attend the unit on a voluntary basis – there was no coercion – and as many as 150 patients a day would be involved with making toys, dolls houses or garden furniture while others would be stuffing envelopes or shrink wrapping products for outside firms. The Manager of the unit for twenty years from 1973 until the closure of the hospital was Ken Toombs and he had a staff of around fourteen, all full time employees including technicians and nurses. The patients were paid a nominal wage of around £5 a week which gave them an incentive to attend and also gave them a feeling of self respect. Ken tried to get work from outside companies, the income of which would go to help defray the costs of running the unit, but this often proved difficult as patients tended to attend when they felt like it, consequently deadlines could not always be met. There was opposition from some of the trade unions who felt that the hospital was using slave labour, but the counter argument was that the work was for the benefit of the patient, rather than the patient being used for the benefit of the work. A survey was conducted among patients in 1984[2] and nearly 77% of them said they liked the work they did. One benefit of the Industrial Therapy Unit was that on discharge patients could find it easier to obtain employment. Two local employers, Standard Telephones & Cables (STC) and the Metal Box Co Ltd were willing to employ discharged patients, although this was not always successful as the routine of turning up for work regularly and on time was often beyond them.

At the Occupational Therapy unit patients would be involved with lighter tasks such as basket making, picture framing or typing and a particularly innovative idea was the creation of a small flat equipped with its own kitchen where patients could learn skills such as cooking, housework and household budgeting. This was part of the Rehabilitation Ward where patient were gradually prepared for discharge back into the community.

A separate Art Hut behind Halliwick House was manned every day by an Occupational Therapist and patients could draw or paint or make pottery as they wished. In 1971 an exhibition of paintings by psychiatric patients was held in London as part of a MIND campaign to raise awareness of the mentally ill. Amongst the paintings were those of a patient who had been at Friern for three years. His early work included two talented drawings of nudes drawn while he was still at art school. The deterioration which brought him into Friern was shown by a frightening self-portrait of his body sunk, black, with sinews and muscles showing and with four arms struggling with each other. The drawing was unfinished because he did not know what the final outcome would be.[3]

By 1948 specialist staff included five Occupational Therapists, a Physiotherapist, an Art Mistress and a Remedial Gymnast.

The benefits to patients involved in the various therapies were that they were able to socialise with others, to learn new skills, to keep to a routine, to learn to be independent and to restore self respect. When Care in the Community took over from specialist hospitals like Friern it was difficult to recreate therapy units of the same quality.

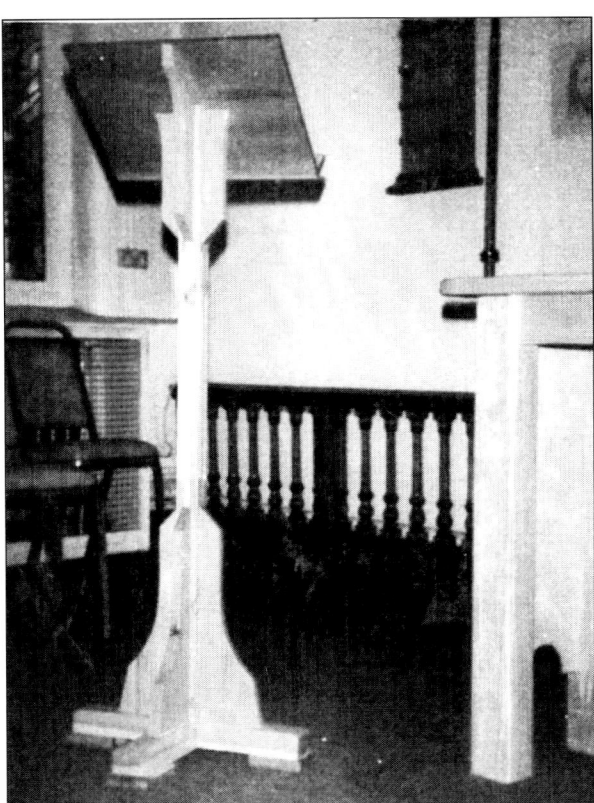 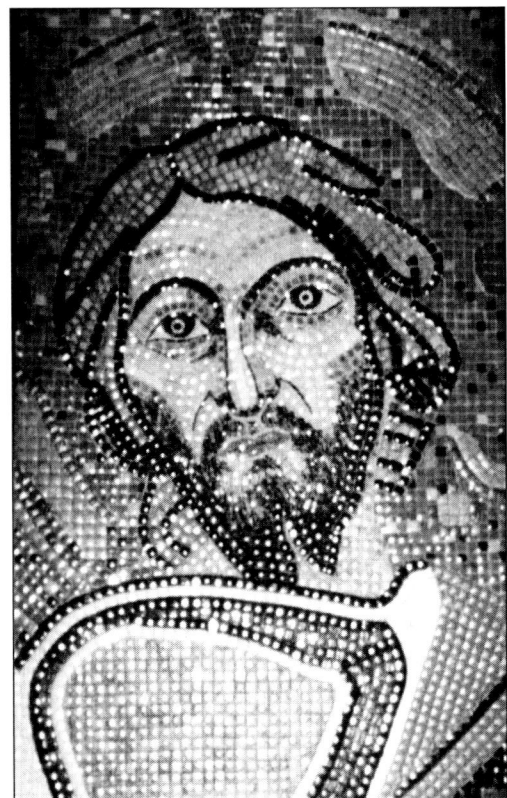

The lectern and the table in the Chazen Room (left) were made by patients in the Industrial Therapy Unit. The mosaic (right) was designed and created in the Art Therapy Unit.
(Jean Crocker Collection)

CHAPTER TWELVE

Taking Care of the Soul

The first religious service was held in the Chapel on Sunday 1 July 1851 and thereafter Divine Service was conducted by the chaplain every morning and evening. From the start emphasis was placed on services of public worship; all other services were ancillary. Sunday morning services were church parade occasions when all Anglican patients were expected to attend. All staff were regular attenders when their duties permitted. All Church of England patients who were considered fit to attend were compelled to do so and the chapel was full.[1] Roman Catholics had their own chapel and had the services of a visiting priest. Patients who requested them were issued with Catholic books and tracts.

From the very beginning, the asylum had been the chief institution for the care of the mentally sick of the Jewish faith. In 1905 about a third of patients were Jews and this had increased to 801 by 1950.[2] Many of these were immigrants and were unable to speak English and had been victims of persecution. In 1854 a Jewish interpreter named Freedman, who was also a nurse, joined the staff and helped the chaplain and later a rabbi who attended the asylum.

One of the most influential and respected men at Colney Hatch was Rev Henry Hawkins who was chaplain for thirty three-years. Henry was born on 25 September 1825 and was privately tutored by a Rev John May who went on to become chaplain at Hanwell asylum. Perhaps it was his influence that aroused Hawkins's interest in the work of asylums, for after graduating from Wells Theological College he was appointed chaplain at the Sussex County Asylum at Haywards Heath in 1859.

He joined Colney Hatch in 1867 and, as well as his religious duties he got involved in the welfare of individual patients. He organised educational classes and helped to find jobs for those who had been discharged. He also set up a library within the asylum for the benefit of patients and produced a number of tracts offering comfort and advice to both

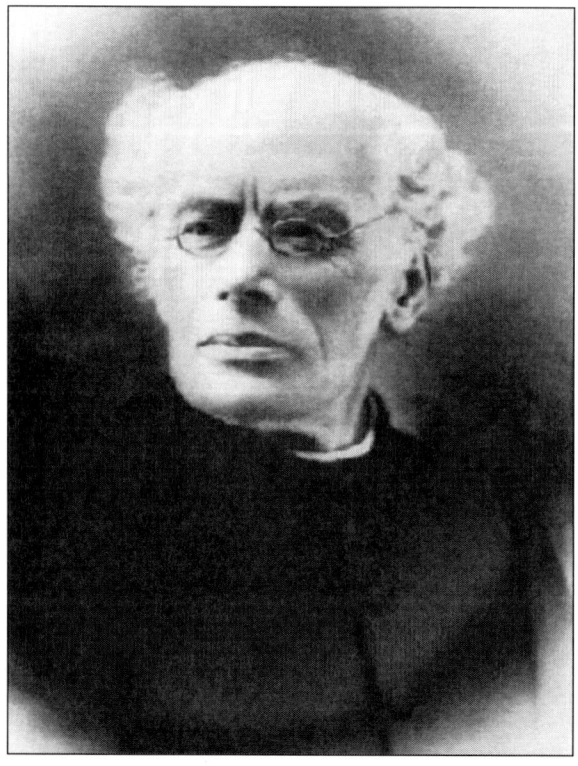

Henry Hawkins. (Together-uk)

patients and staff. Amongst these were *Friendly Words with a New Patient* and *Visiting Day at the Asylum*. He also pioneered the idea of using volunteers to visit and help patients who otherwise had no friends. Hawkins was responsible for arranging community singing and dancing and for seeing that patients had access to musical instruments that had been provided by the Committee of Visitors. He arranged for collecting boxes to be placed in the visiting rooms where relatives and patients would meet and the proceeds from these were distributed to such charities as The Poor Neighbours of the Asylum, Waifs and Strays and Homes for Mental Convalescents.

It was obvious that he was a gentle, humorous and kind man and loved those in his care. He was particularly concerned with those patients, particularly women, who found it difficult to resettle into normal life after leaving the asylum. He wrote an article in *Journal of Mental Science* in 1871 entitled *A Plea for Convalescent Homes in Connection with Asylums for the Insane Poor*. In 1879 he organised a meeting of leading people in the field of mental health and was elected as secretary of the resultant charity, the After-Care Association for Poor and Friendless Female Convalescents on Leaving Asylums for the Insane. In the 1960s this was renamed The Mental After Care Association and in 1998 it changed again, this time to *Together*,[3] a pithier name although not quite as descriptive of its work as the originals.

Hawkins had hoped to arrange separate religious services for the more disorderly patients but the Commissioners in Lunacy insisted that it was better to have a mix of patients in the hope that the more unruly would be calmed down by the saner ones.

Henry Hawkins died in 1904 and a tribute to him was published in the local church magazine *St James Parish Magazine*:

> "To meet him in the street was a privilege and a delight, and one hears on every side how his pleasant little greetings, his humorous sayings, or his tender words of sympathy, have been treasured by all who received them. And then there was that charming humility of disposition, which so persistently refused recognition – in fact, any expression of gratitude almost seemed to distress him."

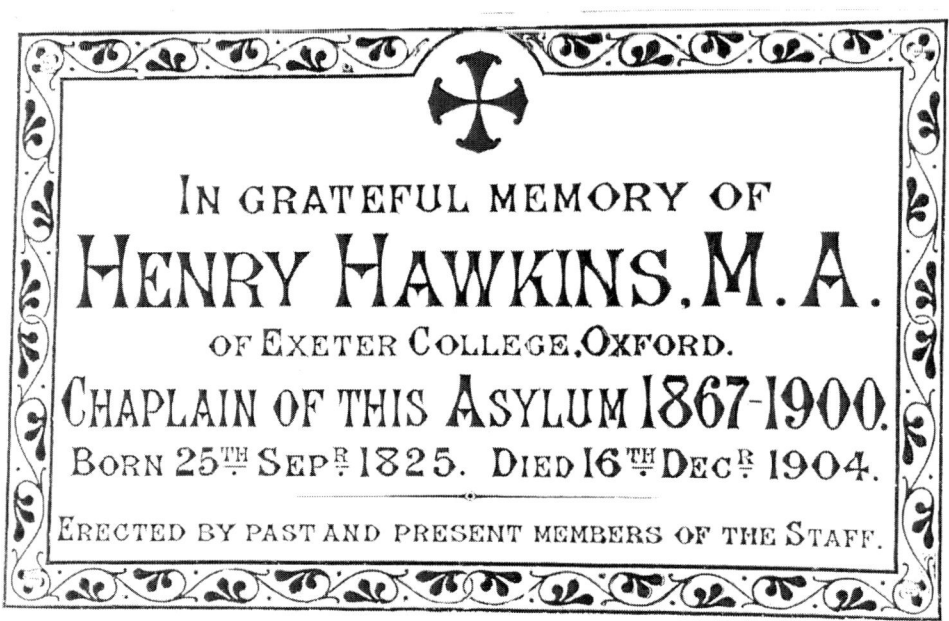

(FB&DLHS Archive)

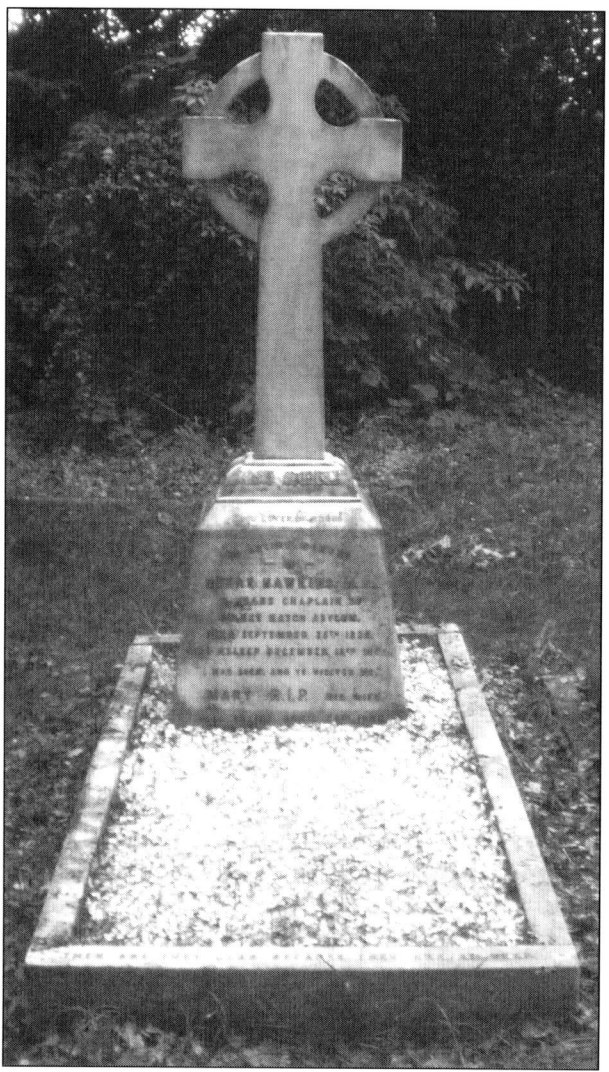
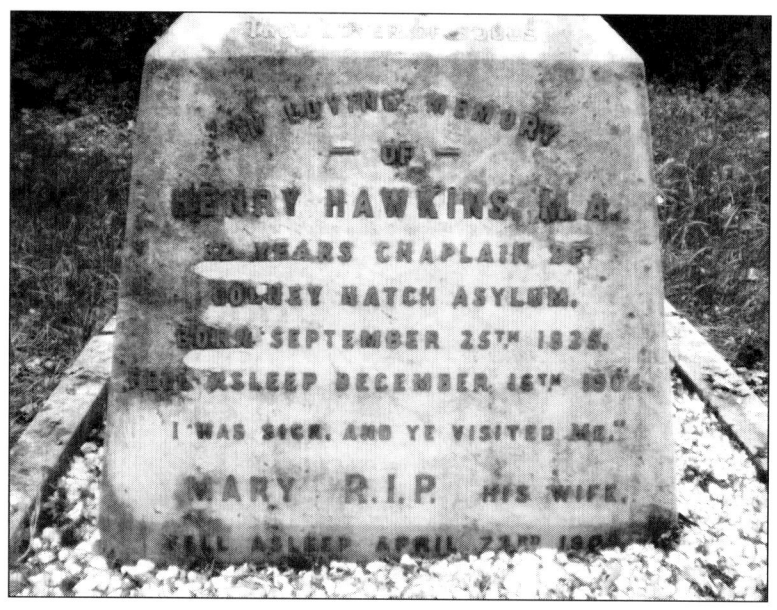

Henry Hawkins' grave in St James' churchyard.
The inscription aptly reads "I was sick and ye visited me".
(Author)

The role of the chaplain in more modern times was slightly different. Vernon Muller was born in South Africa in 1940 and, after coming to Durham University to study, and meeting the English girl that was to become his wife, they returned together to South Africa where he was ordained. Having come across a number of people in his parish in Durban who were suffering from psychiatric difficulties, and feeling inadequate in dealing with them, he sought a solution. He heard of the Manninger Foundation which was a leading psychiatric education institution in the USA and after approaching them was fortunate enough to be granted a Fellowship. He stayed there for a year studying pastoral care and counselling then returned to South Africa. By 1976 the political situation in South Africa and the strength of the problems of apartheid were becoming worse and he decided to come to England on his wife's passport and with his three sons.

With no job and no home, he made contact with the Bishop who covered the North London area and was offered a curacy in Hendon. Whilst there he saw a job advertised in *Church Times* for a chaplain at Friern. He applied and got the job.

His predecessor had been very High Church and had held private Masses in the chapel which was always kept locked except at service time. Vernon told the authorities that he wanted it open throughout the day so that patients could come and go as they pleased. He was told that the place would get smashed up, but in the thirteen years he was there, there was only one incident of vandalism.

A typical day in Vernon's life would involve leaving his house in Consort Close, adjacent to Hallwick Hospital, and walking through the grounds to open up the chapel and say Morning Prayers. The rest of the day would be spent in meeting with patients and staff and a tour of the geriatric wards where he would hold services for those patients unable to visit the chapel. He had a music centre on a trolley that had been donated by the WRVS and would play hymns for the patients to sing along to. He recalled one particular incident:

> "On Ward 9 there was a very demented old gentleman who only used to say "BBC, BBC" and I just knew him as BBC. One day, it was coming up to Easter, and I was playing *There is a Green Hill Far Away* and I noticed he was singing along with the music. The staff were absolutely astounded that this man who was so demented that he could never string any words together, apart from "BBC" was singing the words to the hymn, so there was obviously something there."

He would also take round percussion instruments left over from the time when Friern had its own band:

> "I used them on ward services and sometimes on a Sunday, people would bang tambourines or triangles. An old man on one of the long stay wards had been a drummer, so I brought him a drum, and he played and he was fantastic! Again the staff never knew he had any talent and they were gobsmacked. So I left the drum on the ward for him to play, as long as he didn't disturb the other patients."

Vernon was very ecumenically minded and he worked very closely with the Free Church and Roman Catholic chaplains and had a good relationship with the Rabbi who used to visit. The Jews had their own synagogue in the hospital as well as the Chazen Room for social gatherings. Vernon was invited to the Chanukah meal and after the ceremonial meal there was music and dancing. One of the Jewish laymen grabbed Vernon and they danced together. Vernon said: "For me it was a fantastic experience. I though to myself: 'This is shalom.'"

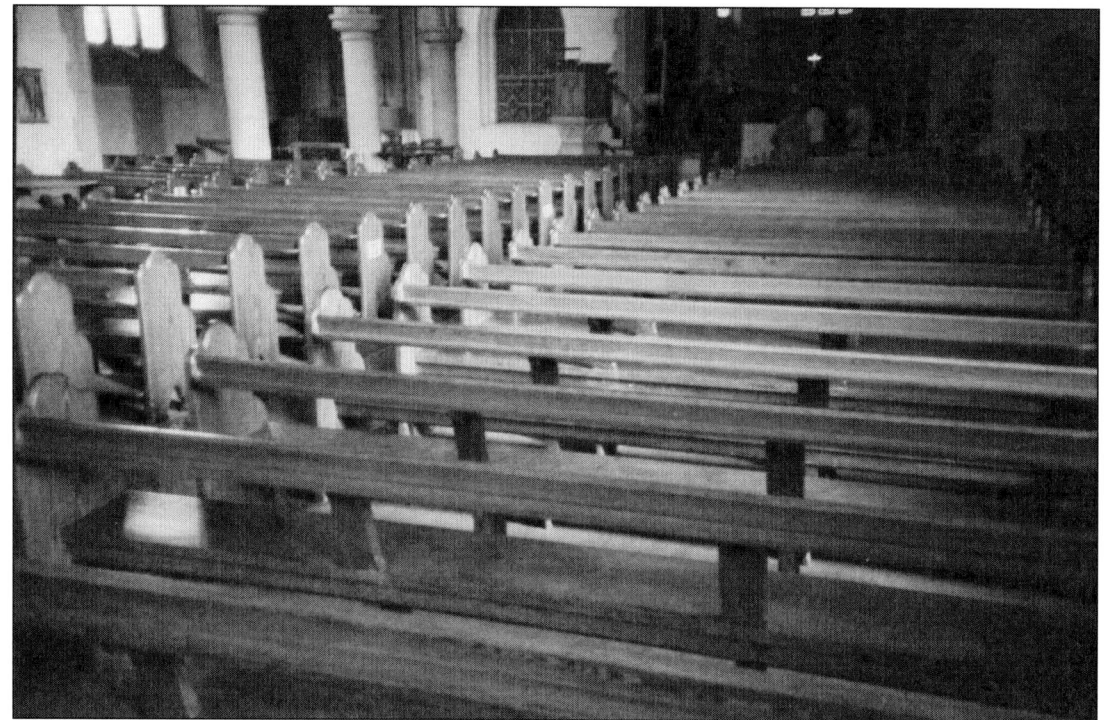

The chapel. (Barnet Local Studies)

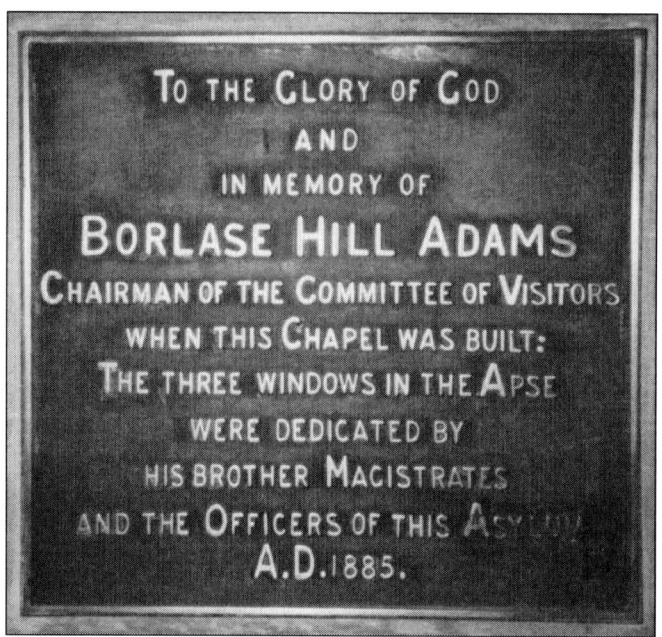

(Barnet Local Studies)

The front third of the chapel itself had been partitioned off for offices before Vernon arrived at Friern and subsequently it was discovered that the beams had woodworm in them and scaffolding had to be erected as a precaution. This meant that services had to be held in the Hall which was very unsatisfactory and Vernon had the idea of setting up a Religious Centre in the synagogue where all the faiths could worship. This was turned down by the Rabbi and his committee until Vernon pointed out that in the synagogue the ark which contained the sacred scrolls was actually on the north wall instead of the east. Since the room would have to be redesigned, they finally agreed to the idea and the new room was dedicated in May 1985 by Cardinal Basil Hume, the Anglican Bishop, the minister from the Free Church and the Rabbi. Thereafter, Vernon would go there on a

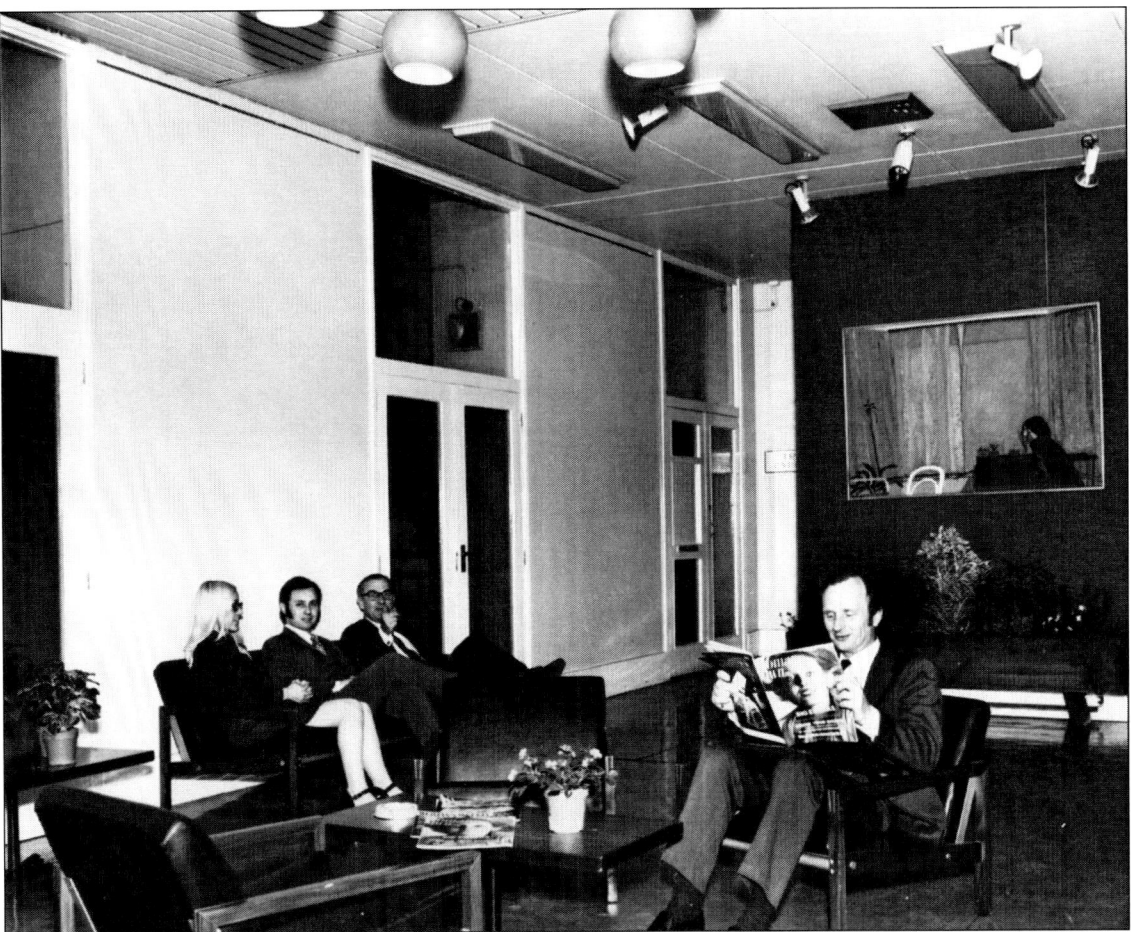

A Reception area was created in the front part of the chapel. (Geoff Smith)

Friday and remove all the Christian symbols, ready for the Jewish service on the Saturday. The Jews would then remove the curtain covering the ark. On Sunday things would be changed round again for the Christian service.

The new multi-faith chapel had two stained glass windows which had been designed by a staff member who worked in the Print Shop and who had worked in a stained glass workshop prior to that.

The Chazen room was named after the Reverend Irving Chazen who passed away in 1975, aged 60. The February 1976 issue of *Pulse*[4], the hospital's in-house magazine carried the following tribute:

> "Mr Chazen had become a firm friend to Jewish and non-Jewish patients alike. He brought kindness, comfort and friendship to so many people who had so few friends. A native of Newcastle, Mr Chazen was educated at Rutherford College at Gateshead Yeshiva, Etzchaim Yeshiva and London and Manchester Universities. He gained a BA in Semitics. His first ministry in London was at High Cross synagogue, Tottenham which he took up in 1952. It was at this time that he first became aware of a vocation to work with the mentally ill and after 10 years at Tottenham he resigned his post and moved to Friern Hospital. Eventually other hospitals under his care included Claybury, Horton, Runwell, and Banstead and during his latter stage he was given the care of Jewish patients in Napsbury. Having no car of his own, he relied solely on public transport to visit all these hospitals which he did regularly and always with a word of comfort for the patients. He always officiated at the services and celebrations in the Synagogue

and was always available when patients wanted to consult him, or when there was an emergency."

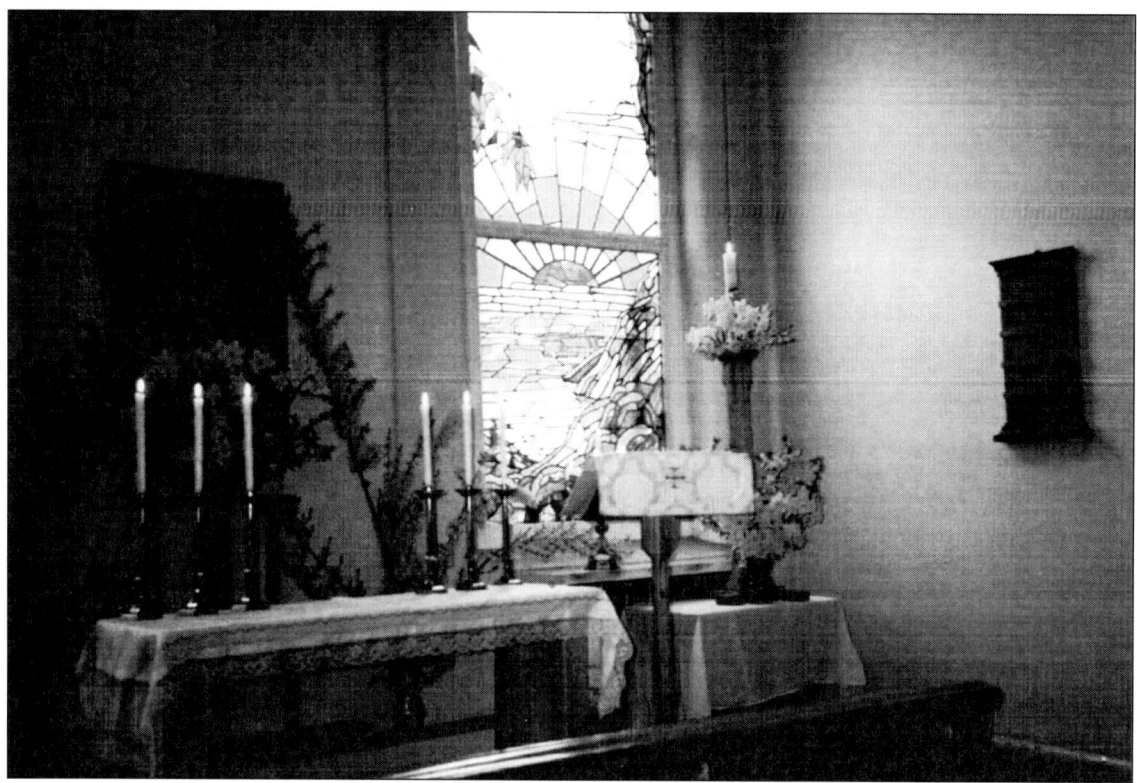

The Interdenominational Room had stained glass windows. (Vernon Muller)

In 1988 a booklet entitled *Out of the Depths* was written by the Rev Pat Thomas, who was Assistant Chaplain at the time. It was " a book of prayers in time of depression." Two of the prayers make very moving reading: The first deals with depression:

> "Lord, I feel so tired;
> - tired of being ill
> - tired of being here
> - tired of being tired
> I'm so tired of just being me.
>
> I want to close my eyes and never wake up.
> My dreary emptiness finds no purpose or meaning.
> I wish I'd never been born, and sometimes I think about ending it all.
> I get so frightened about how I feel.
> I'm so scared – scared of myself.
> Hold me in your love."

The second prayer expresses the anger and frustration that some patients felt:

> "Lord, I feel so angry with you.
> I am tormented by the monsters in the deeps.
> - the monsters of my rage that devours me and destroys me.
> - the monsters of my terror that makes others afraid of me.
>
> I am filled with loathing and disgust for the monster that I have become.
> I rage at you, O Lord, for you have made me. You are the rock on the
> sea-shore and I smash myself against you like a wave from the depths.

You accept all of my anger.
You accept even me.
You **are** my rock."

CHAPTER THIRTEEN

Entertainment

In the early days there was little in the way of entertainment for the patients in the evenings. There was, of course, no radio or television and wards were extremely poorly lit, so reading was almost impossible and in any case the supply of books was very limited and consisted mainly of religious and "uplifting" works. In 1865, however, there was a generous donation of books to the library by a certain Mr W H Smith. In more recent times, in 1921 the Borough Librarian at Hornsey made a gift of books that had been withdrawn from the public libraries.

There were, however twice yearly entertainments which were also open to selected visitors from outside. The September 1858 issue of *The North Middlesex and Southgate Messenger* describes a summer entertainment that took place on 14 July in a field at the west side of the building:

> "The gates were opened for the admission of visitors at 4 o'clock, and at about half past the strains of the band announced the approach of the patients, numbering about 650, who followed in couples, the females taking the precedence.
>
> Immediately upon their arrival they betook themselves to the amusements provided. At the lower end of the field a large number collected together throwing at snuff boxes &c on sticks, which they kept up with great vigour, the sticks flying about in all directions, to the hazard of the attendants, who were constantly employed in supplying the articles for competition: one of the females was highly amused by picking up the articles as they fell and running away with them, to the chagrin of those whose property they legally were. In another spot were nine-pins, which a select few busied themselves with. Cricket also employed others in the centre of the field, while one man, apparently about 50, was amusing himself with flying a kite he had made that morning. Near the entrance groups were engaged in dancing, while solitary individuals were stepping to the music, as if desirous to avoid confusion. Kissing in the ring also afforded great delight, and a laughable occurrence took place on one occasion, one of the visiting justices, having unconsciously intruded in the ring, was seized hold of by one of the female patients who unceremoniously gave him a hearty kiss, which elicited shouts of laughter from the crowd around.
>
> On each side the ground tents were erected for supplying refreshments to the patients, that for the females under the direction of Mr Clark, and one of the deputy matrons, and that of the males under the able superintendence of Messrs Quilton & Shirlaw, who were constantly employed in administering to their wants; the amount of cakes, oranges, beer and lemonade consumed was surprising, while pipes and tobacco were equally in request. A confectioner also had a tent to supply their visitors, of whom there were a great number present.
>
> Under one of the tents near the Band sat an old lady, fantastically adorned with a quality of lace of her own knitting, somewhat reserved, but yet did not hesitate to join in conversation relative to her peculiar notions, who imagined herself to be something more than mortal.
>
> The attendants generally busied themselves to promote their comfort and happiness, and we think successfully; two however were overcome by excitement, and removed to their regular quarters. We heard a sumptuous banquet

was provided for the visiting justices and their friends, but as we were not of the privileged number we can only record such was the fact."

The annual Summer Fairs were to be a feature of Friern right up to the time it closed and one in particular is recalled by Geoff Smith, Manager of Friern in 1981 and 1982:

"They were opened by a celebrity - one year we had Maureen Lipman who lived in Muswell Hill. She had been doing some filming in the morning and she arrived and she said: "I didn't realise how big it was" and she asked to borrow the phone - this was, of course, in the days before mobile phones – and she phoned her husband Jack Rosenthal and asked him to come up with the kids. He said: "The kids are playing with the kids next door" and she said "Well, bring them all" and he eventually arrived with about eight kids. I remember when I gave the opening speech to introduce Maureen she had arrived with a terrible migraine and as she had been the star of a TV series called *Agony* I remember saying that not only was she from *Agony*, but that she was actually in agony. We had side shows, tug of wars and we even got the local fire brigade involved but we would also arrange for the visitors to go on a conducted tour, obviously recognising the privacy of the patients. This was to try and dispel some of the myths."

The Open Days also provided an opportunity for the local community to experience the asylum at close hand and helped to dispel some misconceptions. Geoff Smith remembers:

"One of the things that I did while I was there was to invite the editors of the local newspapers and, because of the catchment area, you had the *Islington Gazette* and the *Ham and High*. One of the editors was Dennis Signy who was involved with Tottenham and later with Barnet FC and who has written books on Spurs and we had this lunch and we got a couple of the nurses and consultants to do a little presentation on what the hospital was all about and how we saw the future. It resulted in some quite positive articles in the papers. And also how it helped was when there was a story about a missing patient or a suicide, despite our attempts to prevent things like that happening, so rather than sensationalise things they understood the hospital and they would have a better take on it. We did a lot with the local press and for a year or two we gave an open invitation to reporters to come in at any time and have a look. We had also knocked four feet off the walls as well. We introduced a staff magazine, *Neurone*, not only to tell the local community what was happening, but also to improve internal communication as well – we didn't want to tell the community things that we hadn't told our own staff. And half of our staff were local people anyway. The article that I wrote was called *Personally Speaking* because as manager of the hospital I wanted to write as a person. The radio station was for patients as well."

In the early days there was also a winter entertainment held in the main hall as this article in *The North Middlesex and Southgate Messenger* of February 1858 relates:

"On Tuesday evening Jan 19th 1858, the annual entertainment to the patients in the above asylum was given in the exercising hall of the establishment, under the superintendence of the visiting justices. The hall was fitted up in a most tasteful manner. Two alcoves were erected at the south end of the room, supported by pillars neatly marbled and gilded, as also those supporting the gallery at the north end; the whole being festooned with evergreens. Banners floated from the side walls, and about twenty Chinese lanterns suspended from the ceiling, together

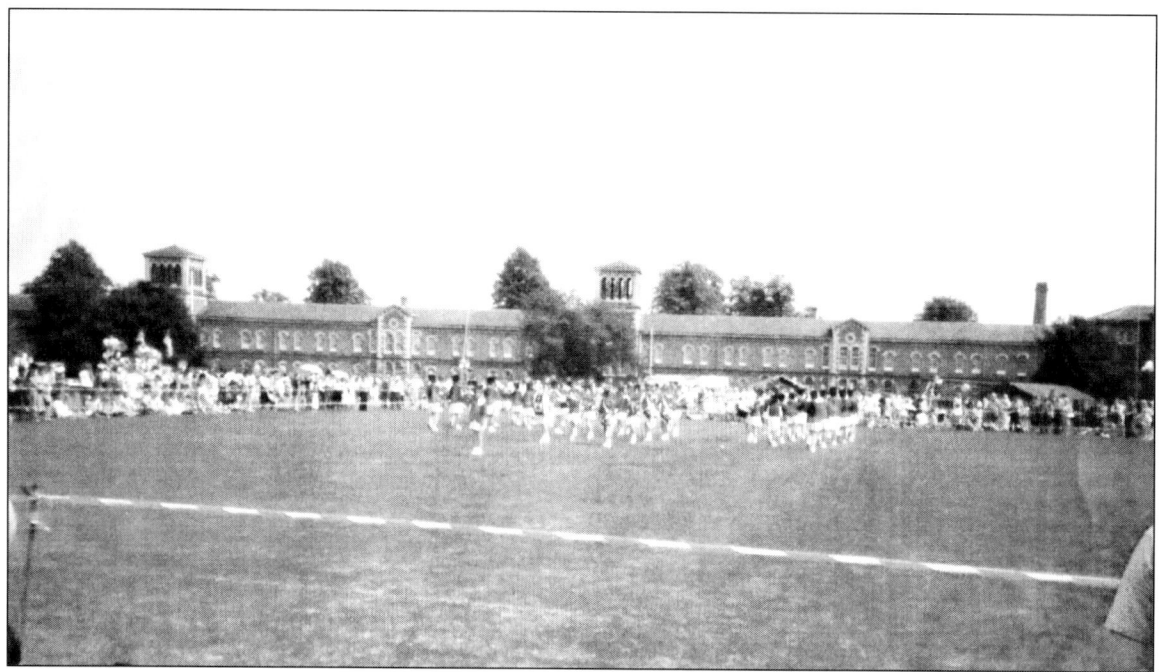

The Open Day on 4 July 1982, with the west wing in the background. (John Donovan)

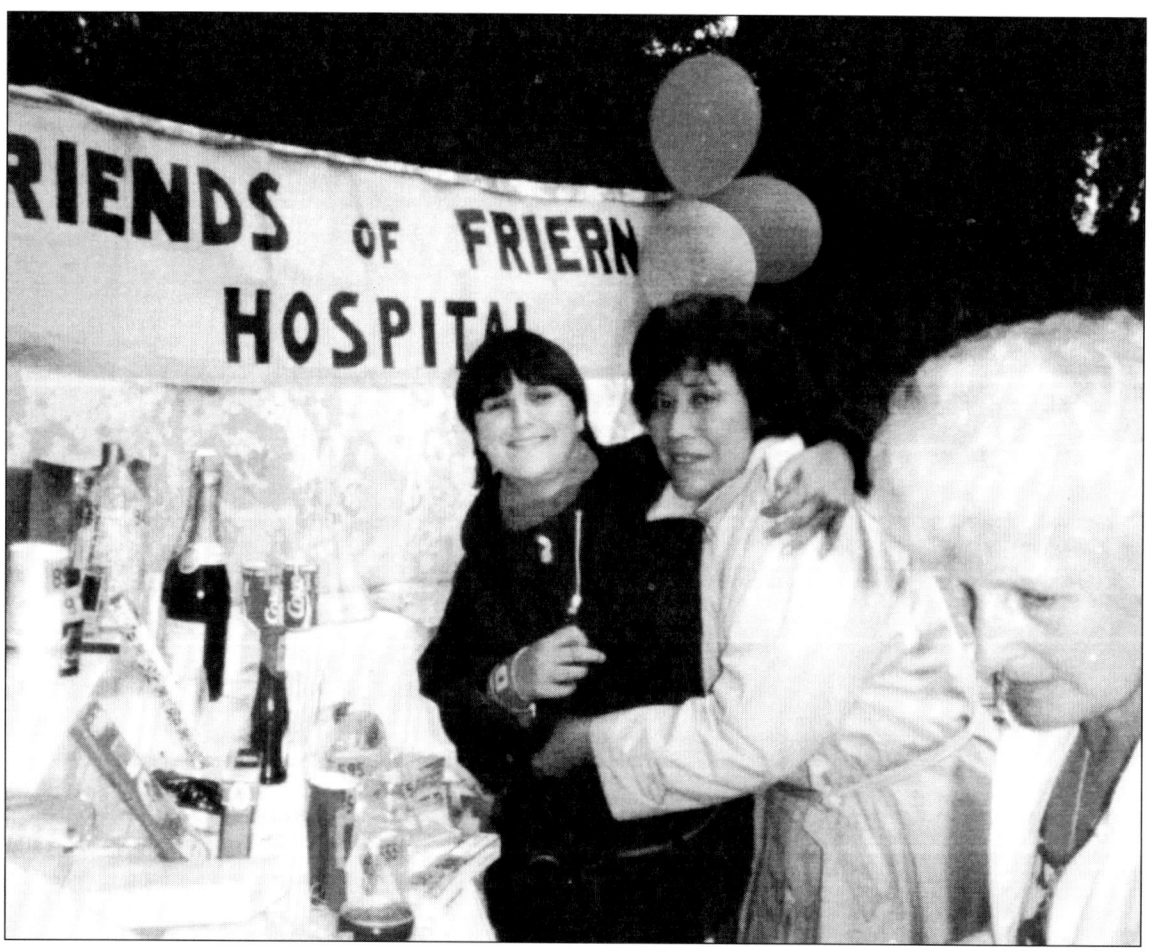

The Friends of the Hospital had a fund raising stall at the Open Day. (Vernon Muller)

with the gas, illuminated the spacious area. The amusements commenced soon after six o'clock, with dissolving views, exhibited by Mr Cox, of Chiswell-street, consisting of views of Interlachen, Ratisbon, Rhodes Harbour, Thames Tunnel, Santa Saluta, Castle of Chillon, Temple of Tivoli, Ruins of Palmyra, Village of Haarlem (summer), Do (winter), Fall of snow, Interior of York Cathedral, Ship at Anchor, Exterior Palace (Delhi), Entrance Do, Holyrood Chapel, Dryburg Abbey, Loch Leven Castle, Street in Madrid; followed by Chromatropes, or artificial fireworks, exhibiting an endless variety of changes and colours, with a final representing the Queen and Prince Albert in medallion. An excellent band was provided for the occasion.

The entertainment appeared to please the patients, if we may judge of their approbation by the continued clapping of hands. The cakes on the present occasion, three in number, were of the same dimensions as those we spoke of last year; one measuring four feet in diameter, and weighing three cwt; the other two being severally three feet in diameter, and weighing two cwt each. The largest, we were informed, was in the oven for 13¼ hours. After the distribution of cake, oranges and other refreshments, dancing commenced, and was continued with untiring zeal until half past 9, when the band played the National Anthem. We were struck with the orderly and willing manner in which the patients separated from their friends and left the hall – in number about 200 males and 250 females.

The hall was completely filled during the evening. Many of the visitors joined in the dance, and endeavoured to promote the amusement of the patients – the chief amongst whom were the medical officers of the institution, who laboured assiduously to keep them in good humour. A large number of them, however, sat merely as spectators; some of their countenances wearing a melancholy aspect, others equally vivacious and talkative. On one side we observed and elderly lady in possession of several dolls, and which at times she was heartily chastising. Another lady was seated by the fireplace with a canary bird in a cage, her constant companion, and which was singing in obedience to her request. Another was diverting her auditory by stating that she had consumed sixteen glasses of rum on Christmas Eve, just one-twenty years since, and from which cause she attributed her being an inmate of the asylum; and then commenced snapping her fingers, and dancing and singing with astonishing vigour, and evident satisfaction to herself. A bald-headed male patient was dancing with great delight, and might be heard exclaiming "promenade" with all the confidence of an accomplished performer. A short man, who we learnt was by profession an organist, was heartily enjoying the amusement, and moving about with alacrity. We cite these few instances, among many others, as having attracted our special attention; but the tout ensemble was striking, and we have seldom witnessed a scene so calculated to humble the pride of man was presented on this occasion – to mingle with the individuals created by the same Almighty Power as ourselves, and yet devoid of that greatest of all blessings, reason"

In 1971 a hospital radio station was started with a donation of £500 from the pupils of Minchenden School. Radio Friern 350 (350 being the phone number of the station by which patients could place requests) was run by volunteers who would play records from their own collections. Activities within the hospital were also featured as well as news and sports. One of the presenters was Pete Abbott, nowadays a broadcaster on TalkSport and who hosts the television programme at Tottenham Hotspur on match days. Pete recalls that when he started at the station it only broadcast on Saturdays and Sundays and

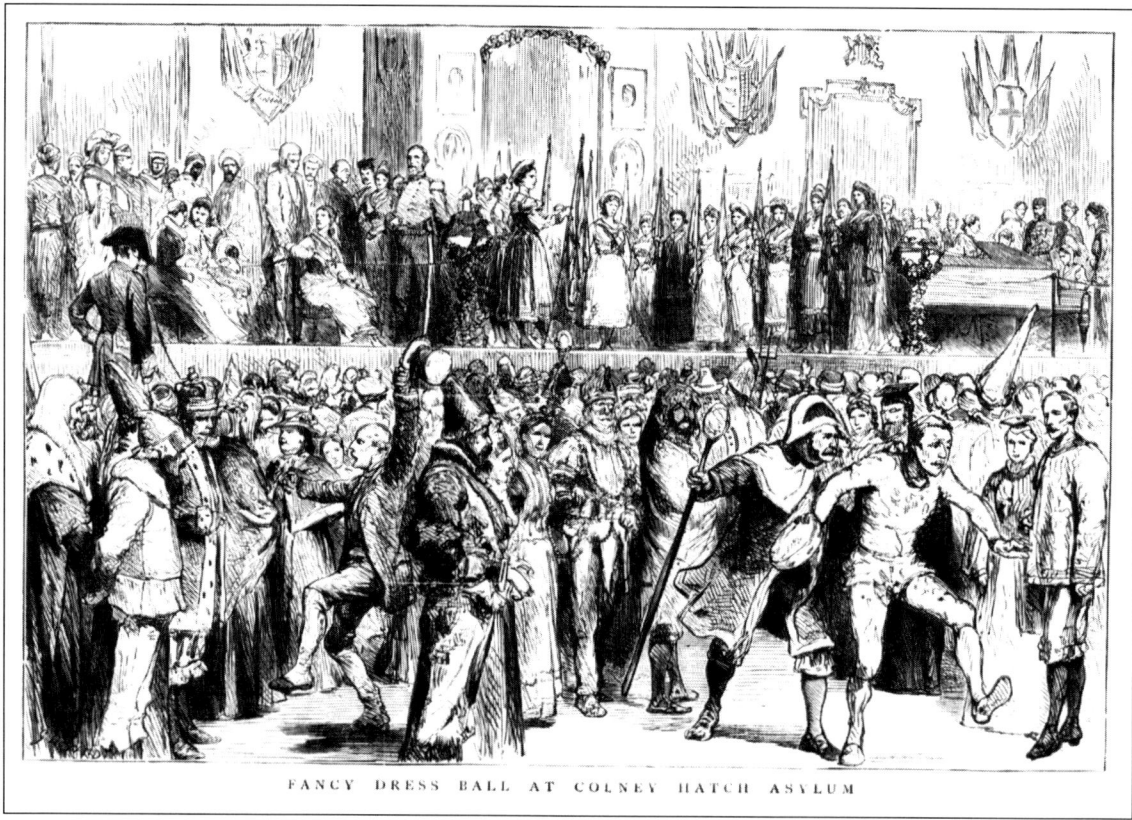

Illustration from The Graphic of 29 November 1879. (FB&DLHS Archive)

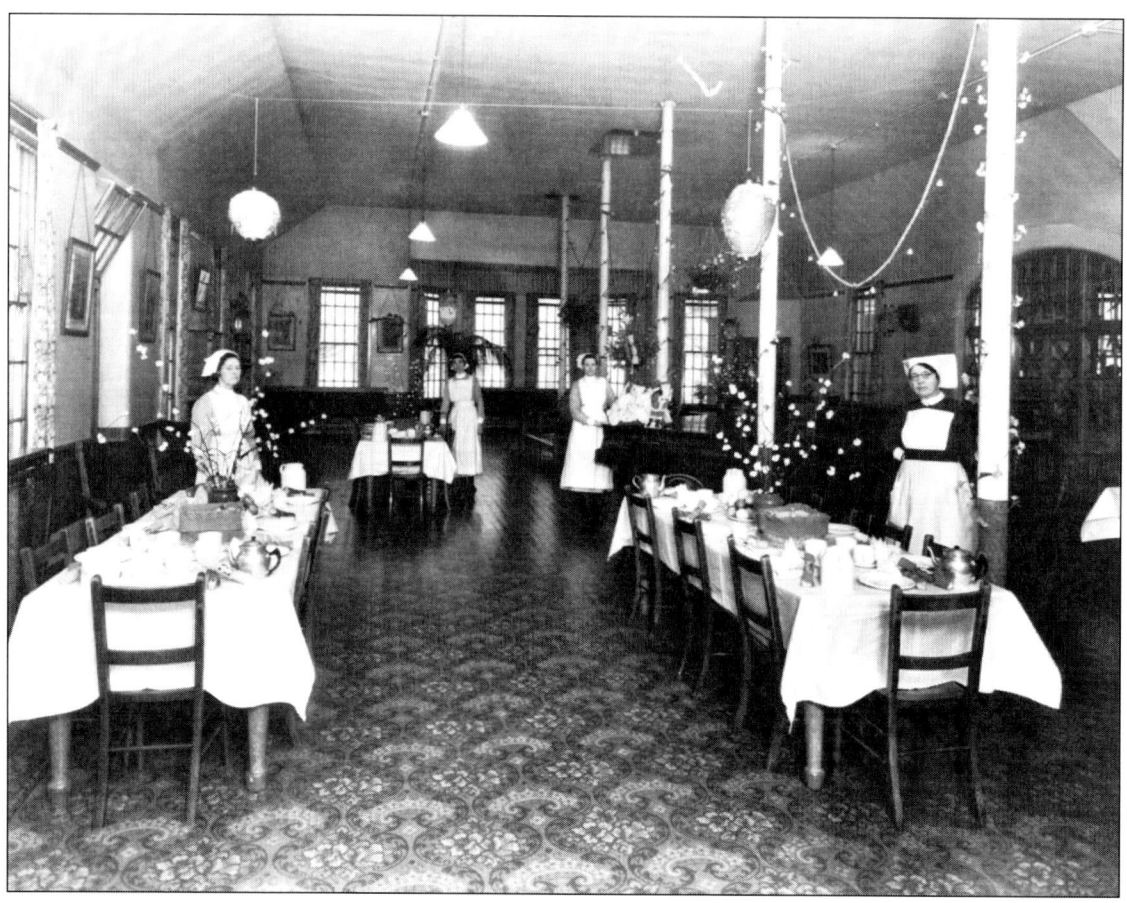

Christmas decorations in 1938. (City of London. London Metropolitan Archives)

he did the Sunday morning stint. Later on the there also were programmes on Mondays, Tuesdays and Thursdays. Pete remembers that the studio was in a tiny room up a steep flight of stairs in the main building and there was only room for three people. They used to broadcast music, all on vinyl in those days, and they had many requests from patients for music of their choice. The last radio programme was broadcast on Saturday 13 March 1993 by which time there were only one hundred patients left in the hospital.[1]

KALEIDOSCOPE

ENTERTAINMENT ★ EVENTS ★ INFORMATION ★ ENTERTAINMENT ★ EVENTS ★ INFORMATION

ORCHARD CLUB CINEMA

Every Tuesday, 7 p.m.

Forthcoming Attractions

2nd March — GAMBIT
9th March — ROBBERY
16th March — BRIEF ENCOUNTER
23rd March — ASSAULT ON A QUEEN
30th March — BACK STREET

ORCHARD CLUB

Mondays — DISCO
Tuesdays — FILM
Thursdays — BINGO

All at 7 p.m.

THE CHAZEN CLUB

Every Wednesday, 7 p.m.

Bingo — Entertainment — Singing

REMEDIAL ENGLISH

Classes are held in The Olive Room
9 a.m. to 10 a.m. and 10 a.m. to 11 a.m.

Patients are referred from the ward

FRIENDS OF FRIERN HOSPITAL

BINGO PARTIES

These are held on Wednesdays alternately in Wards 13 and 17, and fortnightly on Mondays in Ward E2. All patients able to come are welcome.

FRIENDS OF FRIERN HOSPITAL

250 CLUB DRAW

December
£6   No. 95   Mr. F. Farmer
£5   No. 131   Mr. G. Nicholas
£3   No. 191   Mr. R. Lazama

January
£6   No. 1   Mr. K. Lait
£5   No. 6   Mrs. Willsmure
£3   No. 68   Mr. K. Smith

February
£6   No. 44   Mr. S. Sheaf
£5   No. 85   Mr. G. Samuels
£3   No. 61   Mr. E. Kavanagh

Radio Friern 350

PROGRAMMES

Mondays
7.00 p.m.   The Paul Sparrey Music Gallery
8.30 p.m.   The Late Show, with Tony Adams

Tuesdays
7.00 p.m.   Mick Maan's Music Show
8.30 p.m.   The Darren Fogel Show

Thursdays
7.00 p.m.   Vic Groves Vibes

Fridays
7.00 p.m.   Barry Staffa's Motley Collection
8.15 p.m.   Friern on Friday
8.45 p.m.   Claire Walding

Saturdays
7.00 a.m.   Alan Shaier's Early Morning Show
9.00 a.m.   Pete Hill's Saturday Special
11.00 a.m. Vick Elton's Sackful of Soul
1.00 p.m.   Martin Rosen and Sounds Good
3.00 p.m.   Roundabout, by Andy Hunter
5.00 p.m.   The Jon Hirons Show

SPORTSCENE begins at 2 p.m. with a preview of the day's sport. The Half Time Report is at 4 p.m. and at 5.30 p.m. there is a half-hour roundup of the day's sporting news.

Sundays
9.00 a.m.   In The Mood, with David Frome
11.00 a.m. Pete Abbott's Breakfast Cereal
1.00 p.m.   Cheryl Holt, with Popular Sounds
3.00 p.m.   Keith Rowe's Much More Music Show
5.00 p.m.   Tea with Malcom Tims
7 p.m.   William Martin

If you would like a request or a dedication, telephone 350 during broadcasting hours, 209 during office hours or write to Radio Friern.

★ ★ ★

A NEW PROJECT

is afoot to provide amenities for elderly people's wards. It is hoped to revive the sponsored walk this year to start the fund raising. More details next month.

(Neurone, Friern Hospital house magazine 1981)

In 1880 it was reported that some 200 men were taken for country walks by members of staff every fortnight and smaller parties on three days a week. Fifty female patients were taken out weekly and a few daily. In later years a dozen or so patients would be taken for days out in a minibus to such local places as Broomfield Park and Hadley Wood, with the chaplain driving, accompanied by a member of staff and a volunteer from one of the local churches. Venues further afield included Woburn Abbey and Southend, the latter trip in 1978 consisting of two coach loads of patients and staff.

In later years the hall was used at Christmas time for the presentation of nativity plays, often written by the chaplain and with patients and members of staff not only acting but painting and making the scenery. The stage was fully equipped with curtains, flats and professional lighting.

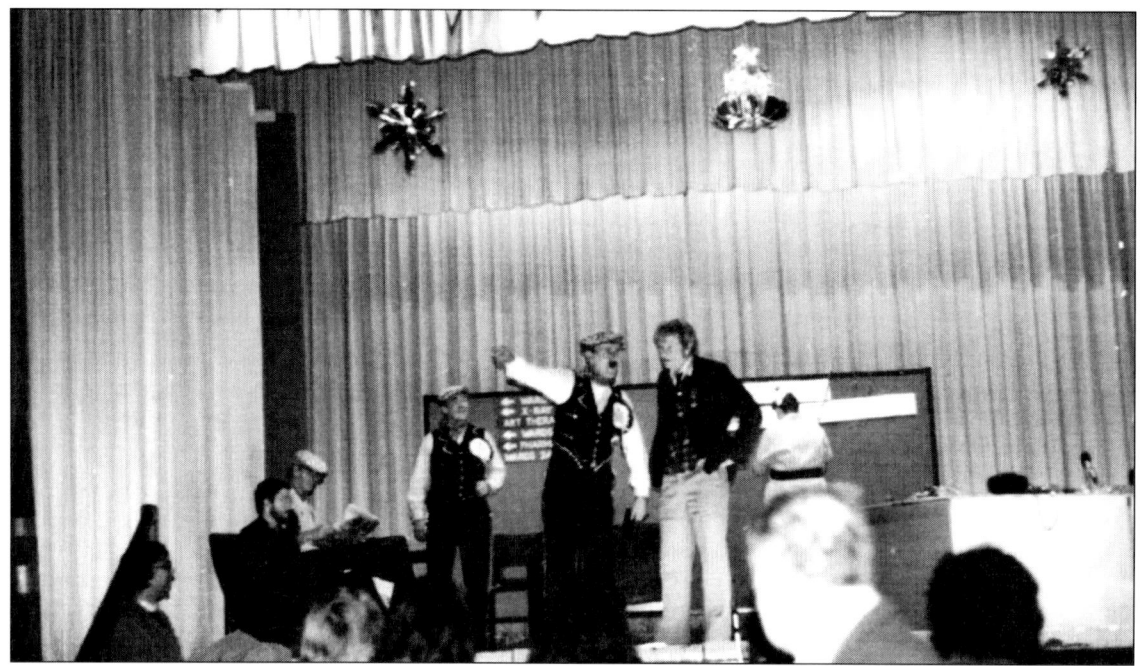

A Nativity play in the Hall. (Vernon Muller)

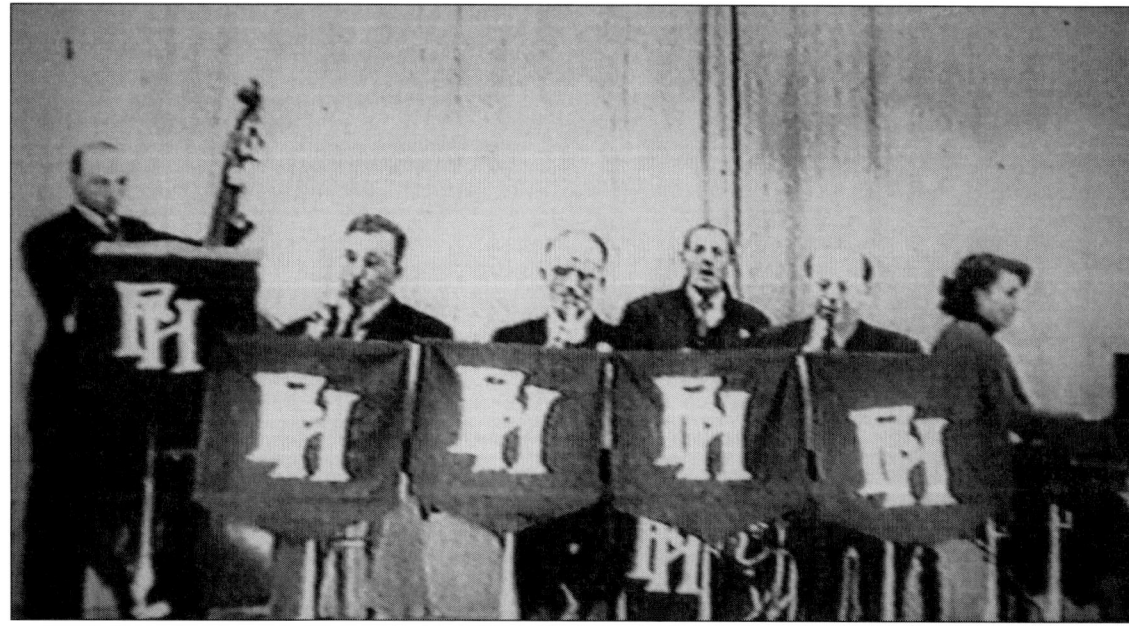

The hospital even had its own band. (Time Marches on at Friern)

CHAPTER FOURTEEN

The Staff

As we have seen, when the asylum first opened it was at a time when the old methods of restraint of patients had been abolished and staff were being expected to cope with disturbed or dangerous patients without the aid of drugs to calm them down, apart from bromide. The work of nurses was extremely hard; in 1859, for example, almost half (36) of the 75 patients who died that year had been bedridden[1], which meant that they would have needed almost constant attention. Epilepsy was common among patients and epileptics too needed a high level of care, particularly at meal times when a fit could have led to them choking. Some patients had to be forcibly fed, another time-consuming operation that would require the use of two members of staff.

It is not surprising therefore that relatively untrained and inexperienced staff dealt with seriously disturbed patients by using some degree of physical force, as the following extract from the *North Middlesex and Southgate Messenger* of September 1860 shows:

> "During the past month an investigation has taken place before Mr Henry, at the Bow Street Police Court, relative to the death of a patient named William Swift, who it was alleged, had died through injuries received from the hands of two of the Warders in that establishment, as far back as the 12th of May last, and which from some information received, the Commissioners in Lunacy considered necessary should be inquired into. From the evidence adduced, it was discovered upon a post mortem examination that the deceased's breastbone, and eleven of his ribs were broken, and the coroner's jury at the time returned an open verdict. The result of inquiry has terminated in the committal of the Warders, Slater and Vivian, for trial at the Old Bailey, and in consequence of an application by Counsel, the same has been postponed until the September Sessions. Any comments therefore, until that has taken place would be premature, when probably the evidence will be more complete, and the public acquainted with the true facts of the case."

A month later they were acquitted:

> "The two warders, Messrs Slater and Vivian, who were committed for trial on a charge of having been instrumental in causing the death of a patient named William Swift, as far back as 12th May last, surrendered to take their trial on Wednesday 19th ult. and after a full inquiry, the jury acquitted them. The only evidence that at all affected them, as to any ill usage having been manifested by them towards the deceased, was that given by two of the patients, who were in the same ward with the deceased, and which the Counsel engaged, argued it would be unsafe to rely upon, and from this cause it would appear the Jury thought it expedient to give them the benefit of the doubt."

Allegations of ill-treatment of patients continued to be made throughout the life of the asylum, particularly by those from outside who did not appreciate the difficulties in dealing with mental patients. Whilst there would have been some staff that were less then sympathetic to their patients, it must be remembered that many patients were volatile and unpredictable. Vernon Muller, the chaplain at Friern:

> "There were abuses, I wouldn't deny that, and some of the things that went on were really awful. Not active abuse, but passive abuse - they were treated as a nuisance, as stupid. I would speak out on occasions because they didn't take much notice: "You don't understand; you're not on the ward for twenty-four

hours." So there were abuses, but there was also a lot of excellent rehabilitative work going on."

Vernon also recalls how patients could be violent towards staff:

"On one occasion I was walking through the grounds of the hospital and there was a big patient who was beating up a smaller, elderly patient and he had him on the ground and he was kicking him so I shouted at him and he ran off. I picked up the old man and took him back to his ward. A few minutes later I resumed my walk across the grounds and I saw this patient who had been attacking the old man and I very foolishly approached him and he then set upon me and, I can tell you, I ran! It was very foolish of me. I could so easily have kept my distance and summoned a member of staff and we could have approached him with reinforcements."

In his moving autobiography *Sectioned: A Life Interrupted* John O'Donoghue, who spent some time as a patient at Friern in 1979, gave this description of an incident that happened at Halliwick Hospital:

"I walk down the little corridor leading from the TV lounge to the office. There's a toilet just beyond this and I need to go. A Rasta girl stands in the corridor, talking to the charge nurse who's on tonight, a Nigerian nurse I've not seen before. Maybe he's from the agency. Sean comes out of the toilet just as I'm about five steps from the office. He goes up to the charge nurse and in one quick movement launches himself at his neck, both hands around him, squeezing as hard as he can.

They fall to the floor. Sean squeezes and squeezes and the nurse yells for help. The Rasta girl looks up at me and starts screaming at me to get Sean off. "He's strangling him!" she shouts at me. "Don't just stand there – do something!" A nurse from Cedar Ward comes belting across and into the corridor. Sean is still choking the charge nurse with all his strength but the nurse from Cedar Ward pulls him off and leads Sean away. As suddenly as he attacked the charge nurse, just as suddenly Sean is calm and under control. But the charge nurse is breathing hard and rubbing his neck. His eyes are wild and red. The Rasta girl looks at me sharply. She thinks I should have helped the charge nurse. But I was so shocked I couldn't move. Now I go up to the charge nurse. "Are you all right?" I ask. "He tried to kill me!" gasps the charge nurse. "What is wrong with him?" "He hears voices," I say.

The Rasta girl is disgusted with me. She takes the charge nurse into the office and shuts the door.

I go into the toilet and look in the mirror. This is not who I wanted to be."

The asylum was nearly always understaffed but the ratio of staff to patients gradually got better as the years passed:

Year	Patients	Nurses	Ratio
1852	1236	91	13.5:1
1858	1295	145	8.9:1
1890	2248	257	8.7:1
1937	2700	454	5.9:1

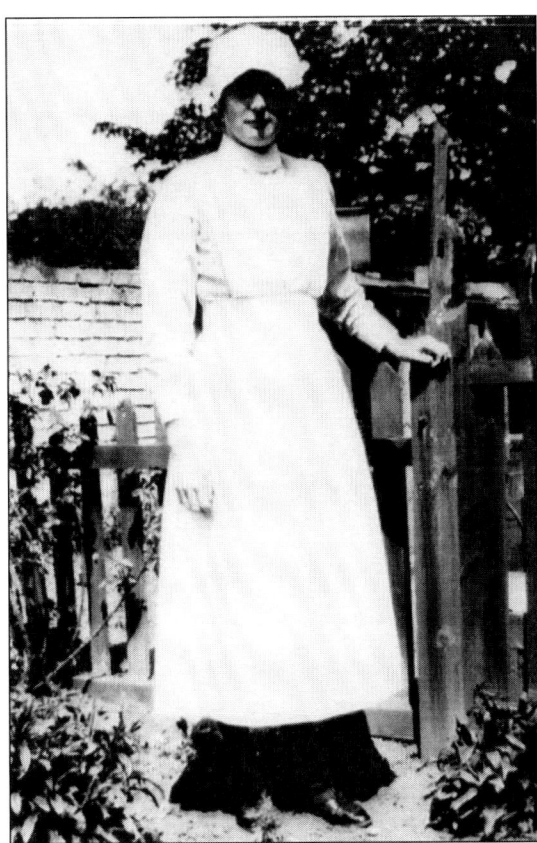 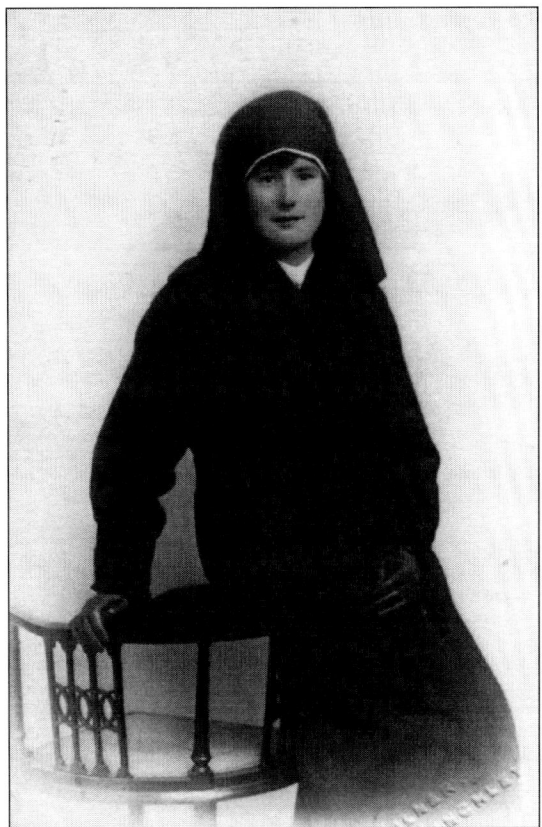

One of the nurses at Friern, Hilda Collins, photographed in 1927. (Pamela Brown Collection)

On 13 Aug 1851, a mere month after the Asylum opened, the following scale of fines to be imposed on female attendants was issued:

Leaving the ward without an attendant	2s
Leaving a patient unlocked at night	2s
Not providing them with clean clothes at the stated times	6d
Neglecting to bathe them according to the Rules and Regulations	6d
Keeping the room doors closed in the daytime	3d
Not having the cleaning done by half past 10 o'clock	3d
The night watch neglecting to turn off the gas	1s
Allowing a patient to escape from the ward	2s
Cleaning not done by ½ past 10 o'clock	6d
Dormitory doors not being open in day time	6d
Not being up in time in the morning	1s

The matrons' job was largely a supervisory one; they did little nursing themselves, although they were expected to know all the patients in their care and to see that they were being treated properly. In addition they were responsible for keeping records of the stores in their department, so a knowledge of accounting was a prerequisite, and to help with the administrative workload matrons were each given an assistant.

The nurses' daily routine involved waking the patients at 6am, helping them to get washed and dressed in time for breakfast at 8am and making sure the wards were cleaned by 10am. Patients would have to be in bed by 7.45pm. Nurses and other staff would be allowed to take exercise in the grounds between 8 and 9pm, providing that they did not communicate with the other sex.

A report in the *North Middlesex and Southgate Messenger* of August 1857 shows that it was not all work at the asylum:

> "Colney Hatch asylum. On July 6 an interesting and exciting cricket match played at Colney Hatch between eleven Carpenters of the County Asylum and eleven Odds and Ends in the different trades and callings of the same institution and which terminated in favour of the latter who had five wickets to spare. The play on both sides was extremely good."

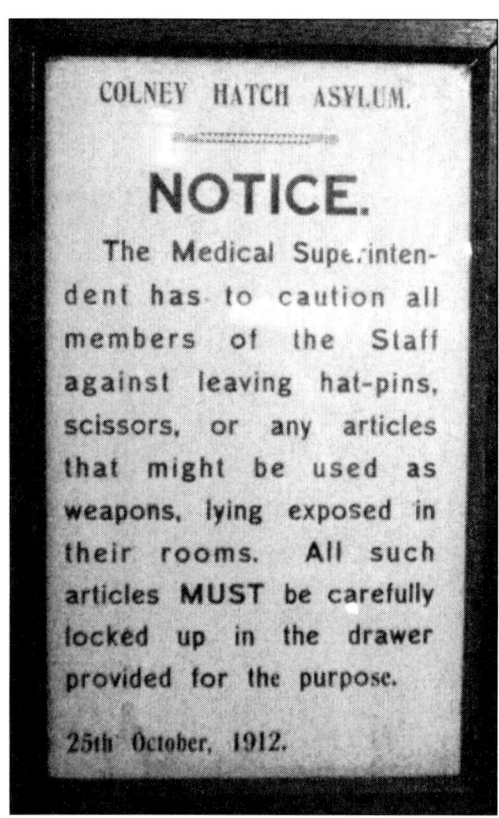

The stories of two of the attendants at Colney Hatch make interesting reading. Both of them were ex-military men who, having completed their service decided on a career tending to the patients. Thomas Edwards was born in 1863 in Brill, Buckinghamshire, the son of an agricultural labourer. At some point between after 1871 the family moved to Yorkshire and Thomas, too, became a farm labourer. In 1880 he enlisted in the army at York. He must have been eager to join because he overstated his age by three years – at that time the minimum enlistment age was 18. He was transferred to the 1st Batallion Royal Highlanders (The Black Watch) in August 1881 and a year later he was in Africa and was involved in campaigns in Egypt and the Sudan. It was in the 1884-85 Nile campaign that he won the VC. The citation[2] reads:

> "For the conspicuous bravery displayed by him in defence of one of the guns of the Naval Brigade, at the battle of Tamai, on 13th March, 1884. This man (who was attached to the Naval Brigade as a Mule Driver) was beside the gun with Lieutenant Almack, RN, and a blue jacket. Both the latter were killed, and Edwards, after bayoneting two Arabs, and himself receiving a wound with a spear, rejoined the ranks with his mules, and subsequently did good service in remaining by his gun throughout the section."

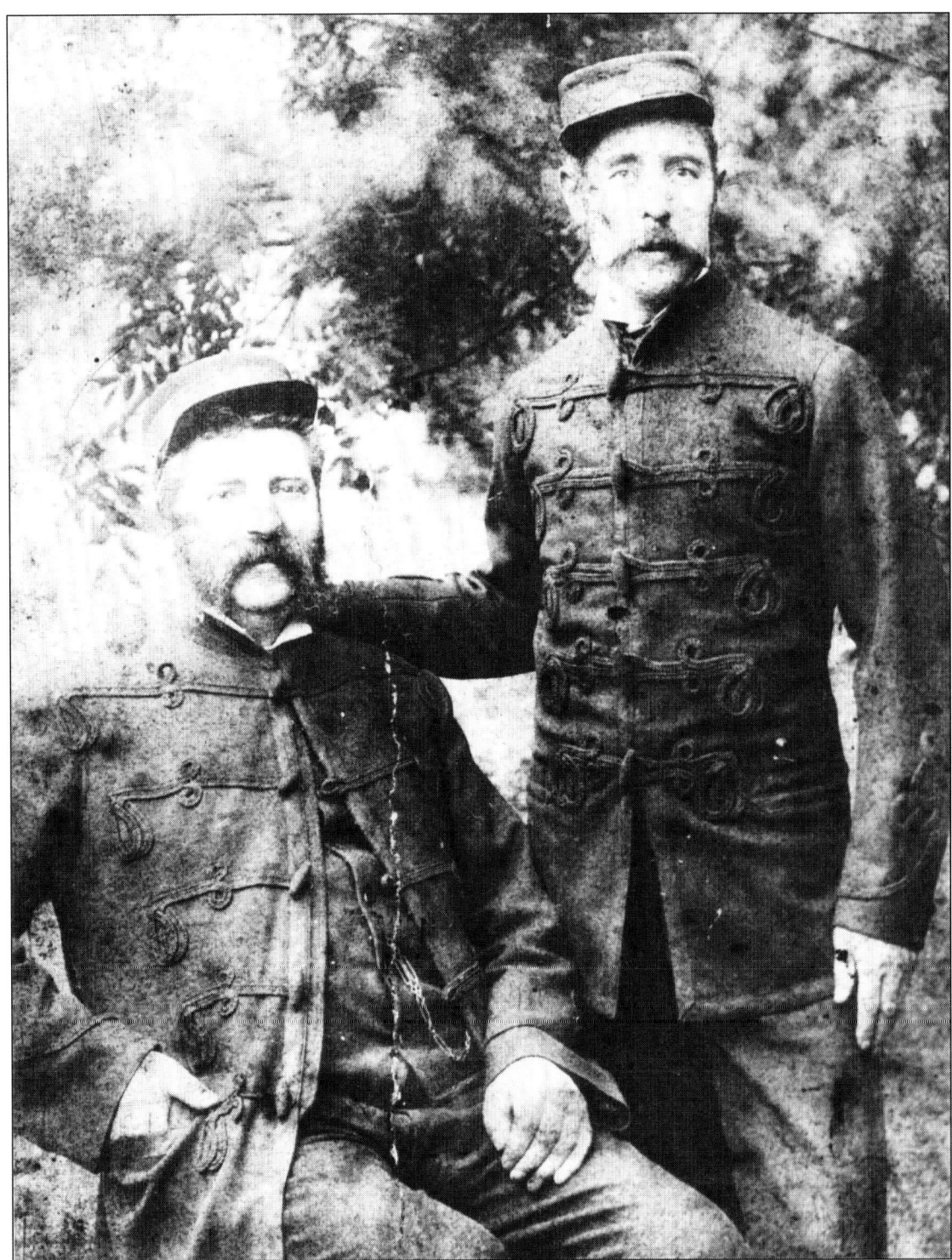

Early attendants with their smart uniforms. (Barnet Local Studies)

He completed his active service in Malta and was discharged to the Reserve at the end of 1886. He started working as a 2nd Class attendant at Colney Hatch in March 1888 and was promoted to 1st Class Attendant in February 1904. In 1892 he married Ellen Roseanna Stone, who had also been an attendant, and they lived at various times in the asylum and also in New Southgate until at least 1914. He retired from the asylum shortly afterwards and he subsequently moved to Woodford Bridge in Essex and died there at the age of 90 on 27 March 1952.

The other story concerns a man who was a nurse at Friern for twenty six years. Robert Berridge was born locally in 17 Bawtry Road, Friern Barnet on 6 March 1897. He later moved with his family to 37 Pembroke Road and attended school at Brunswick Park School. On leaving school he joined G J Lines & Sons Ltd of Down Lane, Tottenham who made wooden toys such as rocking horses and dolls houses. Lines later went on to become Lines Brothers, makers of Tri-ang toys. Robert was an apprentice sawyer and he worked at Lines until 1916 when he enlisted on 10 October 1916 at the age of 19 years 7 months at Mill Hill barracks and was sent to the Army Service Corps at Park Royal where he spent six months training.

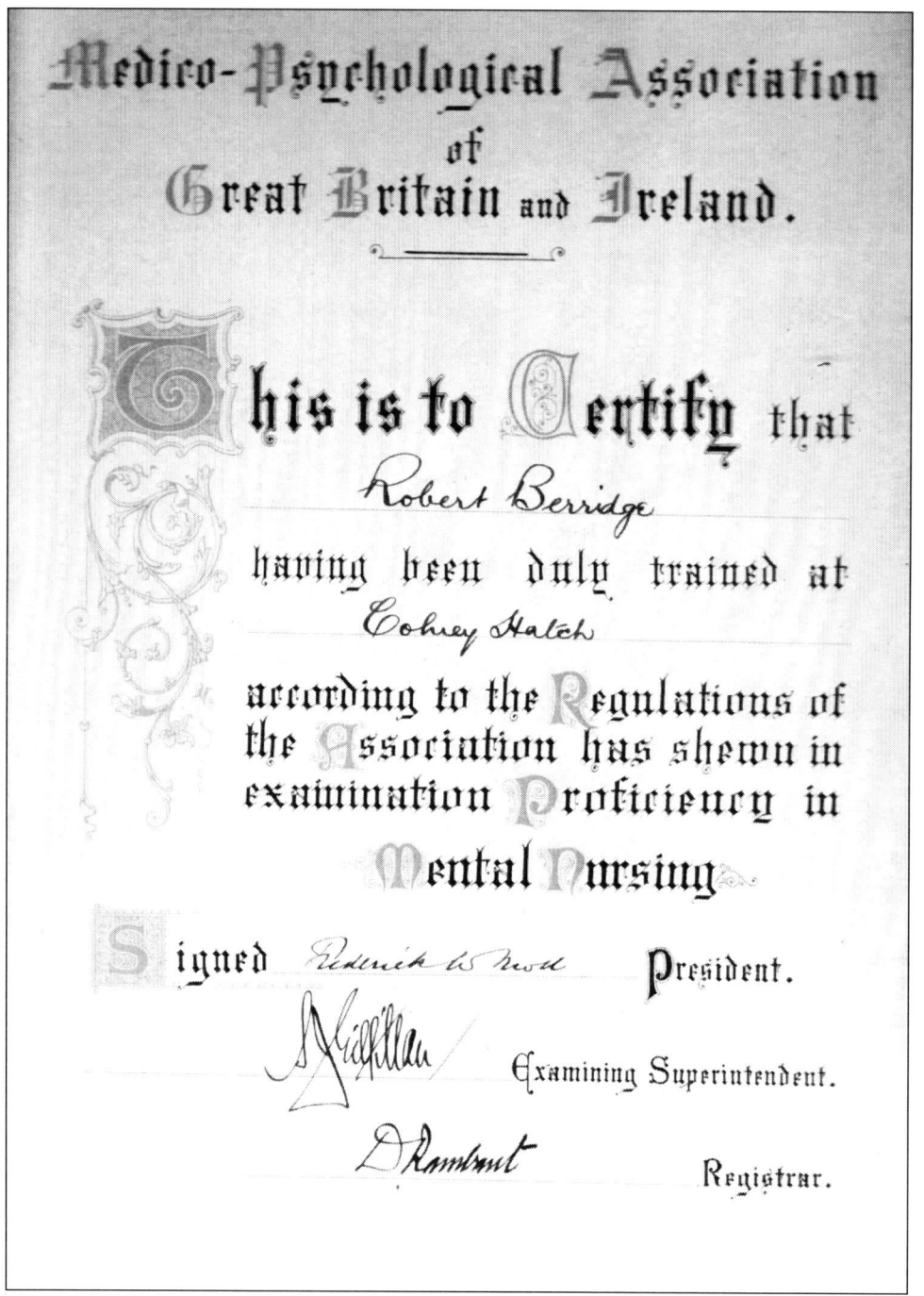

Robert Berridge's certificate from May 1925. (John Rampley Collection)

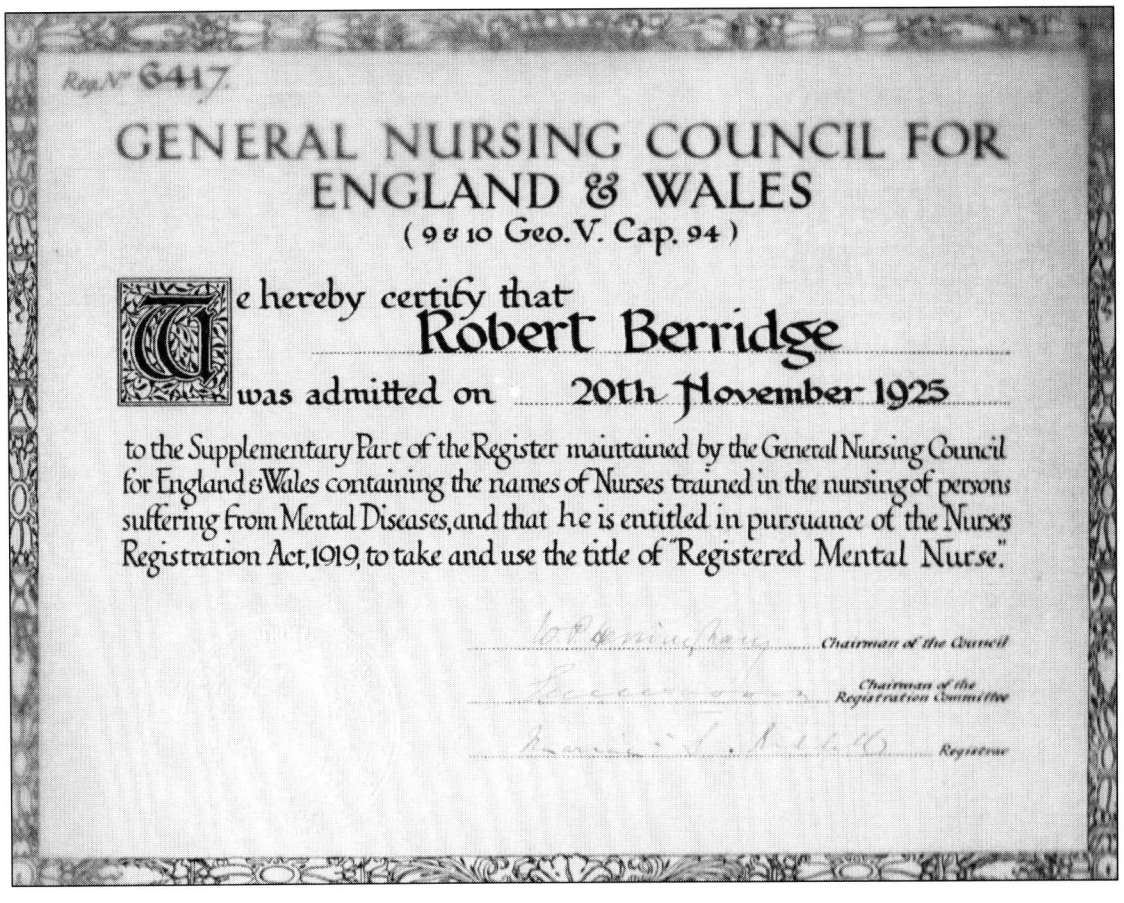

Robert Berridge's certificate from November 1925 confirms that he was a qualified Registered Mental nurse. (John Rampley Collection)

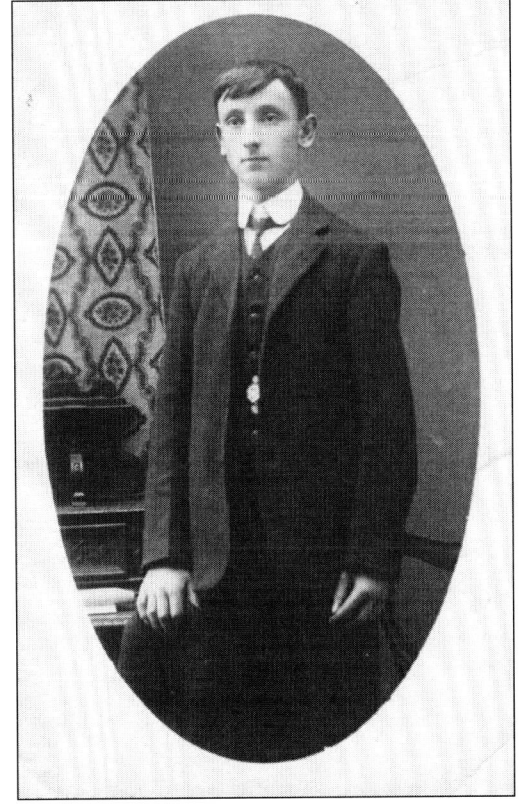 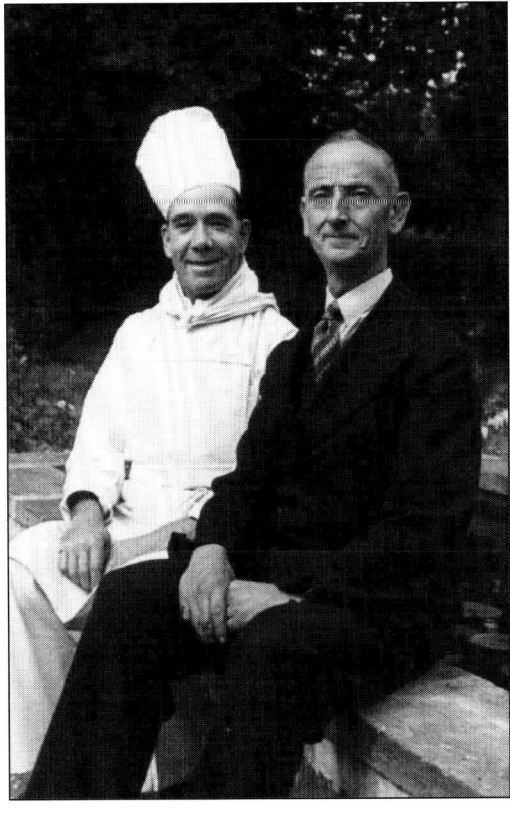

Robert Berridge shortly after joining Friern and on his retirement in 1951. (John Rampley Collection)

After being transferred to Edinburgh where he joined the 104th Training Reserve, he was transferred to the East Kent Regiment, "The Buffs", in Canterbury. On 2 August he embarked from Dover to the reserve area at Mazingarbe and then to the French/Belgium border at Steenvoorde. At the first battle of Passchendale at Ypres on 12 October 1917 Private Berridge was listed as "Missing in Action" but he had, in fact, been taken prisoner by the Germans and, after peace had been declared, he was released unharmed on 19 December 1918. On returning to the UK and, despite having letters to secure employment back with G & J Lines, he decided to join Colney Hatch Mental Hospital and train as a mental nurse. The reason for his change of career is not known, but it is interesting to speculate whether his experiences in the War, and his possible exposure to cases of shell shock, made him sympathetic to mental illness and created a desire to do something to help. Robert Berridge became a fully qualified Mental Nurse in 1925 and remained at Friern until his retirement in 1951.

In common with many hospitals at the time, nurses were given accommodation within the hospital, in the early days they slept in rooms adjacent to the wards. As the number of staff increased it became more difficult to find rooms for them all. A report in 1931[3] stated that out of 254 female staff, 220 actually resided inside the hospital and that it would be impossible to find rooms for more, particularly as many of the 238 existing rooms were below the standard aimed at when the hospital was opened. The need for a nurses' home was considered to be so great that in 1914 Beech House, which had been built in 1865 as an isolation ward for fever patients was converted into the first nurses' home. The breakdown of female staff at the time was:

	Staff living in	*Staff living out*
Sisters	10	2
Chief charge nurses & charge nurses	44	23
Staff nurses and probationers	154	3
Hospital assistants	1	4
Domestic staff	7	4
Laundry staff	3	15
Workmisstresses		1
Assistant workmisstresses	1	

In 1937 a four storey building, Blythe House, was completed to the west of the main hospital and was used as a nurses' home with single bed sitting rooms and a large lounge area and a guest lounge where the nurses could entertain their friends.

In August 1981 a new Nurses Education Centre was opened in the former Villa 5. Up to thirty students at a time were trained to be psychiatric nurses in a course that lasted three years. For the first two months there was only class room work with conducted visits around the hospital; after that nurses would go on to the wards. The centre consisted of four classrooms and a demonstration room and was converted at a cost of £280,000.[4] By the 1970s more nurses were living off site and travelling to and from work by car so the ornamental gardens in front of the main building were converted into car parks.

As well as nurses there was a large number of support staff: cooks, kitchen maids, laundry maids, porters, artisans, gardeners and labourers and secretarial staff. By 1950 there were over 950 people working at Friern and the total wage bill was £293,838.[5]

Ken Dunthorne was an engineering fitter employed at Friern between 1978 and 1996 and he kept meticulous records of all his jobs. The variety of tasks he performed show what a valuable contribution people like him made to the smooth running of the hospital:

WARD	NO	JOB	HRS	DATE
Paint Shop	64748	Turn knob for blow lamp pump stem	1½	11-5-81
Ward E3		Attend to staff locker	½	11-5-81
Medical Records	9973	Repair wheels on No 2 swivel chair	2	11-5-81
Ward 19	67142	Repair wheels on ward mobile screen	1	11-5-81
Ward 13	63497	Repair wheels on dinner trolley	3	11-5-81
Ward 24	65814	Attend to wheels on No 1 commode	3	12-5-81
Builders	60158	Overhaul step ladders - stays & pivot bolts	4	12-5-81
Personnel Dept.	60159	Inspect fire escape (Ward 16)	1	12-5-81
Ward 24	65814	Repair 2 dining chairs	1½	13-5-81
Gardeners	60160	Repair cable drum on strimmer m/c	2½	13-5-81
Ward 9	66680	Repairs to AR50 elevating bath chair	2½	13-5-81
Supplies Office	59571	Fit locking device to staff locker	1½	13-5-81
Butchers Shop	67122	Attend to trolley wheels. New ones ordered	2½	14-5-81
Main Stores	59540	Fit locking device to 3 staff lockers	2½	14-5-81
C.S.S.D.		Drip tray for roller conveyer	2	14-5-81
Fitters		Cut up flat iron as required	1	14-5-81
Main Kitchen		Finish off mixing bowl trolleys	3	15-5-81
C.S.S.D		Make & fit drip tray for roller conveyer	3½	15-5-81
Boiler house		Attend to fire door	½	15-5-81
Builders		Sharpen cutting tools	1	15-5-81
C.S.S.D.		Drip tray	4	16-5-81

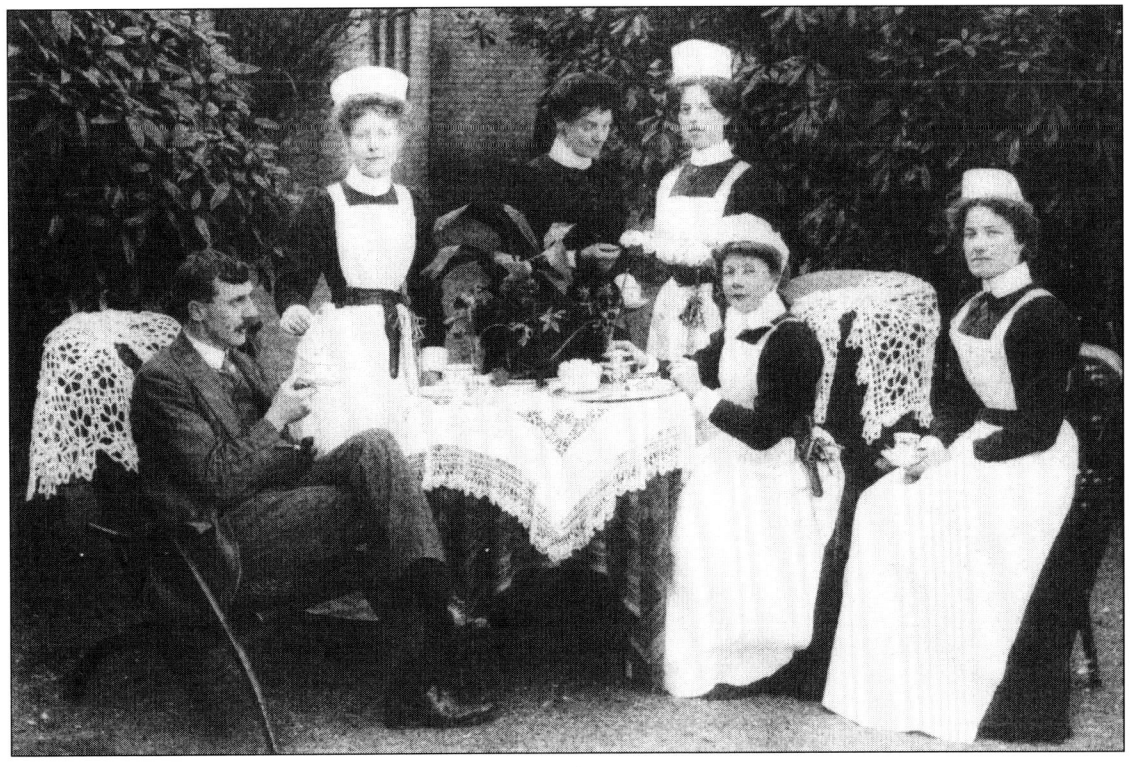

A doctor takes tea with the nurses in the early 1900s.
(City of London. London Metropolitan Archives)

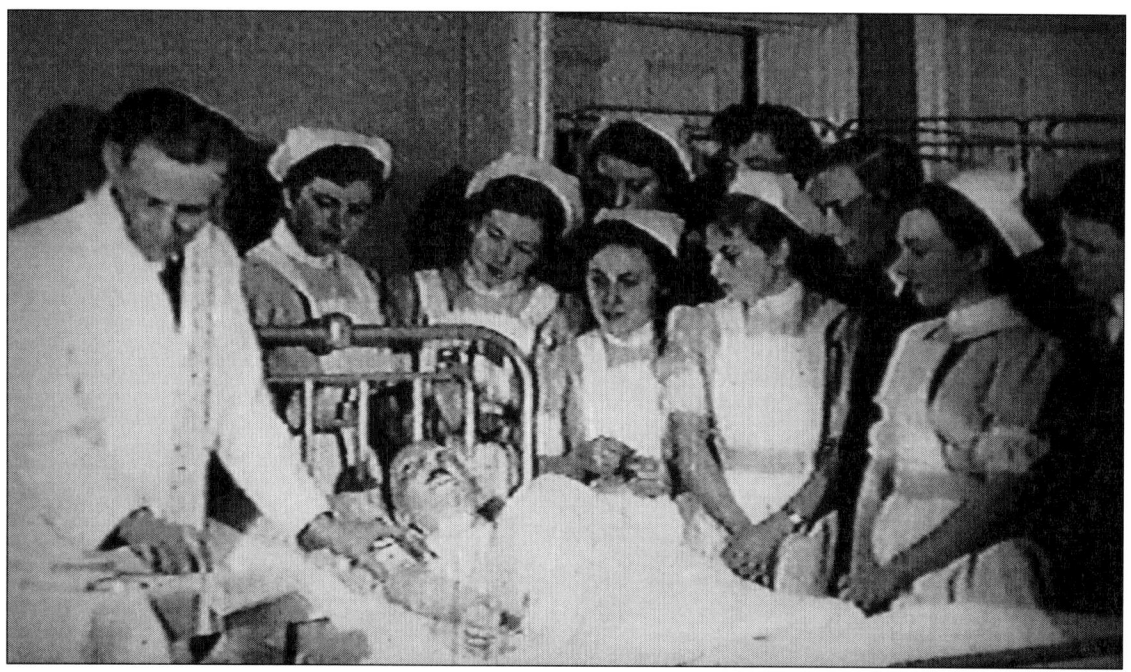

Student nurses at Friern in the 1950s (Time Marches on at Friern)

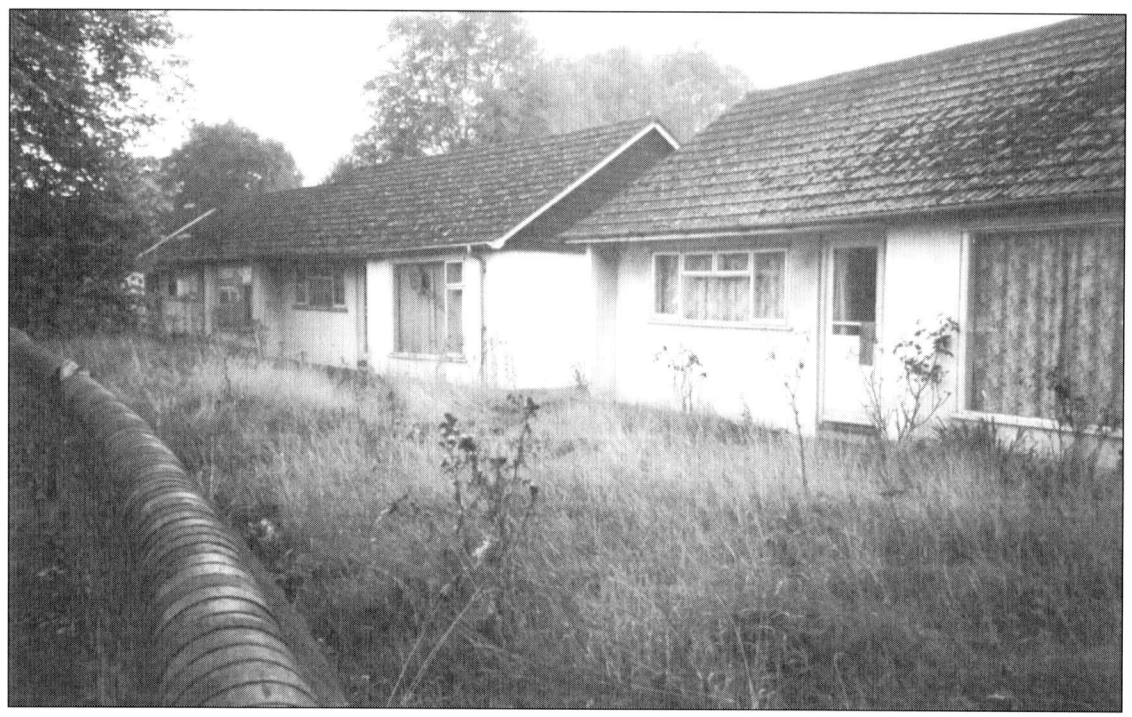

Staff bungalows at the northern end adjacent to Friern Barnet Road photographed in October 1994. (John Donovan)

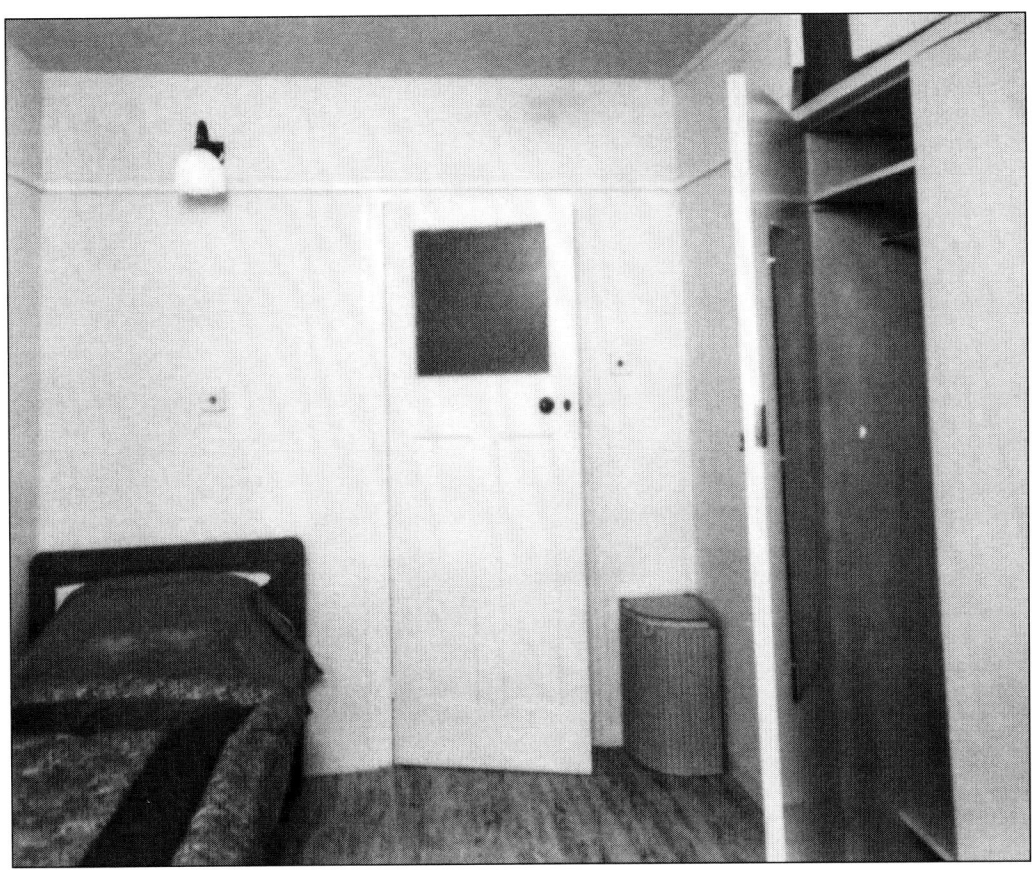
This photograph from 1938 shows how austere the nurses' bedrooms were.
(City of London. London Metropolitan Archives)

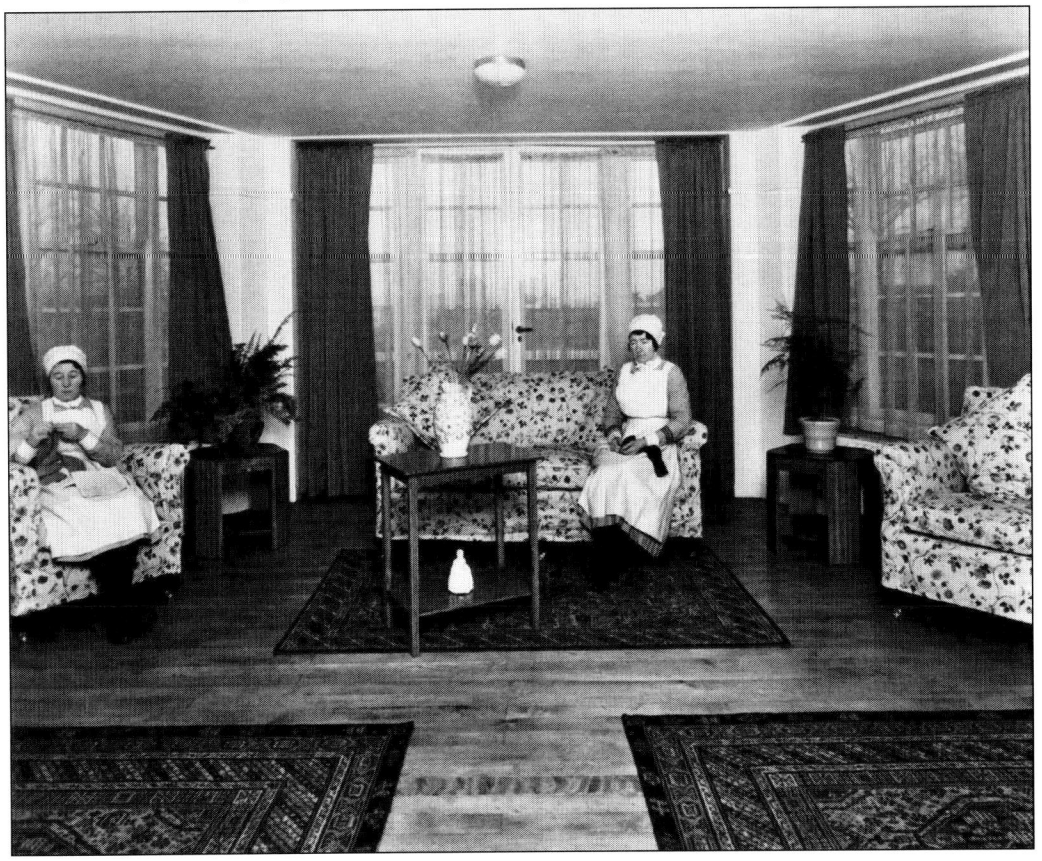
In comparison with the bedroom the nurses' lounge was positively sumptuous.
(City of London. London Metropolitan Archives)

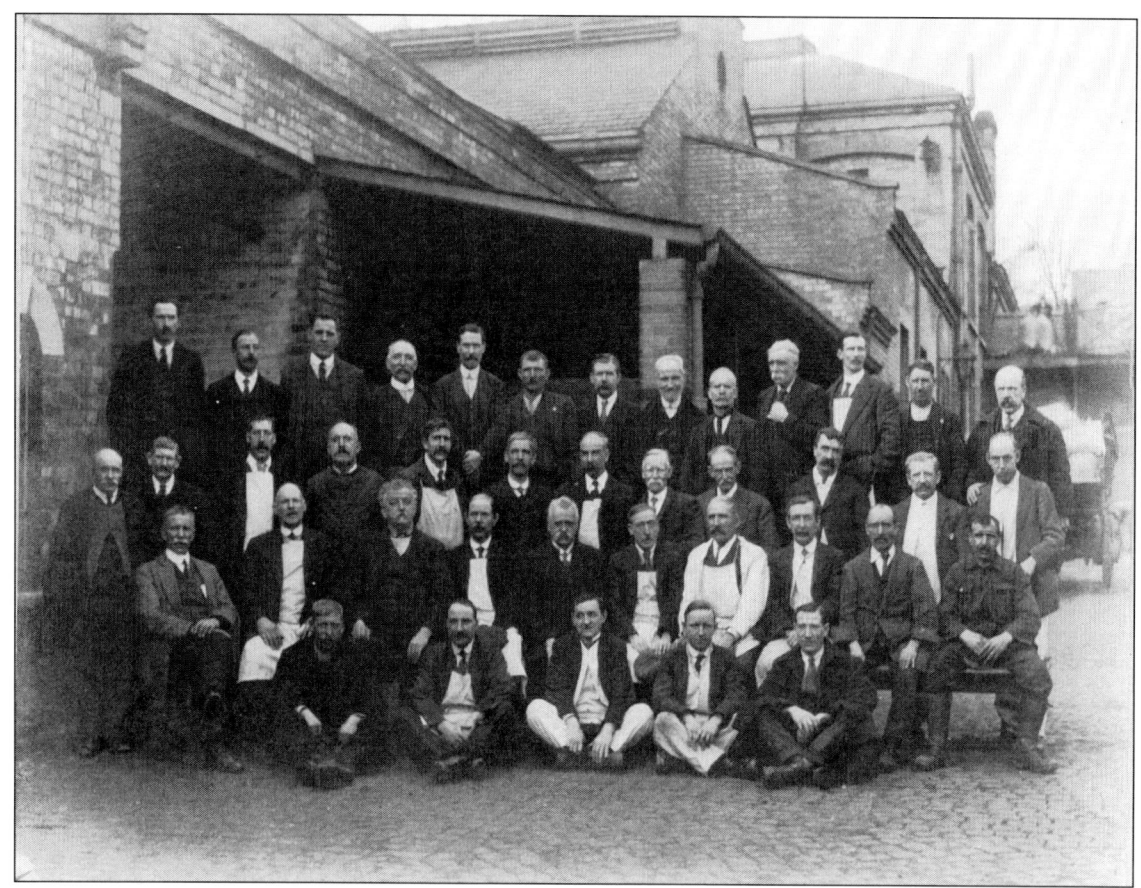
Building and engineering staff. (Colin Barratt Collection)

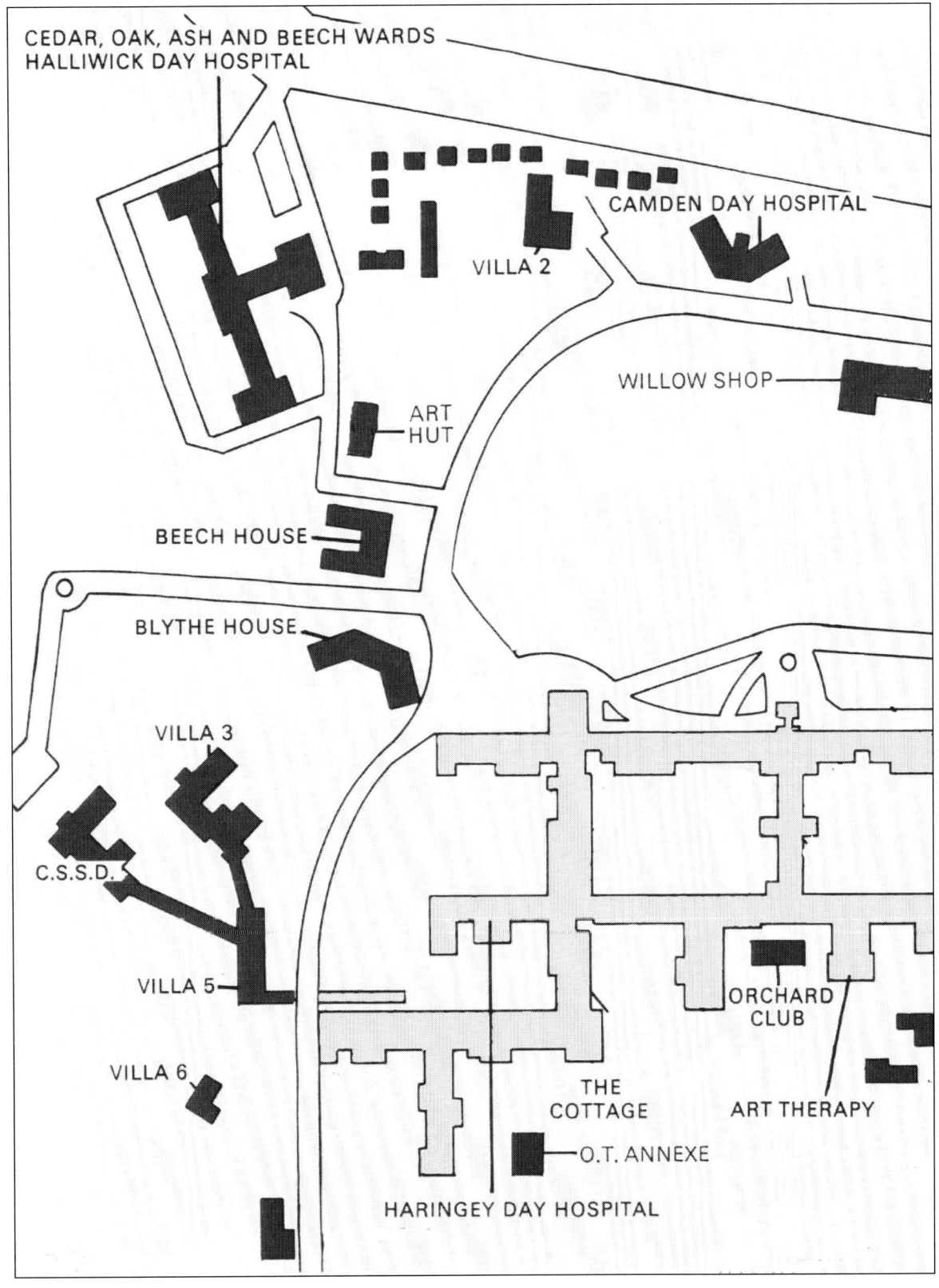

The western side of the site, showing the number of separate buildings that were in existence around 1979, including the nurses' homes at Beech House and Blythe House and Villa 5 which was the Nurses Education Centre.
(FB&DLHS Archive)

CHAPTER FIFTEEN

Fire!

At approximately 5.30 in the morning of Tuesday 27 January 1903 the siren sounded at the asylum. Fire was sweeping through five temporary wards which had been erected at right angles to the main west, female, wing in 1896. The wards were made of pitch pine and corrugated iron on a foundation of brick and were connected to the main block by a corridor, also made of wood and corrugated iron and about 150 yards long. The fire had apparently started at the southernmost block, ward X5 and, it quickly spread from ward to ward. By the time adjoining Ward X4 had caught alight the ironwork in X5 had become white hot. As the wards were constructed with timber frames lined with match boarding they offered little resistance to the flames which were being whipped up by a strong south westerly wind.

The fire was discovered by the nurse on night duty in Ward X5, which was next to the boiler house. The fire first appeared from the angle of the ward nearest the corridor. On the other side of the ward at this point was a small room measuring about ten feet which contained a linen press and store room for the patients' clothes. This, as it turned out later, was the seat of the fire. The nurse sounded the fire alarm and rushed to the nearest hose. At about the same time the fire was spotted by the fireman on duty in the boiler house, on the other side of the store room. He sounded the fire alarm which brought the asylum's fire brigade, numbering seven men and nine auxiliaries, and other staff to the site.

Some local residents had scaled the asylum walls and offered to try and help but they were turned away. The asylum's fire brigade were unable to do much to quell the blaze, particularly as they did not have enough water. Eventually fire brigades from Hornsey, Finchley and Wood Green arrived with their steam fire engines and although they were able to dam a stream at the bottom of the hill this was some 400 yards from the scene and the intense heat meant they were unable to make much impression. The blaze lasted little over an hour and in that time all five of the temporary wards had been destroyed. Particularly distressing to the staff was that some of the patients became disoriented and ran into the fire instead of away from it, whilst others were found wandering distractedly in the grounds.

Once the site had cooled, the remains were searched by the fire brigade and asylum assistants, assisted by police from Church End, Finchley. Of the 320 patients, all of them female, 51 of them perished. Some of the dead were found lying close to the remains of the iron bedsteads in which they had been sleeping, while others were found some distance away, while several heaps of charred bones were found in the corridor. Only one body was in recognisable human form.

The victims' ages ranged from 19 to 77 with forty seven being reported as members of the Church of England, and four were Roman Catholics. They were all buried in a common grave in the Great Northern Cemetery. It was the worst disaster in peacetime in English hospital history.

A series of Coroner's inquests were held on 31 January, 5 and 12 February and in each case the verdict was "fire or suffocation by fumes and smoke, by building known as "The Annexe" catching fire from some accidental cause." The jury found that the plan and construction of the buildings, as well as the materials used, were unsuitable even for temporary buildings and they condemned them as unsafe. However, in the official report of the Asylums Committee of the London County Council (LCC) into the fire there was no such criticism. The Chairman of the Committee suggested that it was easy to be wise after the event but nobody had any idea that a fire could gain hold so rapidly. He pointed out that there had been a hose available with a good supply of water available by merely turning a wheel; there had been someone on duty in the dormitory and that it should have been possible to evacuate the patients from the building in under two minutes and outward opening doors had been designed to facilitate this. It appeared that two things had contributed to the rapid spread of the fire – the corridor linking the buildings acted as a funnel and the unusually strong winds had fanned the flames. The LCC immediately acted to remove felt and wood from similar corridors at Banstead and Hanwell Asylums and they made sure the corridors were divided up into sections.

The report pointed out that when the LCC had inherited the Asylums in 1888 they could only accommodate 71.9% of the certified lunatics in the county of Middlesex; by 1903 this had risen to 97.4%, largely as a result of the building of additional accommodation such as the buildings at Colney Hatch. The LCC had spent £1,925,000 on additional accommodation and had created space for 1700 extra patients in the London area.

An eye witness report[1] by a reporter throws an interesting light on the fire:

> "Col. Fox was good enough to 'phone me very early, to tell me he was going down by road to the fire, and that I could go with him if I liked. Having an evening paper story to send out first, I told him I would follow later on.
>
> "Well," said Col. Fox, "you may have some difficulty in getting in, but you can say you have to see me on important business, and that you are my private secretary or anything of that kind you like."

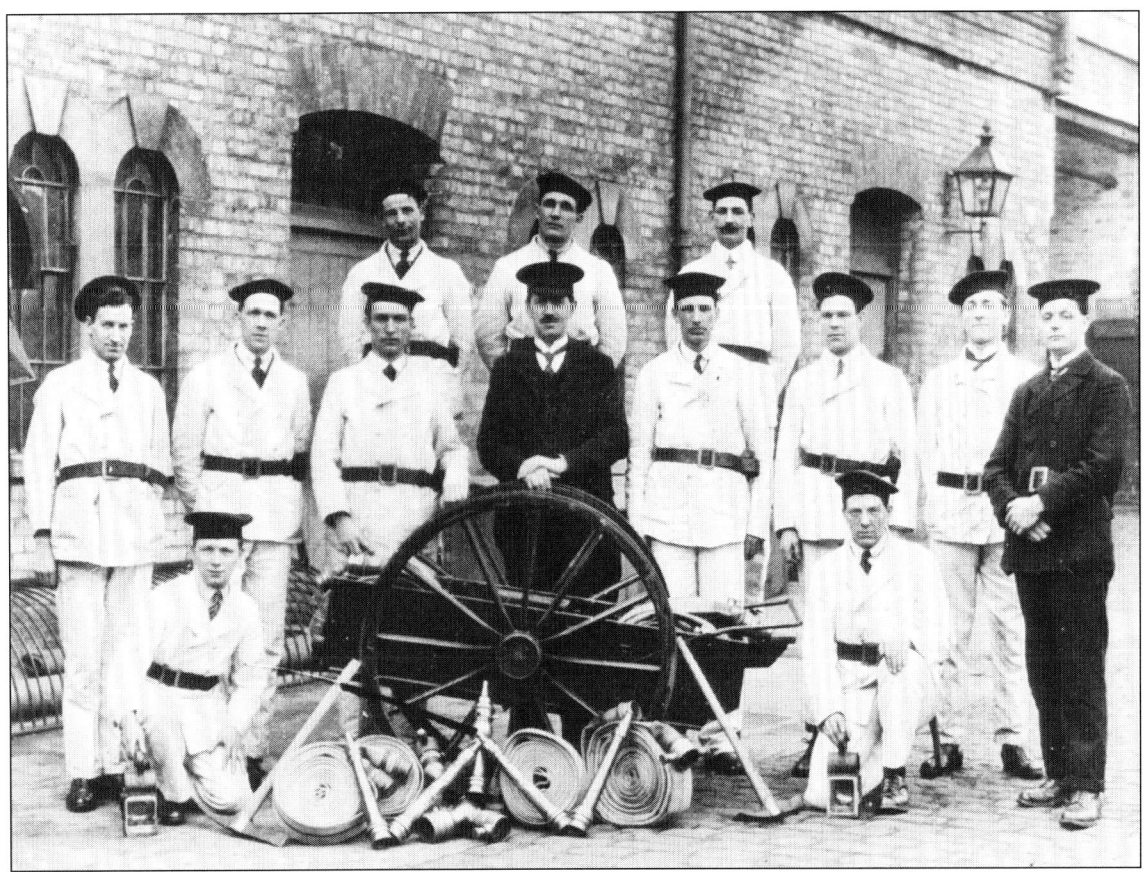

The asylum fire brigade photographed in 1900, before the fire. The apparatus was primitive.
(by kind permission of the Royal Society of Medicine)

I lost no time in getting on the train, and journeyed with Mr. W. G. Fish, then on the Exchange Telegraph Co., afterwards the Editor of the *Daily Mail*, and now a director of Associated Newspapers.

When we reached the asylum we were faced with a hopeless position. There were several reporters gathered outside the big doors of the porter's lodge, but they informed us that the porter was obdurate and would not allow them to pass into the grounds of the asylum.

"Well, look here," I explained, "I am going to say I have to see Colonel Fox on important business, and if I get in I will meet you all out here after I have got the particulars, which I will give to you on one condition – that you don't give me away."

They all agreed to the proposition.

I rang the bell, and that porter opened the grating. "I have an important message for Colonel Fox, the Chief Officer of the London Salvage Corps." "You're not one of those reporters, are you?" he demanded.

"Oh, no," I replied. The reporter then opened the door, and I was in the asylum grounds. Of course, the other reporters outside kept their word. As I walked across a piece of blackened ground one of my fire-brigade friends who was directing the hose on to the smouldering ruins shouted to me.

"Hallo, Jack, you'd hardly believe they were humans, would you?" "What are?" I exclaimed. "What you're walking amongst," he said. To my horror I realised that the blackened heaps, which I thought were charred beams of timber, were the remains of the poor lunatics who had perished in the blaze.

I hastened to get off the ground, and make my way to a group of officials. I interviewed some of them, got the roll call of the names of the unfortunate persons who had been burned to death, interviewed the nurses who discovered the fire, obtained several eye-witnesses' stories, and within a comparatively short time had a notebook full of facts.

I then made my way back to the porter's lodge, where the porter let me out, quite unaware of the fact that I was a reporter, and that I had got all the information regarding the calamity. Instead of finding the group of journalists waiting for me, there only happened to be one, and that was Fish, patient and expectant.

"Where are the others?" I asked.

"I think they have gone to a pub about a quarter of a mile off in that direction."

"Well," I said, "I promised that I would give them the information that I picked up, but I didn't promise that I would search the pubs in the locality for them; and besides, I am in a hurry, for I have to get to Fleet-street to get my story out."

"Quite right," replied Fish. "I'll come with you."

Directly we got into the train, Fish pulled out his notebook.

"Now look here, Fish, I'll be a sport and, of course, give you all the facts I have, but I must make a bargain with you. If you go straight back to your office and put the story on the tapes at once, you will beat me hands down, and naturally my

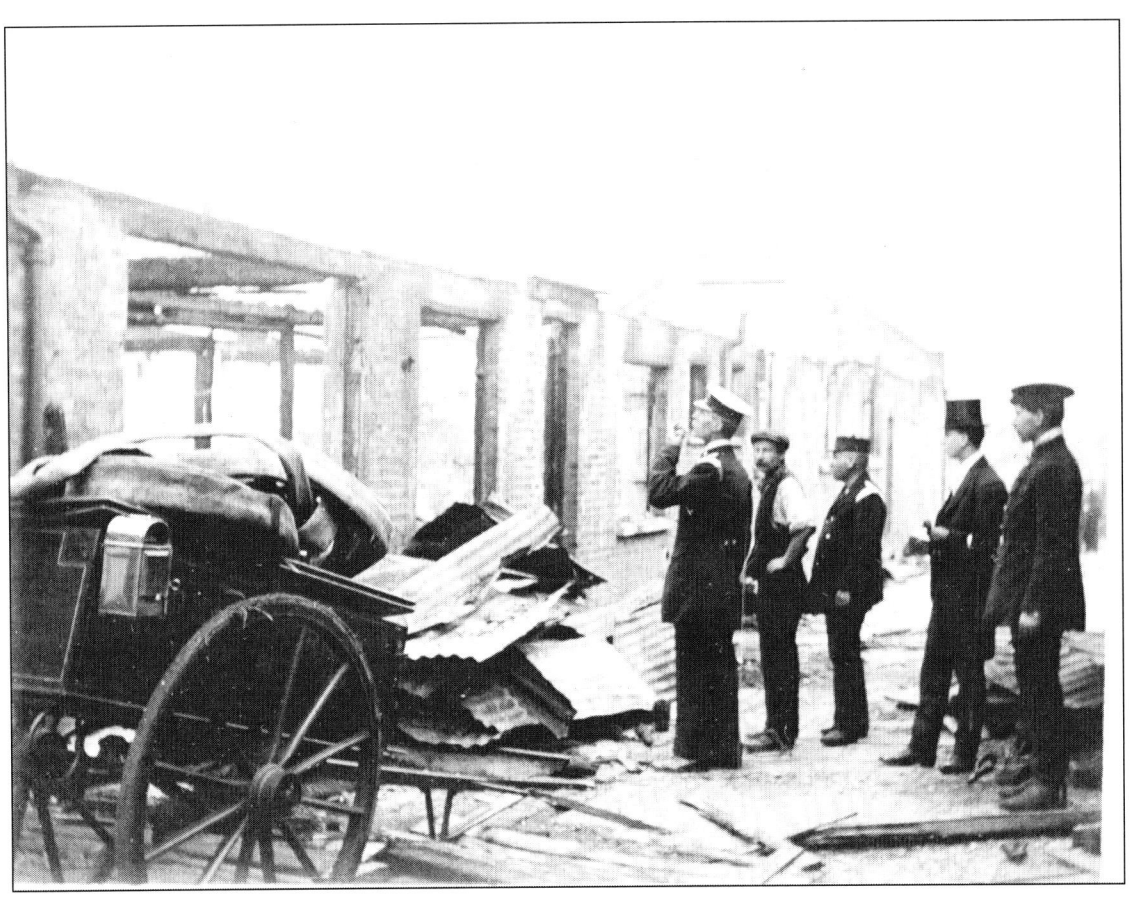

The fire brigade survey the scene after the fire. (Barnet Local Studies)

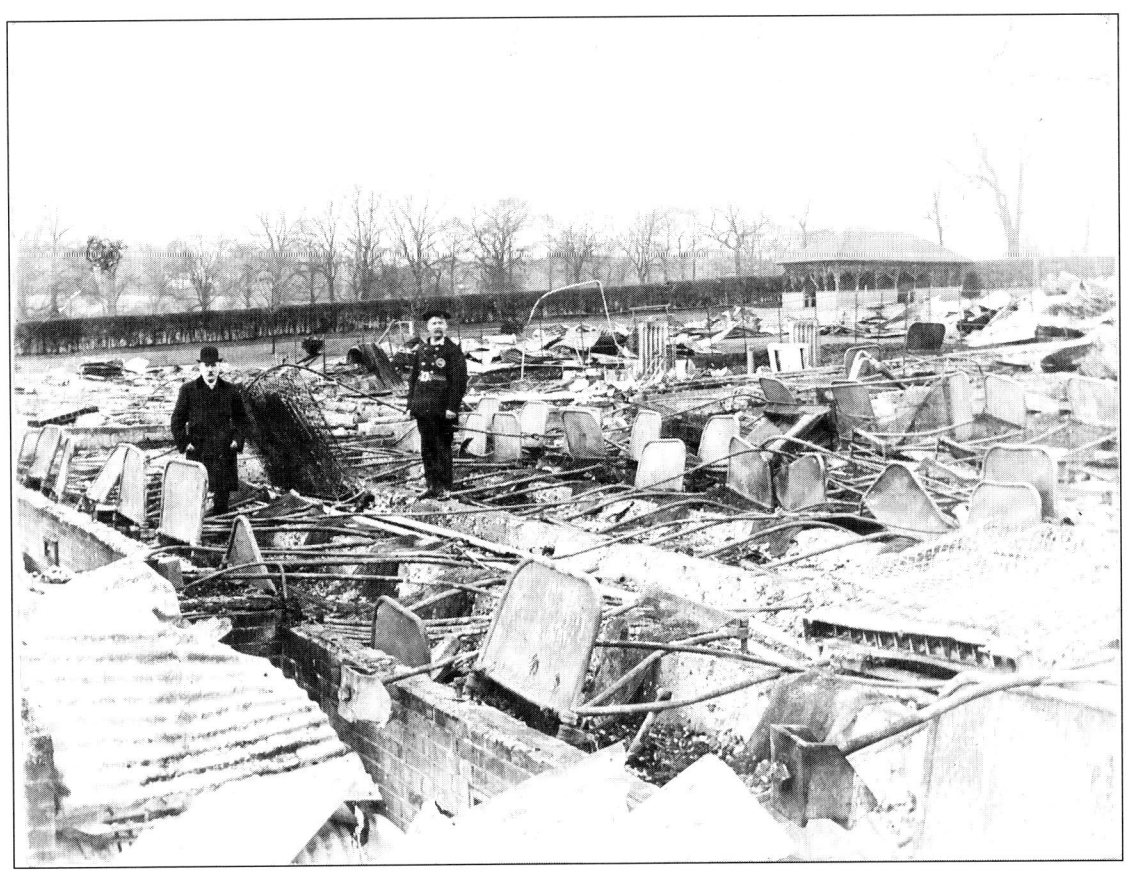

The aftermath. (Barnet Local Studies)

copy will be of no use. Promise me that you won't send anything out from Panton-street for two hours after we reach Farringdon Street, and then you can have everything I have regarding the fire."

He assented, and kept his word. I sent out my detailed information in quarter-of-an-hour batches by special messengers, and had a very good show in all the evening newspapers in London, as compared with three at the present time.

That was the most terrible asylum fire London has ever had."

The victims were buried in New Southgate Cemetery under a simple cross:

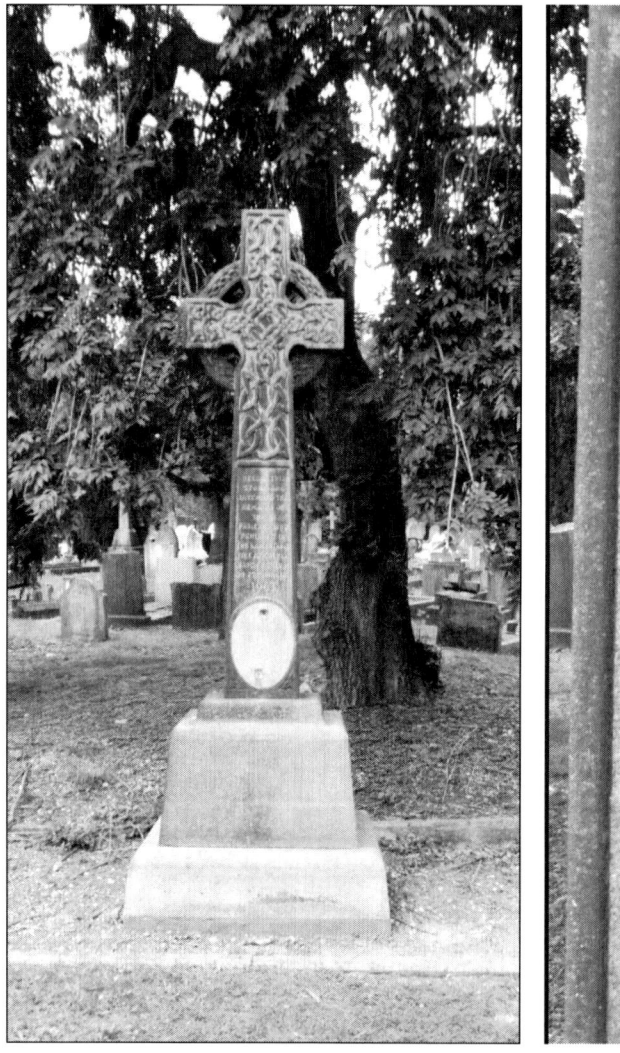 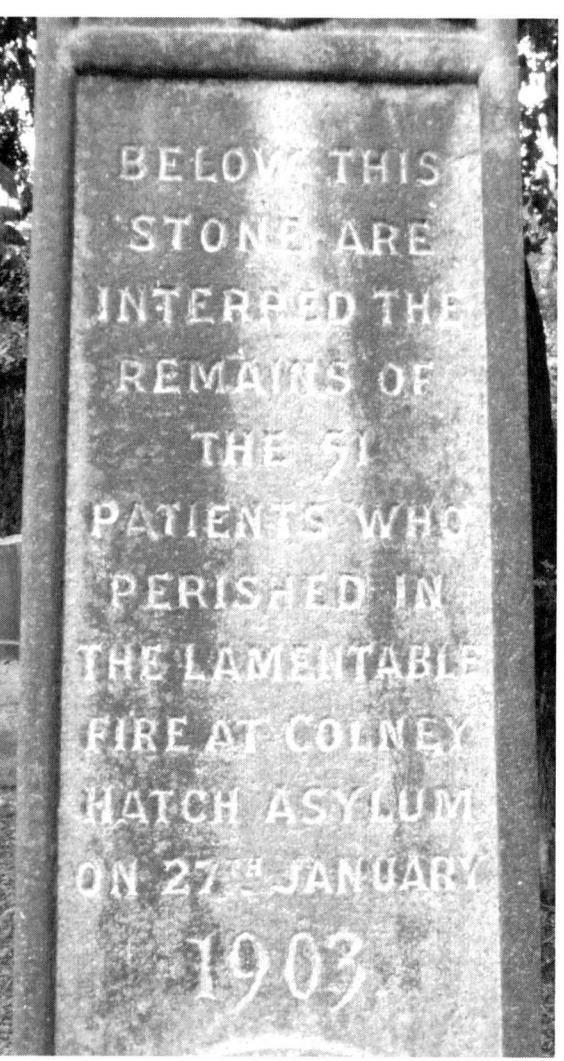

The mass grave in New Southgate Cemetery (Author)

The following touching poem was written by F. E. S, an inmate of the Asylum, in appreciation of the great heroism of the members of staff:

> Only Asylum workers,
> But a truly noble band,
> That cannot be dispensed with
> Throughout this mighty land.
>
> Those without rhyme or reason
> Are placed within their charge.

It would be very dangerous
For such to be at large.

A few words to you, friends,
About the terrible fire.
To say too much upon it
I have really no desire.

'Twas in the early morning
The Asylum staff were awoke,
And what they had to encounter
Was volumes of flame and smoke.

They rushed to the wards of the helpless
And tried to find them there,
But the flames were soon upon them
Before anyone was aware.

> IN APPRECIATIVE COMMEMORATION
>
> OF THE HEROIC CONDUCT
>
> AND
>
> SELF-SACRIFICING DEVOTION
>
> TO DUTY
>
> DISPLAYED BY MEMBERS
>
> OF THE
>
> STAFF OF COLNEY HATCH ASYLUM
>
> IN RESCUING FROM THE FLAMES
>
> 269 LIVES
>
> OF PATIENTS IN PERIL BY FIRE
>
> ON
>
> JANUARY 27, 1903.
>
> THIS TABLET IS PLACED
>
> BY THE
>
> ASYLUM WORKERS' ASSOCIATION
>
> HON SECRETARY — G. E. SHUTTLEWORTH, M.D.
> PRESIDENT — SIR JAMES CRICHTON-BROWNE, M.D. F.R.S

Now think of it for a moment –
Midst fire, water and smoke;
That those they were trying to rescue
Were treating it all as a joke.

But the dead are free from suffering.
And will know no more sorrow or pain.
But the sight and sounds were so awful
May it never occur again.

Doctors, attendants and nurses,
Were nearly done to death,
But they worked away like Trojans,
Each moment fighting for breath.

A word of appreciation
Is surely due to such.
Just to simply praise and thank them
That cannot be too much.

England has many heroes,
But none more brave than they,
For daily they're facing danger –
Protect them, Oh God we pray.

There was one other serious fire at Friern which resulted in loss of life. On 17 November 1988 at 3am a fire was discovered by the only nurse on duty in Ward 15, the Rehabilitation Ward. Over a hundred firemen fought the blaze for three hours and one of the firemen said that the smoke was so thick that they could not see the actual building. Twenty four patients were in the ward and sadly two elderly men, one aged 82, the other 60, lost their lives and a third was critically injured and taken to Barnet Hospital. Over 150 patients had to be evacuated from the building. In a subsequent report[2], London Fire Brigade said that mattresses and covers were easy to ignite and continued to burn after ignition and the material had given off large quantities of black smoke and toxic gases.

The damage amounted to £500,000 and the hospital, being Crown Property, was not insured against fire, so the Hampstead Health Authority had to find the funds.

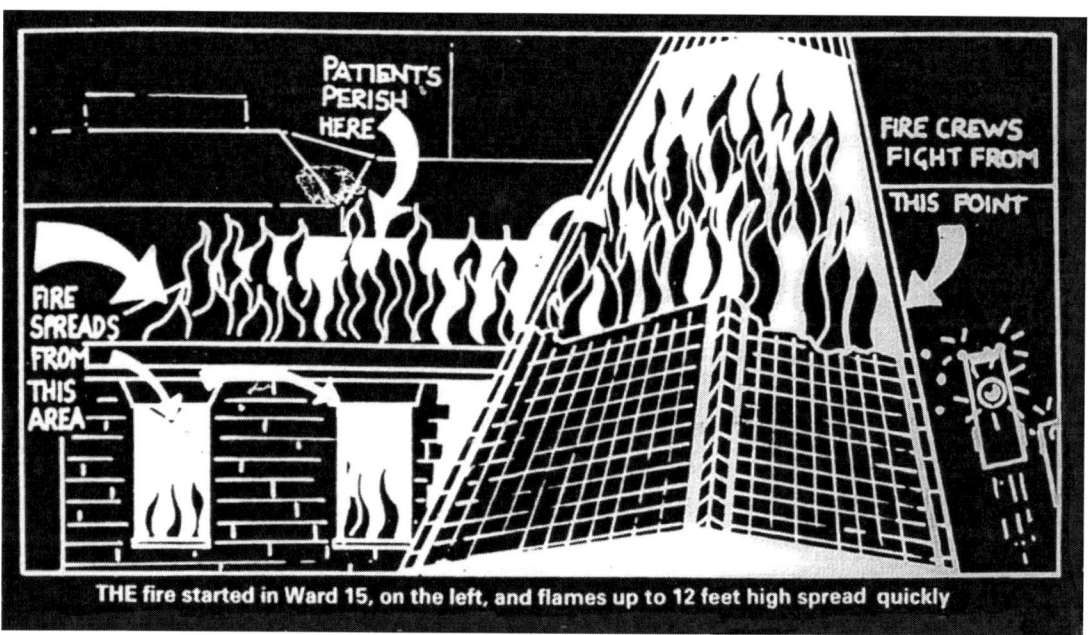

(Barnet Times 24 November 1988)

FIRE ALARM ZONES

Zone	Location	Zone	Location
001	Academic Centre, Social Work, Nurse Education Centre	021	Ward 35, Chazen Club
002	Wards 2, 5	022	Ward 36
003	Wards 3, 6	023	Ward E4, Old Treatment Centre
004	Wards 7, 9	024	Wards E2, E3, Haringey Day Centre
005	Ward 15, Pharmacy, North Workshop, X-Ray	025	Camden Nursing Office, Occupational Health Centre
006	Wards 16, 19	026	Patients' Bureau, Finance Office
007	Wards 17, 20	027	Printing Department
008	Wards 21, 23	028	South Workshop (I.T.D.)
009	Wards 8, 10, 11	029	Camden Day Hospital
010	Wards 12, 13, 14	030	Villa 2, Metabolic Unit
011	A1, Resocialisation Unit, Fellowship House	031	Villa 3
012	Wards A2, A3	032	C.S.S.D.
013	Wards 24, 25, Haringey Out Patients	033	Old Pathology Laboratory
014	Wards 26, 27, 28, Occupational Therapy Annexe	034	Main Stores
015	Wards 29, 30	035	Bakehouse Boutique, Olive Branch Coffee Bar
016	Wards 31, 32	036	Main Kitchen
018		037	Upholstery Store (old Senior Training School)
019	O.T. Assessment Centre (C5)	038	Upholstery Department
020	Islington Villa	039	Haringey Nursing Office, Haringey Doctors, West House
		040	Willow Pavilion, Social Club
		041	Boiler House
		042	Engineers' Yard

Hampstead Health Authority
FRIERN HOSPITAL

ACTION IN CASE OF FIRE

ANYONE DISCOVERING A FIRE, OR SUSPECTING A FIRE, WILL

1. Give the alarm *immediately* by breaking the glass of the nearest fire alarm call point, or dial 222 on the telephone and state *clearly* the location of the fire.
2. Make sure all patients and staff are safe, evacuate affected area if neccessary.
3. Unlock doors as necessary for admission of fire evacuation party or evacuation of patients.
4. If possible, attack the fire with appliances provided, *but without taking personal risk.*
5. If you cannot control the fire leave the area immediately and proceed to the other side of a fire/smoke stop door and await further instructions from the Duty Fire Officer or the Fire Brigade.

NURSING STAFF ON DUTY IN THE WARDS

Act quickly and quietly.
Keep all doors and windows closed.
Use the nearest available exit.
Do not move beds.
Do not stop to collect personal belongings.
Do not re-enter the area.

HOSPITAL FIRE EVACUATION PARTY

The designated Hospital Fire Party will receive the location of the fire on the fire bleep and proceed to the area immediately.

IT IS IN YOUR OWN INTEREST

To study this notice to know what to do in the event of a fire and to know how to use the fire appliances.

To make certain that you are familiar with all the means of escape in case of fire and that staircases, corridors, landings and other exits are kept clear of obstructions at all times.

JANUARY, 1987

Fire precautions were already in place a year before the fire of 1988.
(FB&DLHS Archives)

CHAPTER SIXTEEN

Wartime

During the First World War the asylum, in common with many other organisations and businesses, suffered from a shortage of labour due to staff being called up to the colours. The staff who were left were mostly elderly and they were supplemented by temporary staff, so the level of care available was not as high as it had been. Additional strain was put on those remaining by the influx of some German, Austrian and Hungarian civilians who had been interred at Alexandra Palace. There were 3,000 of these foreign nationals at the Palace; they had all been resident in Britain at the outbreak of war and had been required to register with the police. In 1915, the sinking of the *RMS Lusitania* had led to anti-German riots[1] and the aliens were rounded up and put in internment camps. Many of these internees were married to UK nationals and the separation from their loved ones and the lack of privacy and constant noise at the Palace had a terrible effect on the mental health of some of them. Of those who had been transferred to Colney Hatch, 23 died there. The internees were repatriated to Germany after the war and records show[2] during the period February to June 1918, 51 prisoners from Colney Hatch were accompanied by staff to Boston in Lincolnshire where they were put on board the *SS Sindoro*. An additional 40 prisoners had been moved to Friern from other asylums including Parkside Asylum in Macclesfield and Whitingham Asylum in Lancashire and they too were escorted by hospital staff. All prisoners' luggage was inspected by Scotland Yard detectives before their departure and the War Office agreed to pay Colney Hatch staff five shillings for the considerable strain of escorting prisoners at all times of the day and night. In April 1919 eleven prisoners had arrived from internment in the Isle of Man and they were accompanied by asylum staff to Southampton and then all the way to Rotterdam.

During the First World War the asylum lost seven of its workers in action and a plaque that was erected in the main building was a poignant reminder of the tragic loss of life that occurred in the trenches of France:

Colney Hatch Mental Hospital
To the glory of God and in memory of members of the staff of this hospital who gave their lives in the Great war 1914-1918.

William Richard Henderson (attendant), Trooper 1st Royal Dragoons, missing in France 30th Oct 1914.
George Baker (attendant), Pte. 4th Bn. Royal Fusiliers
missing in France, Dec 1914.
Charles Albert Dickins (attendant), Pte. 4th Bn. Royal Fusiliers,
missing in France, Dec 1914.
Maxwell Mark Humphreys (attendant), L/Cpl. South Wales Borderers, missing in France, 18th Dec 1914.
John Lamont (House Steward's 1st Clerk), Pte. 14th Bn. County of London Regiment (London Scottish),
killed in France, 12th March 1914.
John Reynolds (gas stoker), Sapper 22nd. Field Company Royal Engineers, died in France 15th July 1918.
Arthur Clark (boiler stoker), L/Cpl. 1st Bn. Grenadier Guards,
died in France, 2nd Nov 1918

With Germany's annexation of Austria in 1938 it became obvious that sooner or later a war was likely and the Government started to take steps to prepare for it. Ration books were printed, air raid wardens began to be trained, St John Ambulance Corps recruited volunteers and the Auxiliary Fire Service was formed. In September 1938 everyone was issued with a gas mask. In April 1939 the Home Office wrote to all local councils instructing them to prepare for war and civil defence was to take precedence over all other council business. Auxiliary fire stations were set up in a number of locations including the hospital. These were particularly important additions to the regular fire service as they were able to deal with the small fires caused by incendiary bombs and to prevent them from spreading and causing widespread damage.

On Sunday 3 September 1939 following Germany's invasion of Poland, Britain declared war on Germany. The authorities were convinced that there would be huge civilian casualties as a result of enemy bombing so Emergency Medical Hospitals were formed on the outskirts of London to which patients from Central London would be transferred. Friern was told to prepare 700 beds designed for the treatment of war casualties. Twelve wards along the front corridor were made available, which could house 215 male and 409 female patients and these were given over to the Emergency Medical Service. The patients already in these wards were moved to other wards and 350 female patients were transferred to Bexley.

Two days after London's evacuation plans had been carried out, 200 nurses from various London hospitals, plus consultants, house physicians, surgeons and students from St Bartholomew's Hospital were also moved to Colney Hatch. The hospital even became the Final Year Medical School for Barts. The average admissions during the war years were 3000 – 4000 per year, with 5000 being treated in 1944.[3]

The nearby Standard Telephones & Cables plant between Oakleigh Road South and Brunswick Park Road was a target for enemy bombers and the surrounding area, particularly New Southgate, suffered bomb damage. On 26 October, 1940 a villa in the asylum grounds housing female patients was destroyed by bombs and four lives were lost. Three weeks later, on 16 November, a land mine resulted in the loss of Villas 2, 4 and 6, and the death of 36 patients and four nurses. The damage was so severe that 300 female patients had to be relocated. On 22 January 1945 a V1 rocket landed in the grounds near the North Circular Road causing minor damage to the building and to local houses. As a result of the bombings 1800 windows in the hospital were blown out and were replaced by black cardboard. Lack of material, manpower and funds meant that they were not re-glazed until 1947.

As can be imagined, the war led to severe overcrowding at Friern. At the outbreak of war there were places for 1737 patients (827 men and 910 women) but by 1943 there were actually 2032 in residence (992 men and 1040 women).

A local resident, David Marr, who was nearly eleven at the time, recalled that shortly after the Dunkirk evacuation in 1941 he saw a train load of wounded soldiers arrive at New Southgate Station in the siding that bordered the line path and the hospital. He remembers seeing badly injured soldiers being taken off the train into the hospital through the big gates by the footbridge, or being taken off in ambulances lined up on the road leading from the back of the station to Friern Barnet Road. One badly wounded soldier had his steel helmet removed by nurses to reveal bullet wounds in his forehead. The family doctor, Dr Reid, was on the scene and he said "These children should not be seeing this!" Most of the helpers seemed to be busy holding cigarettes for the injured and feeding them mugs of tea.

Another local resident who lived in a house overlooking the hospital grounds remembers seeing shell shocked soldiers marching up and down the outside wall of one of the wards apparently undertaking some kind of guard duty. A former nurse at Friern, Sofie Carr, recalled her brief time there:

> "I walked along that corridor every day for six months. Not as a patient, but I was sent there as a nurse. I trained at St George's in the East Hospital, Wapping which

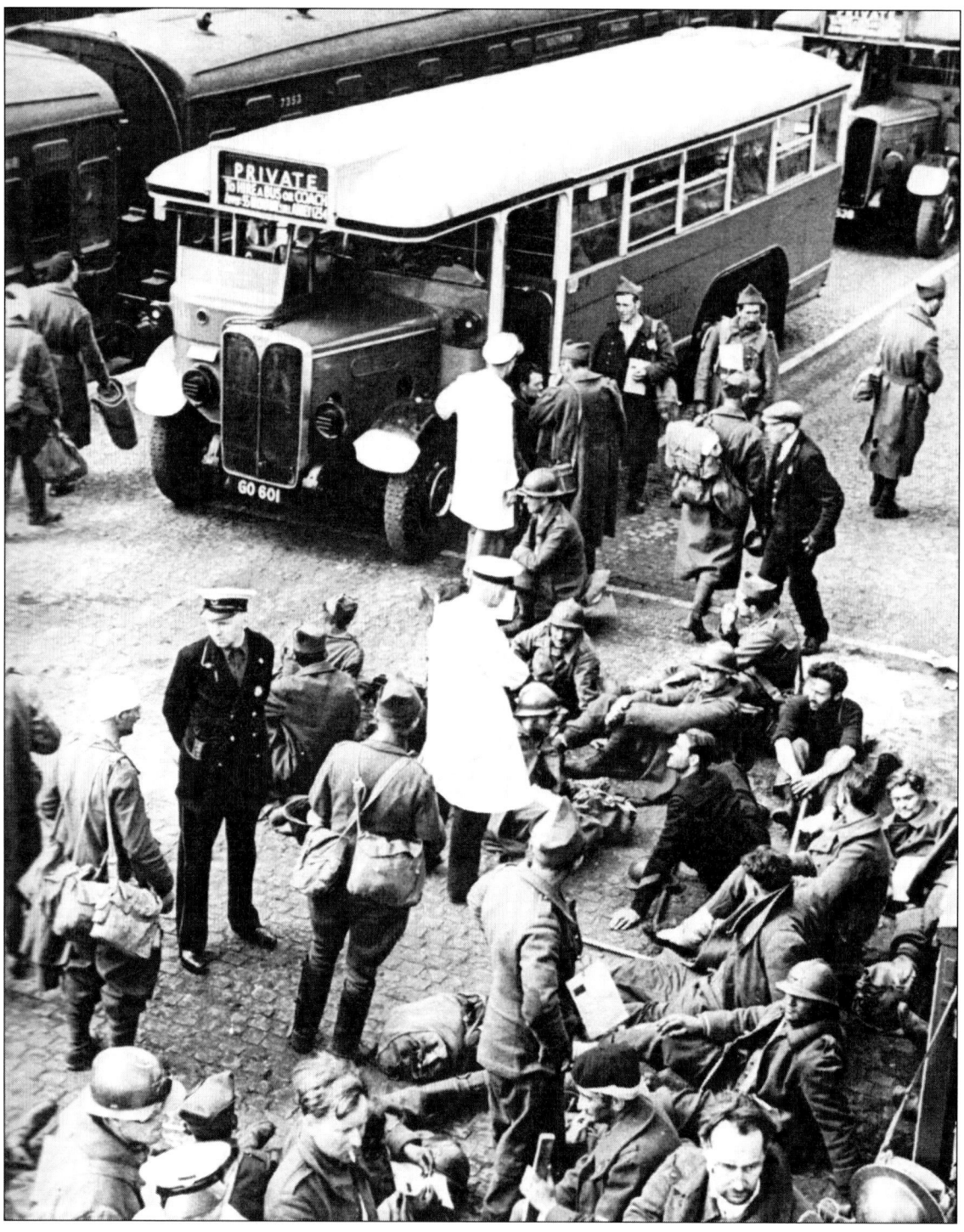

Wounded French soldiers at New Southgate Station on 1 June 1941. The fact that some are still wearing their helmets would indicate that they had arrived directly from Dunkirk. The wounded would have been taken to Friern whilst the able bodied would have gone to a reception and distributing centre at Alexandra Palace.
(F. Cole)

was a London County Council Hospital. During the War all these hospitals had to send their nurses to Colney Hatch to provide staff there for a few months.

I certainly remember the long corridor and I remember the mental patients who walked the corridor. Not only did they walk the corridor – they also worked there. They did all the cleaning and they worked on the wards and in the kitchens. They worked in the pharmacy and delivered food and drugs to the wards.

They were harmless and mild cases of mental illness and they were happy people walking and dancing along the corridor. While I was there we were told one day to get beds ready for German prisoners of war. 500 German prisoners arrived in the middle of the night, all having been badly injured. We nurses had to get ham sandwiches ready for them which we never had due to the rationing. We had to wash and feed them and nobody knew that the enemies were in the middle of London during the bombing – it was a State secret. This is my experience of Colney Hatch."

Irene Warwick confirmed the story:

"I started working at the hospital in Spring 1940. A wing of the hospital had been taken over by St Bartholomew's Hospital for patients to be transferred to the main hospital. These were mostly civilians and my job was to keep the register of patients and record bed numbers daily. Mr Harrison was in charge and we had a small office with two other ladies.

During that beautiful summer we often watched from the grounds the planes overhead, fighting in the Battle of Britain. The blitz started that autumn and I spent several nights on duty, but fortunately not on the night that Bounds Green tube station was bombed (Sunday13 October 1940). When I arrived the following morning it was to hear that several of the lesser injured had been admitted to hospital. It was my job to get their particulars which, for an eighteen year old girl, was a bit disturbing. One lady asked me if I knew where her husband was. I didn't know, so could not help her, but I learned later that he had been killed. I left the hospital the following February."

The hospital suffered, as did many other hospitals, through the lack of staff during the war and a report in 1943 noted the fact there were 23 vacancies in the male staff and 38 in the female staff.[4] In 1941[5] the establishment was:

Staff /Probation Nurses	145
Staff Nurses	125
Chief Charge Nurse (Male)	16
Chief Charge Nurse (Female)	24
Charge Nurse (Male)	20
Charge Nurse (Female)	15
Night Charge Nurse (Male)	26
Night Charge Nurse (Female)	15
Assistant Clerks	22
Assistant Pharmacist	4 (1 part time)

After D-Day, 6 June 1945, convoys of sick and wounded German prisoners arrived and after V-E Day injured British prisoners who had been released were treated. The Emergency Hospital closed on 30 September 1945 and things slowly started to return to normal.

A tribute to the members of the
staff of Friern Hospital who
lost their lives through enemy action
1939-45

Probationer Nurse	Emily McArthur
Probationer Nurse	Janet M. Carlyle
Chief Charge Nurse	Katie C. Smith
Staff Nurse	Dorothy C. White
Probationer Nurse	Wilfrid C. Gibbs
Probationer Nurse	Peter K. Gordon
Stoker	George Swain

CHAPTER SEVENTEEN

Changes and Improvements

Although the creation of asylums at Hanwell and Colney Hatch had relieved some of the problems in Middlesex, the number of pauper lunatics in the county continued to increase and there was a growing waiting list at both asylums. One of the solutions to the problem would have been the creation of a third asylum in the county but this was initially rejected on grounds of cost. The other solution was to enlarge the existing asylum but this was not favoured by the Commissioners in Lunacy who in 1857 issued the following warning[1]:

> "To the cure or alleviation of insanity, few aids are so important as those which may be derived from vigilant observation of individual peculiarities; but where the patients assembled are so numerous that no Medical Officer can bring them in range of his personal examination and judgement, such opportunities are altogether lost, and amid the workings of a great machine, the physician as well as the patient loses his individuality…..the time had arrived to express plainly the opinion that the desirable limit had already been exceeded, that an increase in size would be most prejudicial and that no such proposal ought to be sanctioned."

Despite these protestations it was decided jointly by the committees of Colney Hatch and Hanwwell and the Secretary of State that enlargements would take place and plans were drawn up. At Colney Hatch wards were refurbished, unused rooms were converted and new wings were added which resulted in the creation of 700 new beds at a cost of £150,000 (£9,000,000 at today's values). The work was completed by 1859 and the architect for the project was Lewis Cubitt, a notable architect who had designed King's Cross Station and the Great Northern Hotel.

The addition of two wings at the rear running east to west had a detrimental effect[2]:

> "The new wing for female patients at the western extremity of the asylum overshadows and renders gloomy the yards on either side of it, and by some oversight the roof of the new block on the south had been so constructed as entirely to obstruct all the view of the country in that direction; whilst the new spur on the east still further encloses the airing courts, which were before open

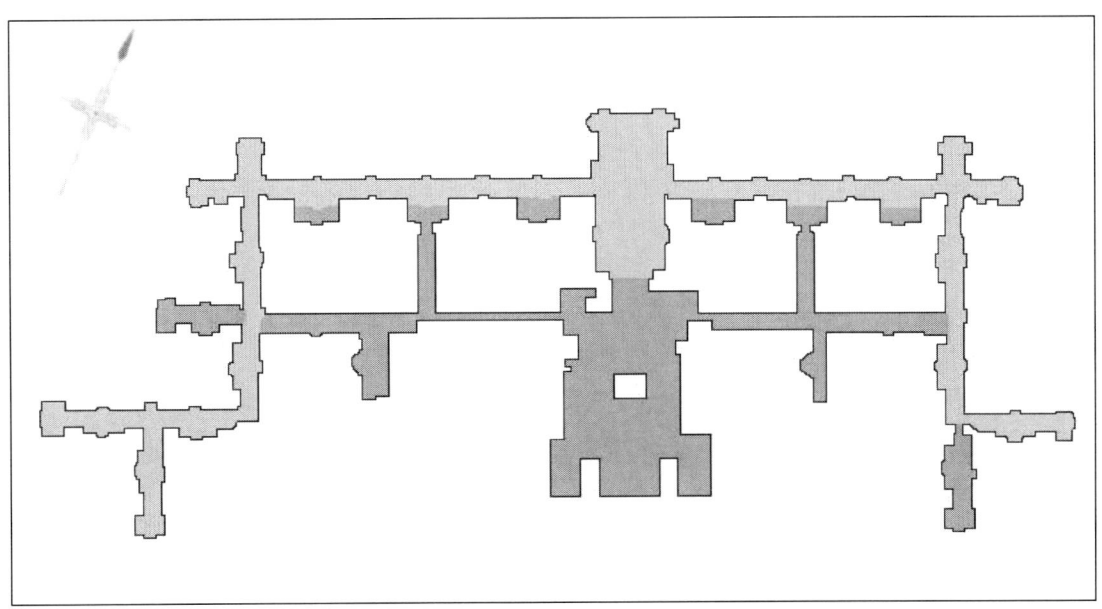

The dark areas are the additions that took place between 1857 and 1859.

and cheerful, and indeed the best belonging to the asylum."

As time went on, the pressure on space became major concern. The overwhelming problem was that it was the last port of call for mental patients, they could not be moved anywhere else, thus elderly and long term patients were preventing the admission of new patients. The only solution was to once again enlarge the establishment and this took place between 1908 and 1913 but instead of adding to the main building it was decided to build a series of separate buildings in the grounds. There were seven of these, named villas, and they ranged in size from single storey to two storey. One villa would be for behaviour disordered subnormal and epileptic boys; two with verandas for tuberculosis patients and the other four for women who had survived the fire in 1903.

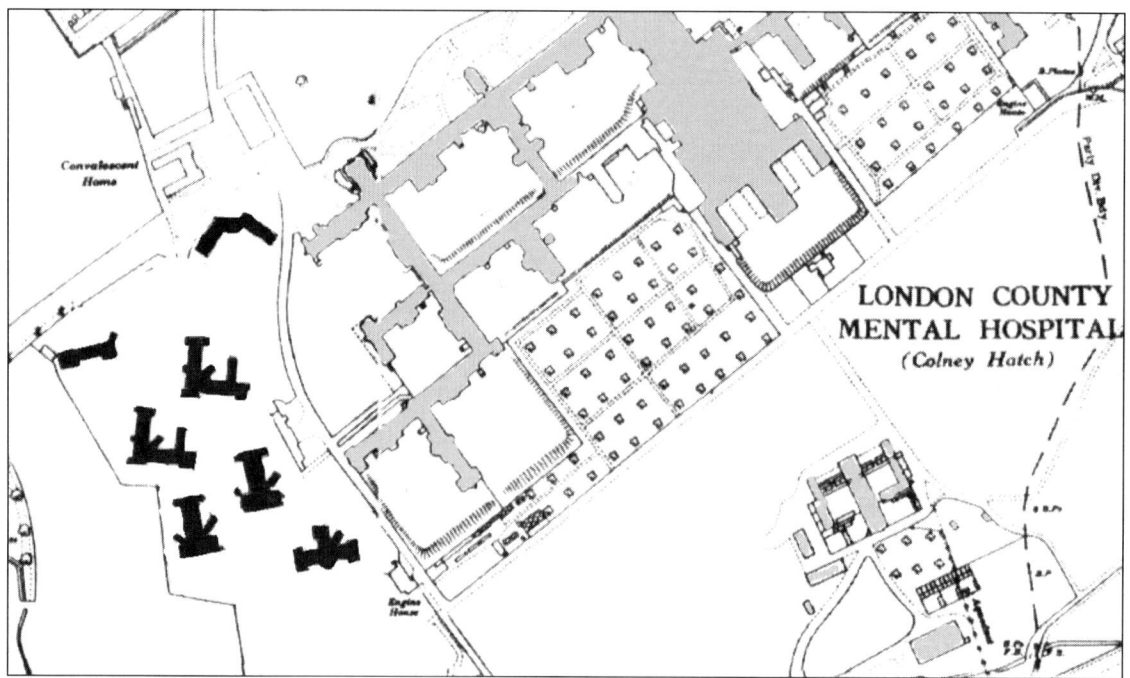

The new villas (here shown in black) were to the west of the main building.
(Barnet Local Studies)

With the huge growth in motor traffic, Middlesex County Council embarked on a wide road building scheme in the 1920s and 30s. Among the projects was the extension of the North Circular Road between Finchley and Palmers Green. The site chosen meant that the new road would have to be driven through the grounds of the asylum. Three parties were involved in this, Friern Barnet UDC was the local authority, Middlesex County Council was, of course, to build the road and the LCC were responsible for running the hospital. At various points both the Ministry of Transport and the Ministry of Health was also drawn into the planning process. Negotiations between the parties started in 1927 and were long and tortuous.[3] In the end a land exchange scheme was devised which involved Friern Barnet UDC giving up some 14 acres of derelict land on part of what was then called the Halliwick Recreation Ground, to the west of Colney Hatch Lane, and the Hospital losing a piece of land on its southern boundary which included part of the old farm.[4] Up until this point the boundary of the hospital had reached as far as Cromwell Road. Part of the original hospital wall can be seen in Cromwell Road to this day, albeit in a lower form. The building work involved constructing a culvert into which Bounds Green Brook would run and the construction of a bridge for the LNER railway at a cost of £92,000. The sewer pipe which had run from the hospital to the sewage works in

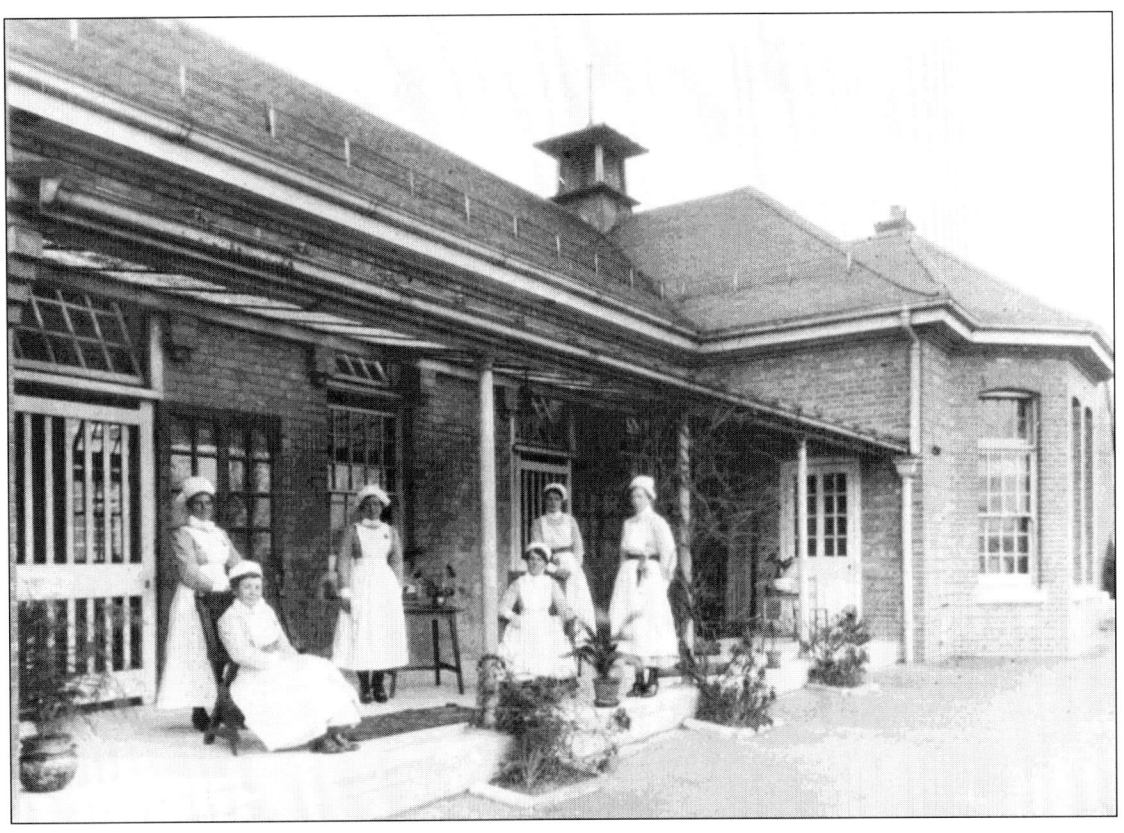

This villa for tuberculosis patients was photographed in 1910. It was one of the ones destroyed in the Second World War. (Barnet Local Studies)

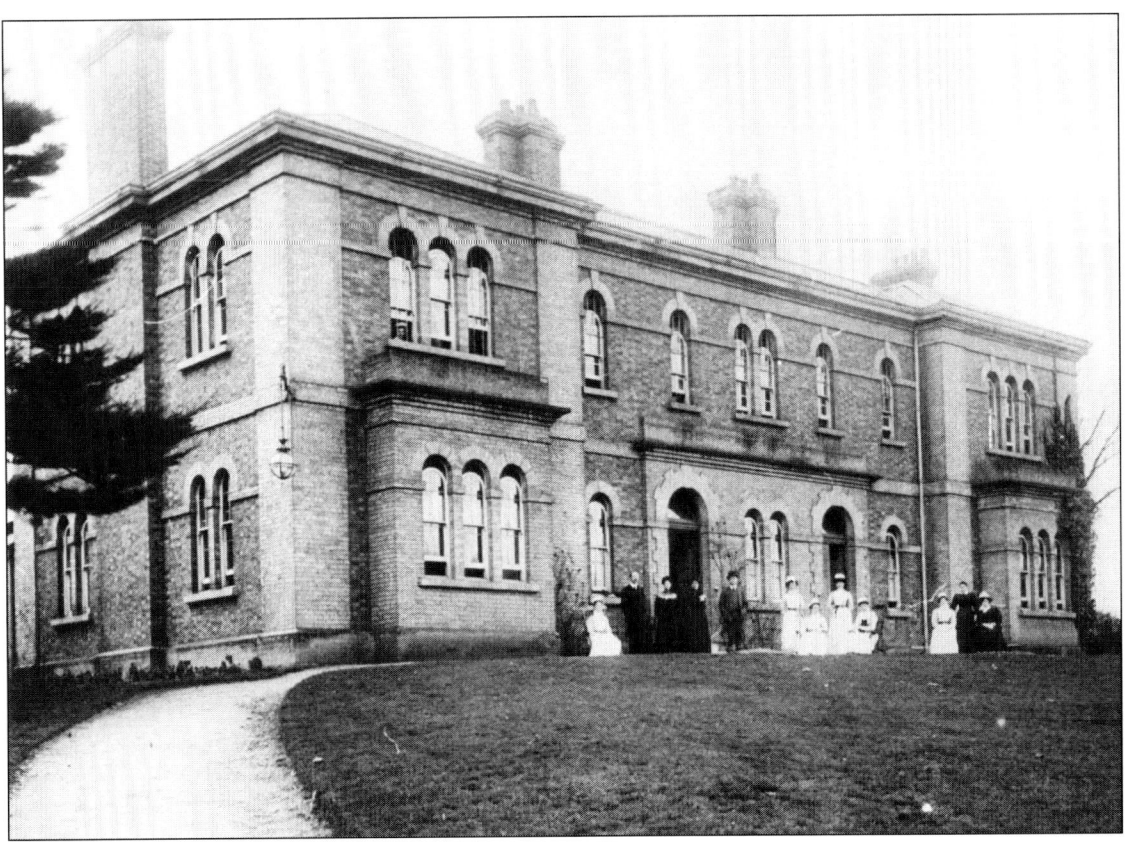

A convalescent home for female patients was opened in 1865 and was turned into a nurses' home in 1914.
(by kind permission of the Royal Society of Medicine)

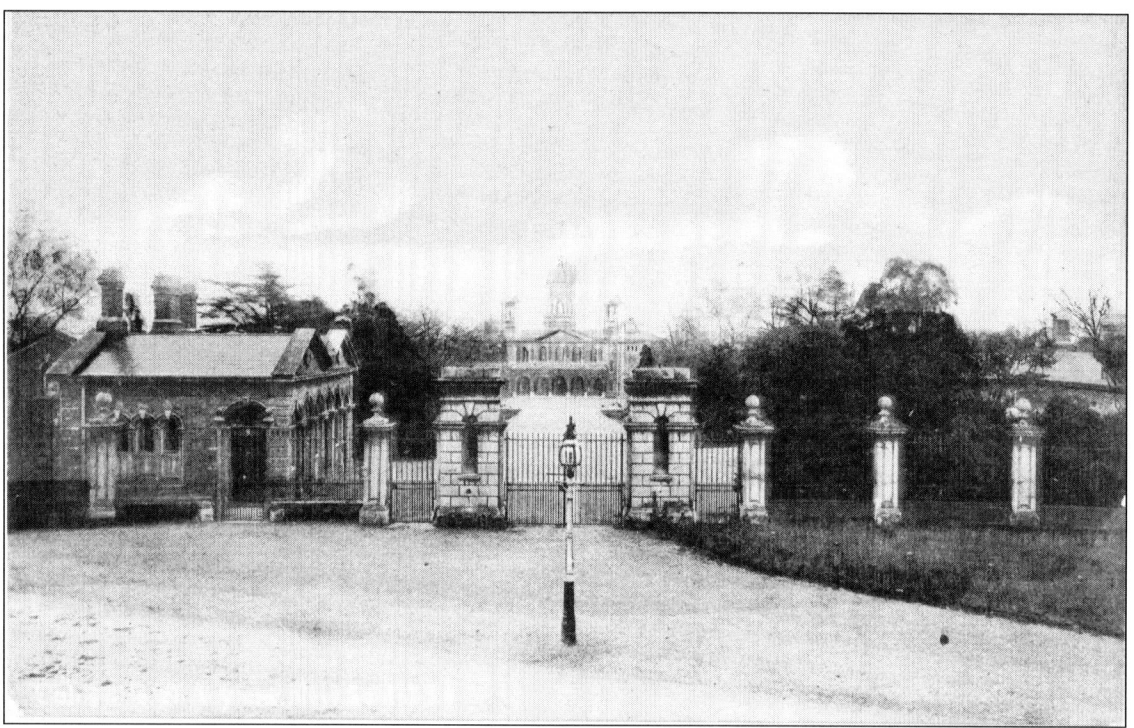

The main gates were closed from 1889 to 1937. (Commercial Postcard)

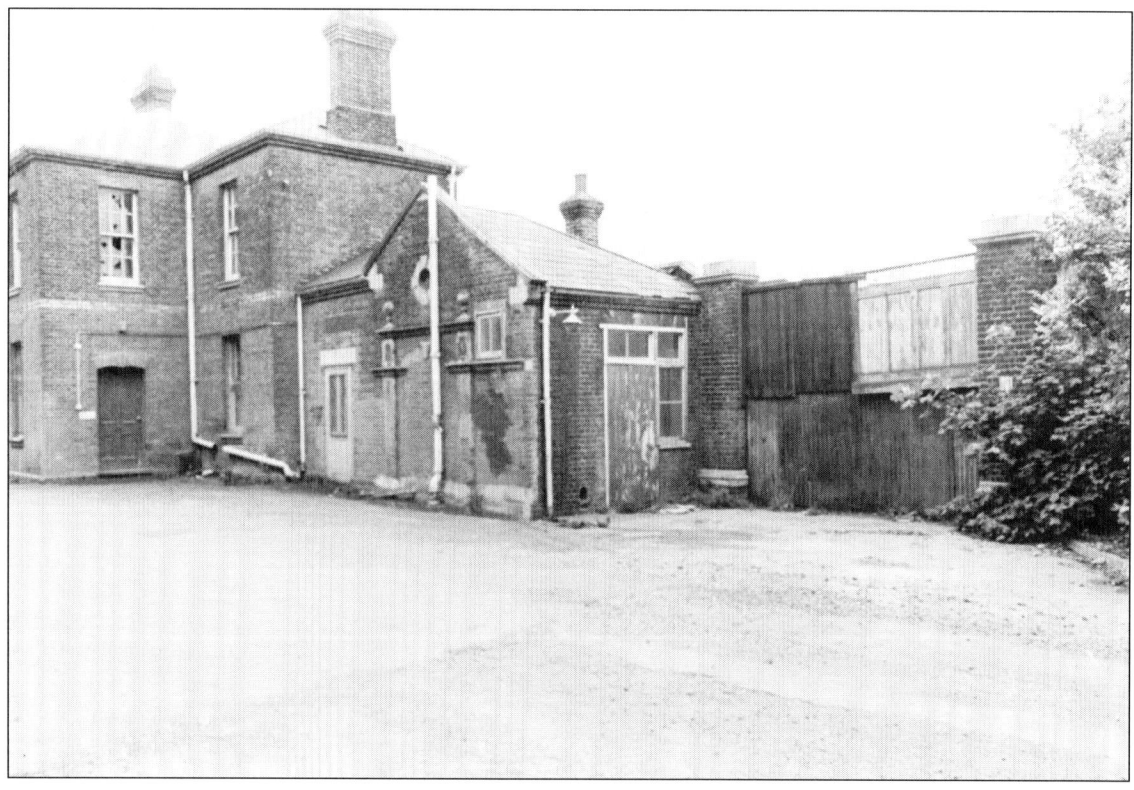

During the period the main gates were closed, the only entry to the asylum was by the South Lodge which was accessed from the line path alongside the railway line at New Southgate station. The gate porter not only controlled the entry of visitors but also prevented patients from trying to escape or to communicate with anyone from outside the asylum.
(by kind permission of the Royal Society of Medicine)

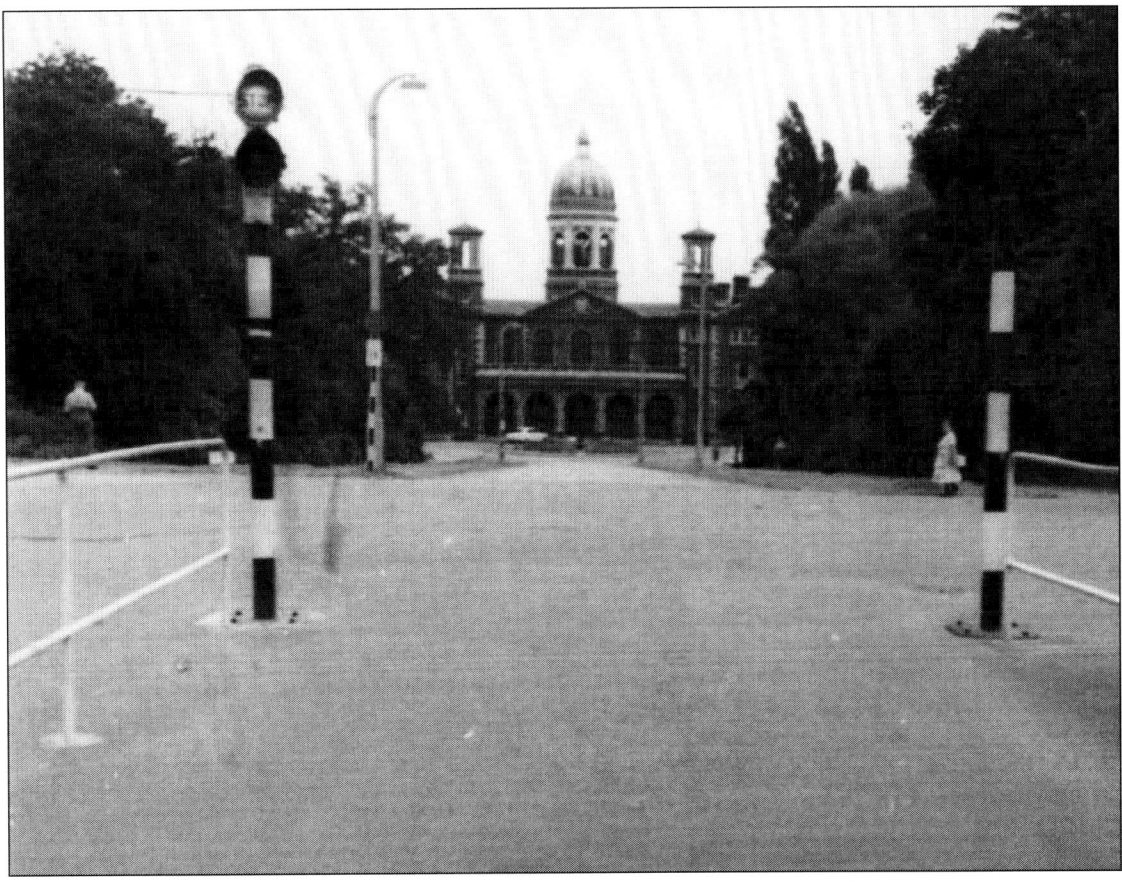

Once the main gate had been reopened, traffic lights controlled the movement of vehicles.
(John Donovan)

Cromwell Road, N10 on concrete piers was replaced by an inverted siphon. The piece of land between Cromwell Road and the new arterial road was later used by the LCC for educational sports. Friern Barnet had wanted to name the stretch of new road Elizabeth's Way, but they were overruled by MCC who opted for Pinkham Way, after Sir Charles Pinkham who had been responsible for many road schemes in Middlesex. The road opened in 1932.

The building of the North Circular left approximately seven acres south of the new road which were still part of the farm and initially cows would be herded across the road but this obviously proved too dangerous and so in 1935 the land was transferred to the LCC who used it as a playing field for schools. With the demise of the Inner London Education Authority (ILEA) the land ceased to be used for this purpose and, despite various efforts to build on it, it still remains unused and is designated as Metropolitan Open Land.

A little recognised problem in a building the size of Friern was the provision of food for the patients. A new kitchen had been built in 1952 at a cost of £22,000 but the transport of food to the wards was criticised in a report by the King's Fund in September 1953[5]. Hot food was being placed in large tin boxes under which hot water was kept. The boxes were then taken from the kitchen on trolleys but the problem was that as there were no lifts, the boxes then had to be unloaded and carried up flights of stone steps to the ward kitchens where they were served to the patients. As the hot water could have been poured in some two hours previously, the food invariably arrived cold. The report recommended that lifts should be installed and that trolleys heated by electricity should be purchased. The Management Committee applied for a grant from the King's Fund and by 1957 two

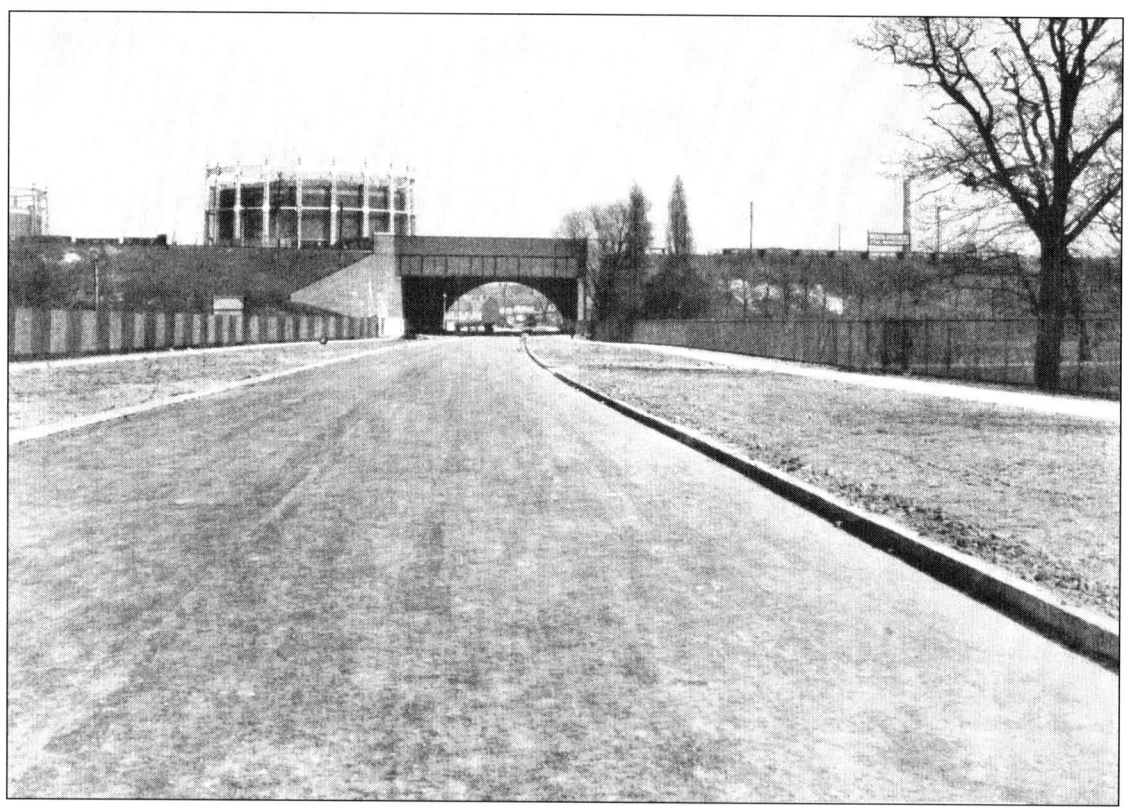

The North Circular shortly after construction was finished. The new boundary to the hospital is on the left. (Colin Barratt Collection)

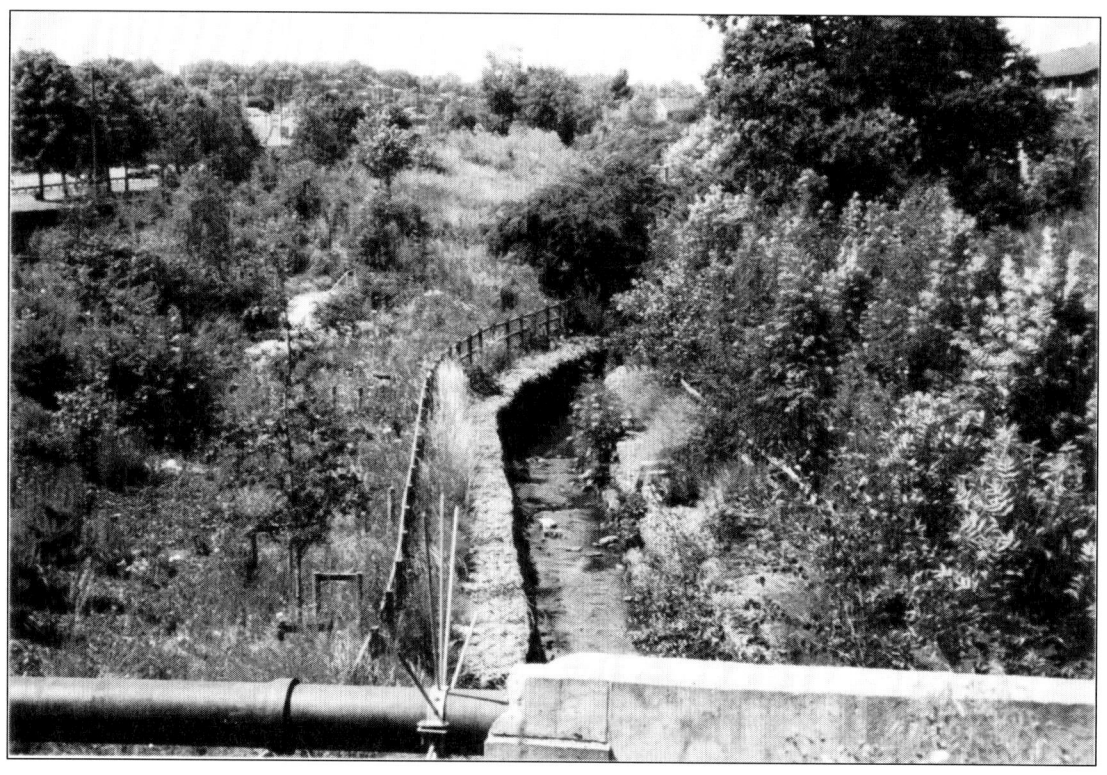

Bounds Green Brook now runs in a culvert. (Author)

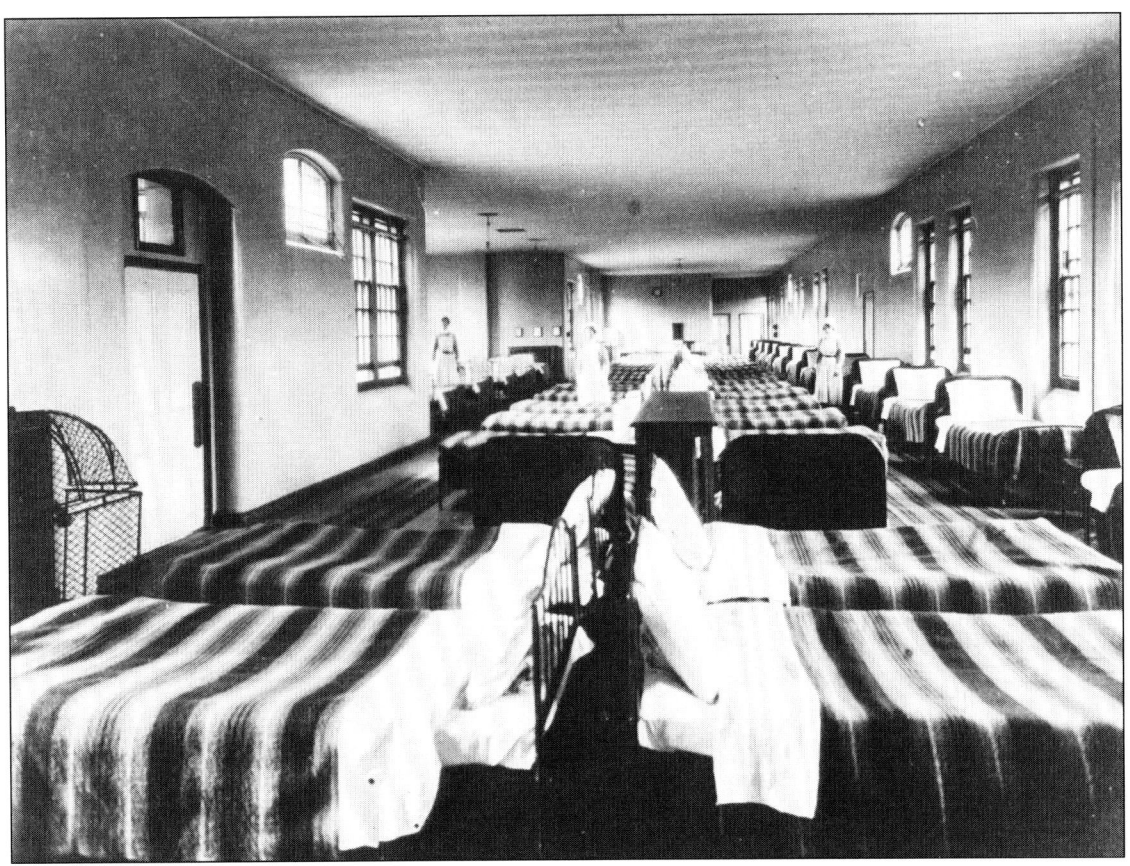

Ward E1 photographed in 1900, with beds closely packed in.
(by kind permission of the Royal Society of Medicine)

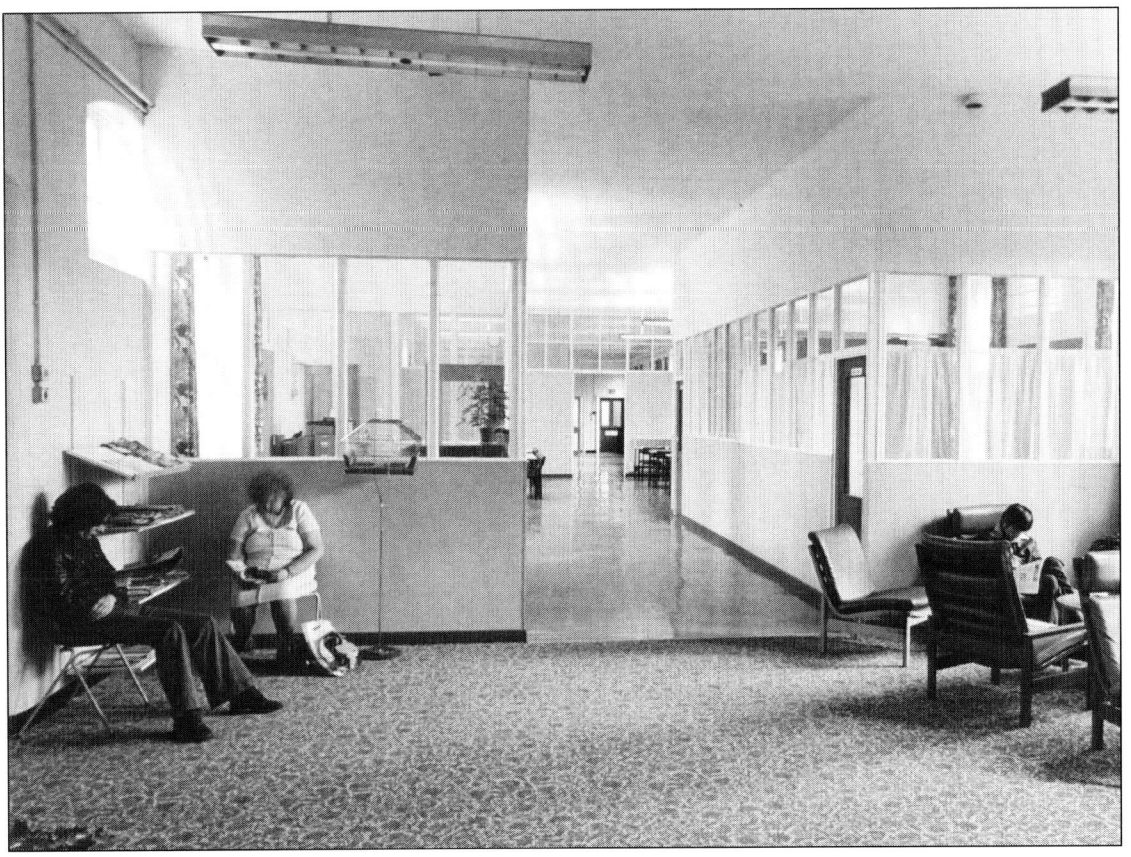

Ward E1 converted into an out patient department photographed in 1973.
Note the bird in a cage! (By kind permission of the Royal Society of Medicine)

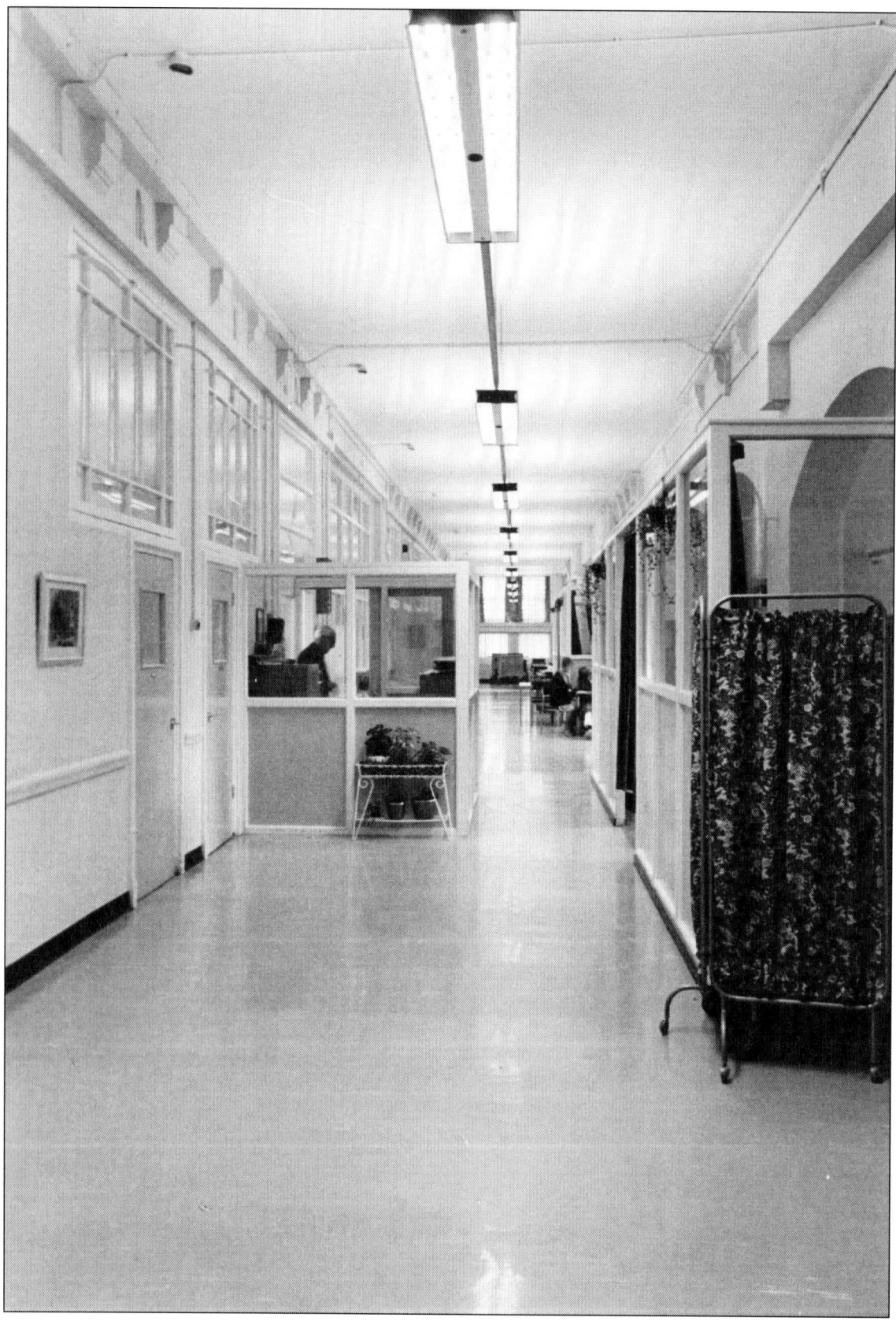

Ward 25 after modernisation. Photographed in 1973.
(By kind permission of the Royal Society of Medicine)

lifts had been put in, one in either wing, at a cost of £4200 and electrically heated trolleys were supplied at a cost of £3500.

In the same report the King's Fund had also commented on the grave shortage of nursing staff, both male and female, and there were only a third of the number of students required. In response to this, one of the Villas that had been damaged in the War was refurbished as a Nurses Training School and opened in December 1954.

The Mental Treatment Act of 1930 made it possible for patients to be admitted voluntarily to psychiatric hospitals and also for outpatient treatment to be given. It was recommended that mental hospitals should have a unit for what was termed "recent cases", wholly separate from the main building, in which patients with confirmed mental disorder should be housed. It was not until 1958 that Friern was able to introduce such a unit.

Halliwick Hospital was opened on Thursday 27 November 1958 by the Duchess of Kent and was situated to the northwest of the main building, near Friern Barnet Road. It had 152 beds of which 18 were for day patients and it included an evening clinic whereby voluntary patients could attend without their employers' knowledge. Halliwick also acted as an admissions unit for the main hospital.

There were four wards, Ash, Beech, Cedar and Oak. Two of the wards were on the ground floor, along with a lounge, and two on the first floor plus a games room, an office, and the patients' canteen. In 1960 day rooms for group and art therapy, were introduced. Halliwick was renamed Halliwick House in 1974 by which time it had 130 beds for newly admitted patients and for those convalescing from the main hospital. Three of the wards in Halliwick were Admission wards which complemented three wards in the main building; the other was a Rehabilitation ward in which patients were prepared for their transition to the outside world. The King's Fund provided money for landscaping the grounds around the hospital.

Friern had its own laundry which dealt with some 30,000 items a week. Initially the work was done by hand by ten laundry maids but in 1874 two washing machines were installed[6]. The laundry at Friern was situated in the rear of the main building and catered not only for its own staff and patients but in latter years also dealt with linen from the City of London Maternity, Hornsey Central, Royal Northern, Southwood and Whittington hospitals. The laundry closed in 1993, along with the main hospital.

There was also a separate Sterile Services department in a separate building to the west of the site which dealt with the sterilisation of goods for the same hospitals as well as Chase Farm, Cheshunt Cottage, Lister Hospital Renal Department, North Middlesex Hospital, Queen Mary's (Belsize Park), St Ann's, St Albans and Hemel Hempstead, as well as Holloway and Pentonville prisons. The Sterile Services department remained open for another three years until 1996.

Once the farm had ceased to exist, around 1971, the large area of land to the south of the hospital was used for tipping of waste and for infilling. A programme of upgrading and redecorating wards was begun in the 1950s and the old "poor law" appearance of the asylum was slowly transformed. The layout of the wards was also changed and the number of open wards rose to 13 out of a total of 46; before the War there had only been five open wards. This may seem a small proportion, but for many years the hospital had admitted most unpromising patients where prognosis was bad and for whom no special treatment was provided, with the result that in 1952 45% of the patients had been in hospital for over ten years. This necessitated a somewhat slower progress in the opening

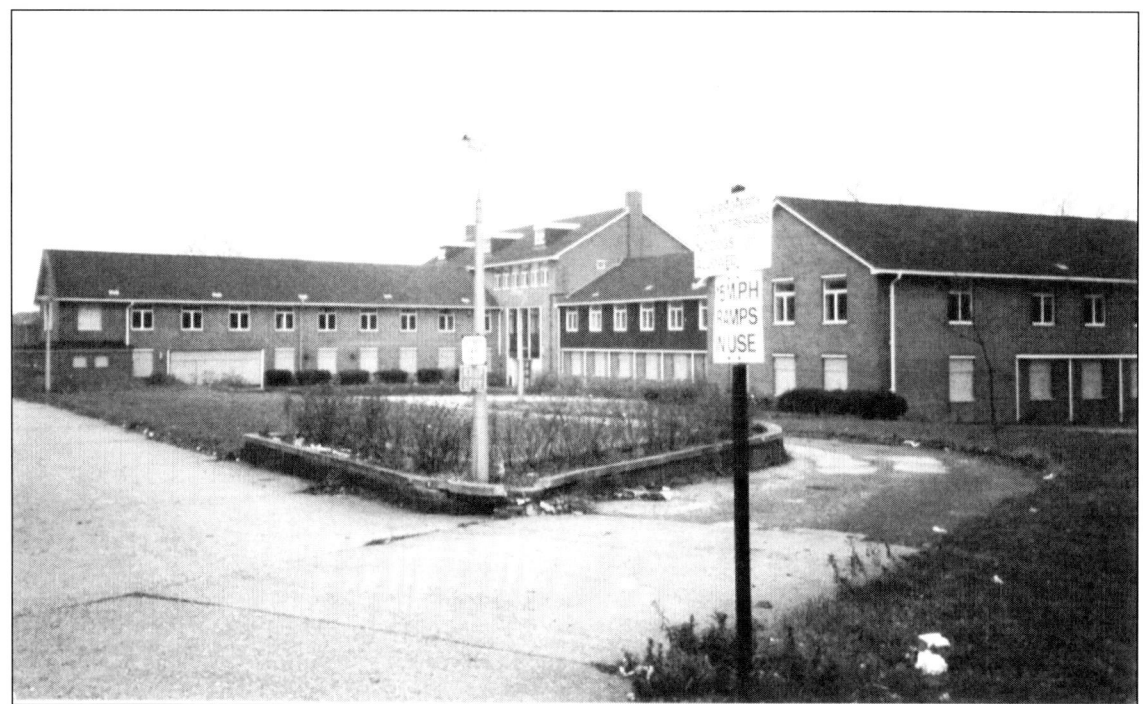

Halliwick Hospital in 1991 after its closure. (John Donovan)

up of wards than would have been desirable, but the result was worthwhile as it gave increased freedom to patients.

As far as chronic patients in closed wards was concerned, there had not been any lack of effort in trying to raise the general level throughout the hospital, even though discharge was more than could be hoped for. Upgrading and redecoration of wards was carried out in just the same way as in wards for new or convalescent patients.

The male and female sides of the hospital were no longer separated by locked doors as before the War, nor were the doors from the corridors to the entrance hall locked. Any patient in the corridors of the hospital could easily leave the building and even the hospital premises, but in fact they did not do so any more frequently than before when to have "escaped" was looked upon as a more serious matter.

Geoff Smith recalls one improvement that took place while he was Manager at Friern in 1981:

> "One of the things we did during my time was to start a personalised clothing scheme. Some of the patients didn't have any money, although some did.. Originally there was like a communal clothing scheme but the personalised clothing scheme meant people had their own clothes which went into the hospital's own laundry and came back and that was developed into a Patients' Boutique which we named The Bakehouse Boutique after the area where it was situated. The clothing scheme was excellent, run by Carol Wright, who had come from the retail clothing industry and she bought in good quality clothing and the staff could also buy them; I bought three or four Mr Harry suits from them. It was just like a shop and the patients would go there on their own or with a carer and they would choose their own clothes."

The Bakehouse Boutique enabled patients to select clothes suitable for their requirements, at a price they could afford, in a relaxing atmosphere and where they could gain confidence in shopping along with the feeling of independence. Geoff recalled one of his meetings with the Prime Minister and MP for Finchley, Margaret Thatcher:

> "There was a lady called Olive Dyke who ran the WRVS and the League of Friends and Olive had known Margaret for years. On the day she arrived the security men were keen that she went straight through but she stopped and chatted and she really impressed me that day. I may not have agreed with all of her politics but as a politician she was excellent. She went into the big kitchen and there were a couple of people there that she called by their first names. She came into the boutique area and after she had drawn the cord to open the Boutique the chairman of the Health Authority asked me to take her into a little room at the back where the catering department had prepared tea and cakes. The idea was that she would get a cup of tea and a cake and come out again but she took her tea and perched on a windowsill and said: "I've been on my feet all day. Do you mind if I sat here for a bit?" I had fifteen minutes with her and we chatted and she asked if we had sold the land at the back of the hospital and if we had got a good price for it. Fortunately, I knew exactly how much. I asked her whether she had had a busy day and she said "Oh, yes, I looked at my diary today and saw that I had a meeting with Pierre Trudeau at 11 o'clock, lunch with the Venezuelan Foreign Minister at 12 and Geoff Smith at Friern." I remarked that she had a reputation for only having three or four hour's sleep and I told her that I sometimes worked late in the evening and had difficulty switching off and she told me that she had her red boxes which her secretary put in order – in box 1 was things she had to look at, those in box 2 were things she didn't need to look at and in box 3 were things she just needed to sign and so she just used to gradually tail off."

Other services provided by the hospital were the Orchard Club, where patients could buy tea, coffee and other refreshments; the Willow Shop which provided refreshments, confectionery etc. and a hairdressing service for patients. The Patients Affairs Department managed money on behalf of individual patients, including DHSS benefits and the operation of patients' bank accounts. Friern had a full time Voluntary Services Organiser who acted as a link with the many voluntary organisations who were dedicated to helping patients. Voluntary help took several forms including donations or gifts to the hospital and arranging outings for patients. Help over the years was also provided by the WVRS, the League of Jewish Women, Jewish Comforts Fund and the Hospital's Friends.

The wall to the north of the asylum remained at eight feet until 1981 when it was lowered to around four feet. The height had not only deterred inmates from escaping but also prevented the public from looking into the grounds. The company responsible for the running of trams along Friern Barnet Road (Metropolitan Electric Tramways) installed a spiked dog collar-like device on each of their traction standards next to the walls of the asylum to deter potential voyeurs from shinning up the poles. These devices were known irreverently by tram crews and later trolleybus crews, as "lunatic spikes".

In 1930 the Mental Treatment Act did away with the term "asylum" and the name was changed to Colney Hatch Mental Hospital, changed again in 1937 to Friern Mental Hospital and finally in 1959 to Friern Hospital. It was in 1937 that the hospital's catchment area was enlarged to include Finsbury, Hampstead, Holborn, Islington, St Marylebone, St Pancras and Shoreditch. Also from this date it was decided that Jewish patients from the whole of the County of London would be concentrated in Friern, as historically there had always been a number of Jews there and the hospital was used to

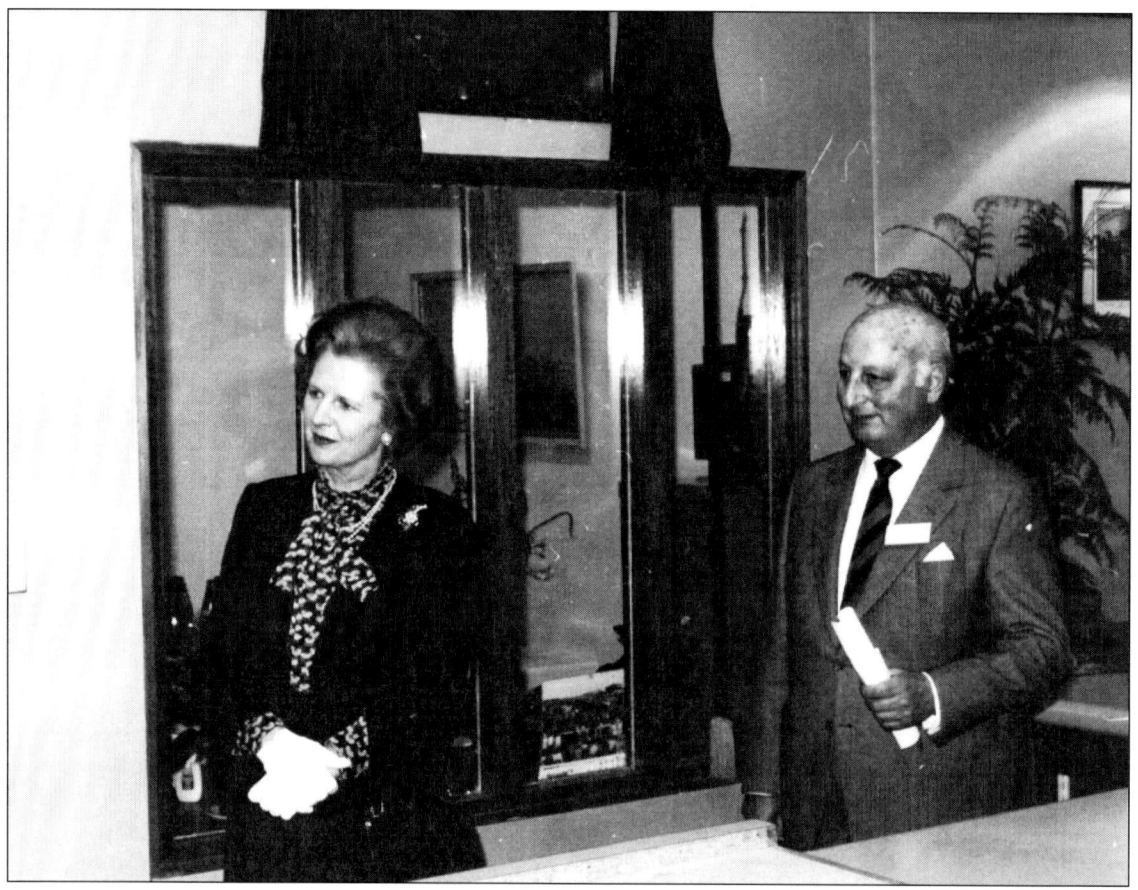

The Bakehouse Boutique was opened on 26 June 1981 by the local MP, Margaret Thatcher.
(Geoff Smith Collection)

ministering to their religious and dietary requirements.

Although the asylum started life as an enterprise of Middlesex County Council, it did not remain so.. When the London County Council (LCC) was formed in 1889 it took over the work of the Metropolitan Board of Works but was also given extra responsibilities including tramways, schools, council housing, hospitals and the "care of the mentally defective and mentally disordered". The running of Colney Hatch Asylum was therefore passed to the LCC who ran it until 1948 when the newly formed National Health Service took over and Friern came under the control of the newly formed North West Metropolitan Regional Hospital Board.

In 1974 the NHS was reorganised and Friern came under the North East Thames Regional Health Authority. A further reorganisation took place in 1982 which saw the abolition of Area Health Authorities, so Friern came under the auspices of Hampstead Health Authority. In 1993 Hampstead Health Authority merged with Bloomsbury and Islington Health Authority to form Camden and Islington Health Authority which managed Friern until its closure.

By 1970 the long-established practice of separating male and female patients was abandoned and from then until the closure of the hospital there were mixed wards which were looked after by male and female staff. At this time the hospital was divided into three divisions based upon the boroughs making up its catchment area, so Haringey patients occupied the west wing and Camden the east wing, with Islington in the centre.

CHANGES AND IMPROVEMENTS

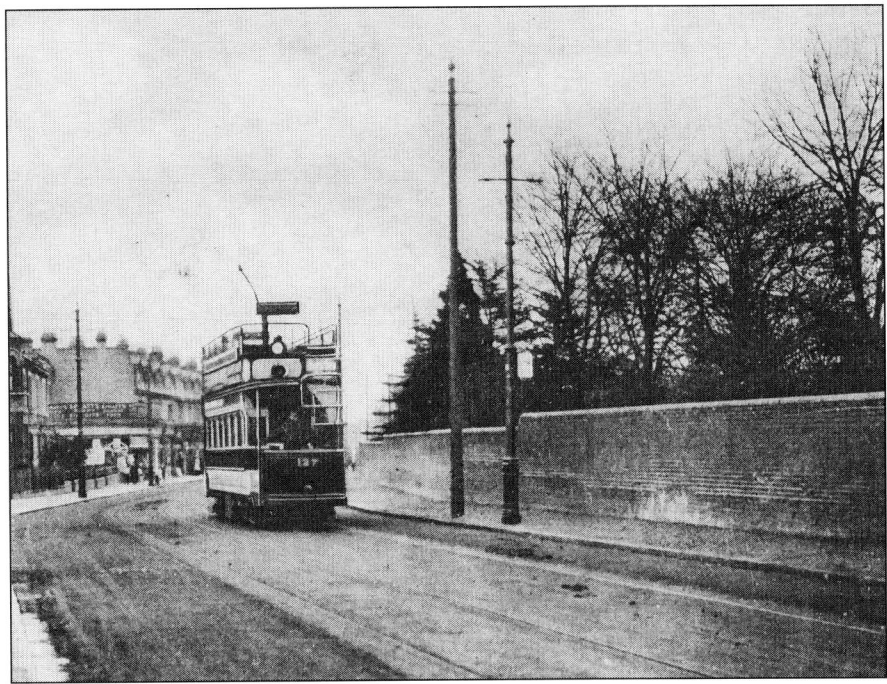

This view of Friern Barnet Road from 1910 shows that the wall of the asylum was approximately eight feet high in places. (Commercial postcard)

In 1991, some two years before the hospital closed, an English and Religious Studies teacher and amateur artist, Andolie Luck, was visiting a friend in Friern and was appalled at the grim and forbidding appearance of the long corridor. She approached the hospital authorities and asked if she could paint some designs on the walls and she was given the necessary permission. Her friend, Margaret Leibbrandt, recalled that Andolie would approach anyone she met in the corridor and ask them what they would like. Among the many requests, a pest controller asked for a cockroach and a rat which he duly got and two of the doctors requested a dinosaur and some zebras. It was most noticeable that all of the patients wanted calming scenes – there were no requests for anything disturbing.

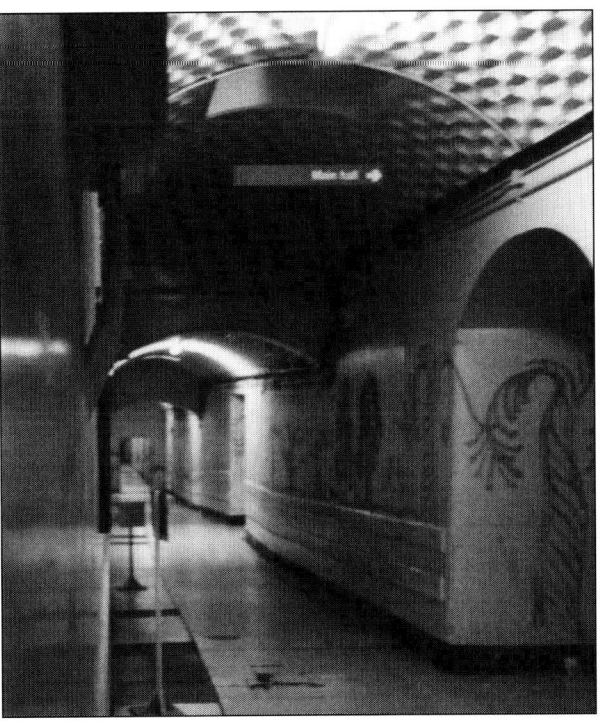

A less depressing corridor (John Donovan)

CHAPTER EIGHTEEN

Sans Everything

In June 1967 a book, *Sans Everything*, was published on behalf of AEGIS, the Association for the Elderly in Government Institutions, in which a number of contributors made serious allegations about care of elderly patients in seven NHS psychiatric and general hospitals, including Friern. The public reaction to the book via articles and letters in newspapers and magazines and coverage on television was such that the Minister of Health requested the various Hospital Boards to investigate the accusations.

In August 1967 the North West Metropolitan Regional Hospital Board appointed a committee consisting of a QC, a nurse, a doctor and a lay member. The committee spent some eleven months investigating the complaints and subsequently produced a report[1]. Of the 83 pages in the report, 32 of them related to Friern.

The committee found that most of the accusations in the book could not be substantiated, either because the complainants refused to be interviewed by the committee to corroborate their claims or because many pseudonyms were used throughout, it was often impossible to verify the accusations. The authors of the book maintained that pseudonyms were used to prevent punitive steps being taken against either patients or staff, however it made the task of investigation extremely difficult. The committee scrutinised the hospital records and interviewed medical, nursing and administrative staff and their accounts were invariably at variance to the claims made in the book. Among the more serious accusations that had been made in the book were:

- There was a lack of entertainment for middle aged schizophrenics and of occupation for the elderly. The committee stated that while many patients may have appeared bored, they were often incapable of animation

- The hospital clothing was inadequate and that staff resented the extra work in providing proper clothes for the patients. The committee stated that clothing was constantly being soiled or damaged by the patients themselves. It doubted that staff resented changing these and that when patients went on outings they had to be properly dressed

- If patients were let out of locked wards for entertainment "we would lose the bloody lot". The committee agreed that this phrase may have been used but it was necessary to keep wards locked to prevent patients wandering out onto the busy public highway (Friern Barnet Road) without supervision

- Everything was arranged to suit the staff. The committee rejected this and stated that patients' welfare was their prime consideration

- The Physician Superintendent was seldom in the hospital. The committee said this was a "false and scandalous accusation" as he had attended the hospital daily between 9.00am and 5.30pm

- There was criticism of the matrons and assistant matrons. Since the author was anonymous, the committee was unable to interview him or her

- Nurses and doctors were idle and doctors seldom went into the wards. The committee said that this was unsupported by any evidence and was in contradiction to visual evidence when they conducted their inspections

- Staff regarded patients as "cogs in the machine". The committee admitted that some may take this view, but not the majority

- Patients were maltreated and were sometimes hit, leading to cases of bruising. The committee found that no specific instances were given in the book. Bruising may have been due to patients falling and hurting themselves. If there was ill treatment it would have been reported and investigated

- Various cases of mistreatment against patients were reported. The complainants refused to be interviewed by the committee so the claims could not be substantiated

- An outside Social Worker had reported a conversation that she had with a doctor. The committee found that the inclusion of this in the book was a breach of professional etiquette on her part

- A doctor had expressed a preference for treating psychotic patients rather than seeing discharged patients in a follow-up clinic. The committee did not consider that this remark impugned the services he had rendered during his nineteen years at Friern

- There were a large number of accusations of poor treatment by a lady whose father had been admitted to Friern in a confused, agitated and deluded state. The woman refused to be interviewed by the committee and they considered that her version of events was grossly distorted

- A number of allegations were made concerning the treatment of a particular elderly female patient, in a chapter headed *"Diary of a Nobody."* None of the complainants would co-operate with the committee and as pseudonyms of staff were used, it was difficult to prove or disprove the accusations. The committee found that none of the accusations of cruelty could be substantiated and that some of the accusations were false and scandalous

An important factor affecting the investigation arose out of the lapse of time since the majority of the alleged matters of complaint arose or occurred, namely the first half of 1965 or earlier. The Committee did not know why publication of the book did not take place until almost two years later, in the late spring of 1967; although this delay had permitted the inclusion of one section of the book (on page 58) which the Committee were able to discover related to an event in August 1966. In assessing the value of the evidence given to them the Committee had naturally borne in mind the effect on people's memory of such a time lag.

The committee presented their report on Friern Hospital in July 1968 and the Minister of Health, Kenneth Robinson, made the following comments in a speech to Parliament on 9 July 1968:

> "All six Committees of Enquiry have now made their reports, and their findings and recommendations are published today in a Command Paper. These independent Committees of Enquiry find most of the allegations in "Sans Everything" to be totally unfounded or grossly exaggerated. They make some criticisms of present conditions in the hospitals and suggest how they might be improved, but in general they report very favourably on the standard of care

provided. I deeply regret the anxieties which have been caused to patients and their relatives, to hospital staff and to the public generally by the publication, which I believe the whole House will deplore, of so many allegations which are now authoritatively discredited."

Although most of the allegations in the book could be dismissed, its publication achieved one important thing – the committee were able to investigate and report on all aspects of the running of Friern Hospital.

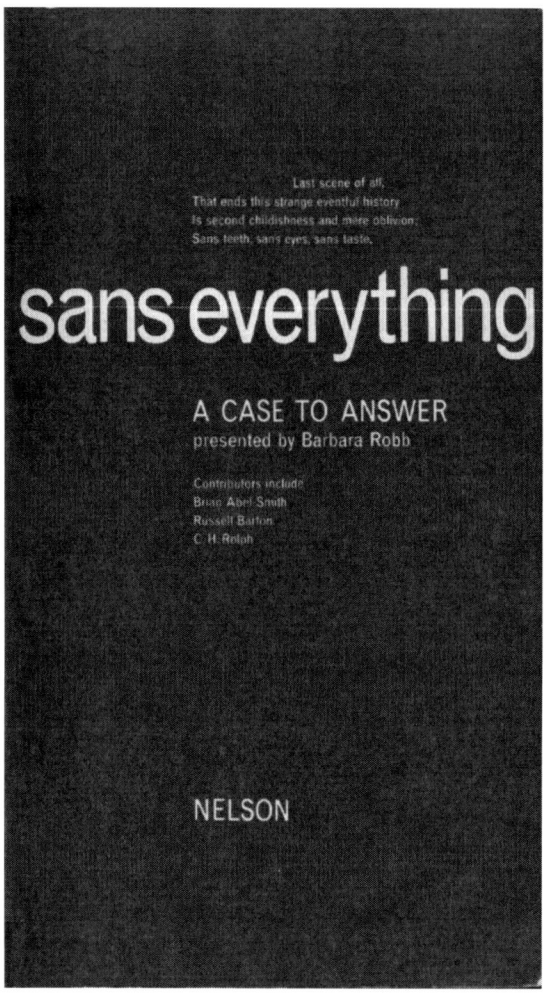

(Barnet Local Studies)

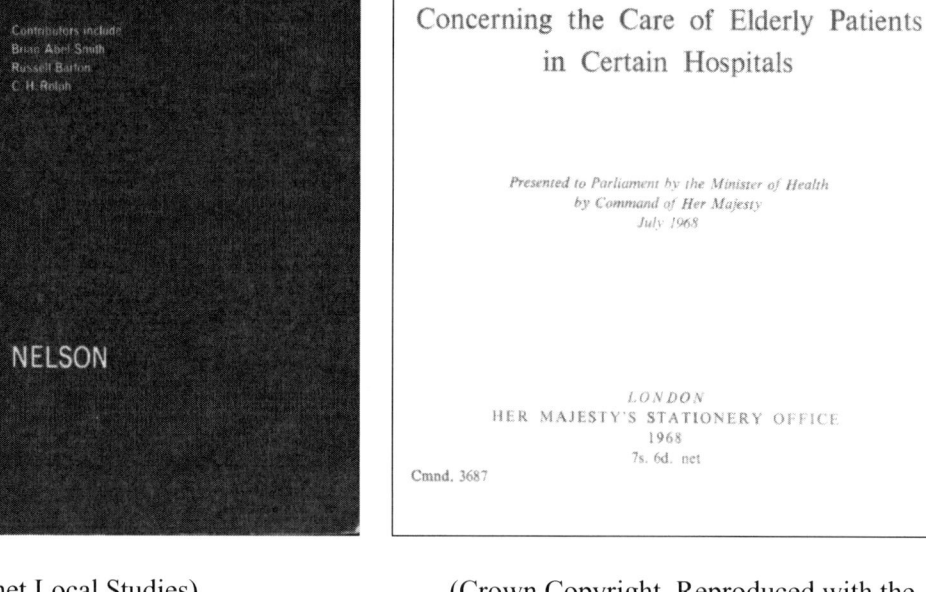

(Crown Copyright. Reproduced with the permission of the Controller of HMSO)

Many of the elderly patients were either being discharged or would die in the hospital, so there was a steady flow of incoming patients, 75% of whom would be women. Most of the permanent patients suffered some form of schizophrenic illness. One problem was that patients who were fit to be discharged had to remain, as relatives were unable or unwilling to take responsibility for them. For those without dependents, a return to a solitary life at home could lead to a relapse. Other patients had become so acclimatised to life in the hospital that it would have been unkind to discharge them.

The medical staff at the time comprised six consultant psychiatrists; ward doctors, of whom three were senior Hospital Medical Officers; one senior Hospital Dental Officer; eight registrars; three part time registrars; three senior house officers and one medical assistant. Outside consultants, including two ophthalmic surgeons, made weekly visits or more frequently if required. There was a full time physiotherapist and a full time remedial gymnast.

The committee were of the opinion that the number of nursing staff at Friern was gravely inadequate, particularly as most wards were overcrowded. The lack of domestic help necessitated nursing staff doing domestic chores. The administrative staff numbered 38 and was considered to be adequate. The overall impression that the committee gained was that there was a lack of finance, a grave shortage of staff, especially nursing and domestic staff and antiquated buildings. It was considered scandalous that one night nurse would have to deal with over 20 incontinent patients, often involving changing clothing and bed linen and washing patients. The severe shortage of staff was responsible for the low morale and sense of defeatism at the hospital and was strongly condemned by the report.

The committee examined the procedure regarding admissions and found that these followed a consultation with the GP or mental health social worker, an interview at the hospital outpatient clinic, or a reference from the police under section 136 of the Mental Health Act 1959; often a referral by the police was for someone who was simply drunk or may have been refused admission at a general hospital. The committee recommended that in future most such admissions should be refused. Elderly patients suffering from depression were admitted without question, but confused or senile patients should, ideally have been dealt with in geriatric wards of general hospitals, however local authorities often failed to provide suitable accommodation so that Friern was overburdened with patients who should not have been there. A particular problem was admissions after 10pm, which sometimes amounted to ten per month, mainly males. Most of these should have been admitted to general hospitals as they were often suffering from physical illnesses, but medical officers who referred them were not always honest with their comments.

The report examined the treatment of geriatric patients and found that many of those who needed care for senility and incontinence were being put in wards with people with psychiatric problems, which was unsatisfactory. They also felt that there was insufficient provision of occupational therapy, notwithstanding the fact that many senile patients were unable to avail themselves of any recreational therapy.

One of the problems associated with Friern was the state of the building. Some of the female wards were described as being in very poor condition, although some had been refurbished and were bright and cheerful. Part of the gloomy appearance was down to the original windows which were set very high in the walls. Unbelievably, there was only one external telephone for the whole of the female side of the hospital and in one ward 47 patients shared two baths and seven sinks and they were bathed without privacy in batches of twelve a night[2].

The committee made 22 recommendations including the extension of visiting hours and the separation of mentally and physically infirm patients from those requiring active psychiatric treatment.

The question of underfunding had been raised in an investigation that the *Daily Mail* had carried out when in an article in their issue of 10 September 1965 they found that Friern needed £30,000 for repairs to the roof but only £4500 had been granted. £33,000 was required for repairs to dangerous stonework but they received only £2500. The newspaper reported that before that, in 1963, the management at Friern had been asked by the Regional Board by how far it was behind with maintenance work. It claimed

£74,000 to improve wards, £13,700 for engineering and £40,000 for fabric repairs. Of the total of £127,700 they received a mere £13,000.

In a Committee Meeting on 8 August 1968 the board of Friern agreed the following:

- An attempt would be made to increase the nursing establishment recruitment through advertising and publicity. Nothing could be done about increasing salaries as they were the responsibility of the Whitley Council

- The medical establishment would be increased by two Consultants and one Registrar

- The Board would be asked for funds to increase the number of domestic staff

- When surplus land at the site was sold the money raised would be used for a geriatric home to be built

- The wards would be upgraded, although the limiting factor was the severe overcrowding which made it impossible to close many wards while work went on

- The separation of patients was desirable but difficult to achieve until the legacy of long stay patients was reduced. It was the policy not to transfer elderly long stay patients as this often proved distressing for them

- Clothing could only be improved if the finance was available

- Improved Industrial and Occupational Therapy required new funds

- A newsletter should be published to improve internal communication

- The salary of psychiatric social workers should be increased

To give some idea of the size of Friern at that time, in 1966 the population of the suburban area was 600,000 from where the majority of the patients came. Out of just over 2100 patients in the hospital, 35% were over 65 (536 women, 202 men) and 292 geriatric patients admitted were suffering from senile dementia, others from serious or mild depression. Most of the geriatric women patients were nursed in 12 out of the 24 female wards. Those 24 wards had a total staff on each day shift of about 80, including sisters, all grades of nurses and students and ward orderlies. The majority of the elderly men were nursed in 4 of the 16 male wards where nursing staff fluctuated between about 38 to 60. Total nursing staff for the whole hospital in November 1967 was only 429, including administrators.

So, although *Sans Everything* was perhaps a flawed piece of work, it did lead to improvements at Friern and other psychiatric hospitals and it brought into the public spotlight the treatment and/or mistreatment of mental patients. The despair at the time can be summed up by a quote by Dr Ralph Emery of Brookwood Hospital:

> "The rising tide of demented old ladies pressing, or being pressed, for admission to the mental hospitals, has to be seen to be believed. It is a sad state of affairs that doctors more or less secretly hope that their patients will not live too long, but in view of the care given by a devoted staff this hope is rarely fulfilled"

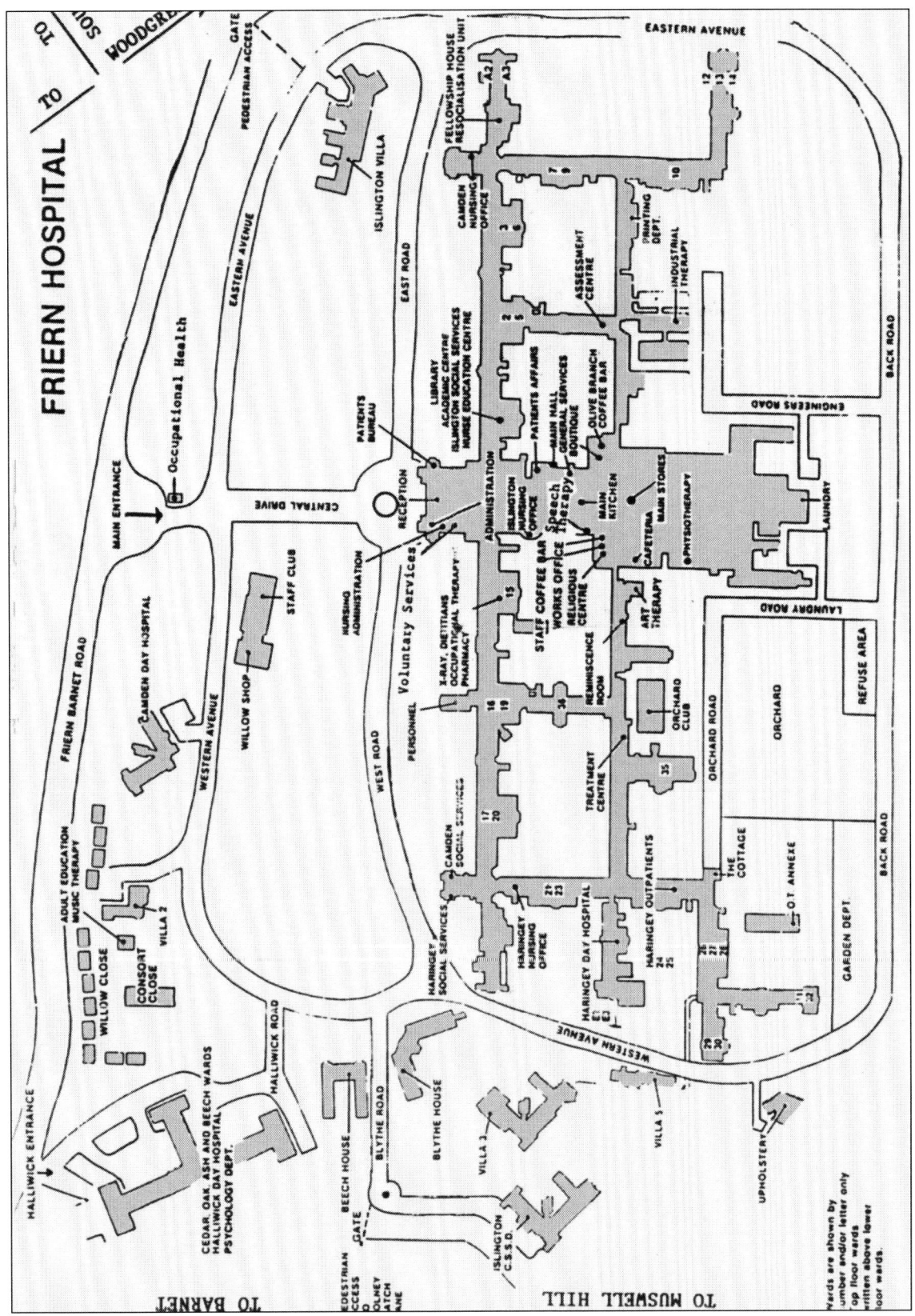

The site in 1989 (FB&DLHS Archive)

CHAPTER NINETEEN

Care in the Community

By the second half of the 20th century it was becoming increasingly obvious that the Victorian way of dealing with mental illness was no longer viable. Institutions like Friern were outdated, overcrowded and increasingly expensive to run and the greater understanding of the causes of mental illness and the introduction of new methods of treatment, particularly through the use of drugs, meant that the whole system needed to be overhauled. By 1955 there were almost 150,000 people in mental hospitals and almost half of the new hospital beds being created were for those suffering from mental illness or mental disability and the cost to the NHS was beginning to become unsustainable.

The Mental Health Act of 1930 had created two new categories of mental patient, voluntary and temporary, and the LCC had established psychiatric outpatient clinics specifically for the examination of applicants as to their fitness for reception as voluntary patients[1] but the first indication of serious changes came with the Mental Health Act 1959, introduced by the Macmillan government and which attempted to bring the hospital treatment of mental patients more in line with general hospitals. This was to be achieved by making admissions to mental hospitals as informal as those for physical ailments and also by making local councils responsible for social care of people who did not need in-patient treatment.

In a keynote speech to the National Association for Mental Health in March 1961 the then Minister of Health, Enoch Powell said:

> "There they stand, isolated, majestic, imperious, brooded over by the gigantic water-tower and chimney combined, rising unmistakable and daunting out of the countryside – the asylums which our forefathers built with such immense solidity to express the notions of their day. Do not for a moment underestimate their powers of resistance to our assault."

This was quite a prophetic statement as the asylums managed to resist attempts for change, however things were starting to move forward, albeit at a snail's pace. Meanwhile, two feature films on the treatment of mental illness had a profound effect on public opinion. The 1972 film by Ken Loach, *Family Life* was particularly harrowing in its treatment of schizophrenia and in 1976 *One Flew Over the Cuckoo's Nest* brought to public notice the conditions in asylums and in particular the inhumane treatment of patients by staff, but there was still resistance to change. However, the major stumbling block to reform was that there was just not the infrastructure in place to allow patients to be treated in the community; this was the fault of successive governments who had failed to provide local councils with the necessary funds.

In February 1970 in a memorandum to the Hospital Management Committee from the Medical Advisory Committee at Friern[2] had recommended the gradual running down of Friern:

> "The primary reason for this being the dilapidated nature of a considerable number of wards and the inability to renovate these to a sufficiently high standard without total rebuilding. Very considerable expense would be incurred if rebuilding to the necessary scale were undertaken. The present construction of the central hospital block effectively mitigates against individual sub-units within the whole. However, the very large number of long-stay patients and the problems in finding alternative old age and hostel accommodation would probably mean that such a run-down would have to be a very gradual process. Needless to say, the

creation of a wholly long-stay hospital would have considerable effects on the recruitment and retention of staff."

In 1971, the Secretary of State for the Social Services visited Friern to open a new patients' social centre which would replace the Willow Pavilion. Dr John Bradley, consultant psychiatrist and chairman of the medical committee at Friern, took the opportunity to announce that they wanted to gradually run down the hospital because there was no excuse for a hospital with nearly 2000 patients. Their aim was to reduce this to 1500.

The gradual closure of hospitals like Friern raised serious doubts in some people's minds, as a letter to *The Guardian* from a Divisional Nursing Officer shows[3]

> "The nonsensical suggestion that hospitals can be done away with in the next ten years is both irresponsible and dishonest. Could anyone tell me where this wonderful caring community is of which they speak? I have worked in Hertfordshire, Leicester, and now Surrey, and in my experience, if you want to start a group home for your patients, it is okay so long as it is not next door to anyone.....we are striving at the hospital in which I work to get our patients into the community but we must be honest; at least 70 per cent will never, and could never, exist in present-day society even if money was available".

In recognition of the need to treat those suffering from psychiatric illness as "just ordinary patients" within general hospitals, in 1959 the Camden & Islington Health Authority Hospital started to design a Psychiatric Wing at Whittington Hospital in Highgate. This was in fact part of a proposed £12m scheme to rebuild the St Mary's Wing of the hospital. The six-storey Psychiatric Wing was opened in May 1976 and had accommodation for 90 in-patients and 50 day patients, along with rooms for various types of occupational therapy such as pottery, carpentry, sewing and domestic services.[4] Once the unit was up and running patients were transferred there from Friern.

In 1981 the Conservative government published The Parkinson Report which highlighted the lack of progress in implementing community care. However, the big breakthrough came when the Thatcher government published a Green Paper entitled *Care in the Community*. The report stated:

> "Most people who need long-term care can and should be looked after in the community. That is what most of them want for themselves and what those responsible for their care believe to be best."

The report covered the care of not only the mentally ill but also the elderly and recommended that as many as 20,000 long stay patients could be immediately discharged if funding was transferred from the NHS to local authorities.

In 1982 the government implemented three measures: 1) The maximum period for which the NHS could pay for joint finance would be extended from seven to thirteen years for projects to move people out of hospital, and the NHS would pay 100% of the money for up to ten years 2) District Health Authorities would be allowed to make guaranteed payments to councils and voluntary bodies for ex-patients they provided for in the community 3) £15,000,000 would be set aside to develop and assess a series of pilot projects.

Some health professionals were still urging caution. Dr Malcolm Weller, consultant psychiatrist at Friern was quoted as saying:[5]

> "In hospitals, some of our patients and staff have been together for 20 years. There is a real sense of community. How will they ever find the same sense of community outside, where they are unwanted?"

In 1990 a group called the Peter Bedford Trust published a paper[6] outlining the results of an experiment that had been conducted into the settlement of people into a community based setting. They found that at Friern in 1983, at the time of the decision to close the hospital, out of 850 patients, 72 had been there for more than 5 years and 60 had been there between 2 and 5 years. The investigation showed that a large number of people had been involved in the trial release of patients into the community. As well as hospital nursing staff and psychiatrists, help from the outside involved community psychiatric nurses, social workers and community pharmacists. The latter were particularly important in order to avoid patients stopping their medication, which could lead to mental breakdown. However, there were two interesting case studies which seemed to question the role of medication. One patient steadfastly refused injections for a whole year with no apparent side effects while another altered the doses of oral medication himself which prompted doctors to reconsider how they should prescribe for him.

Geoff Smith, Manager of the Hospital in 1981-82 recalls the start of the Care in the Community programme:

> "I think it was an amalgamation of things, but certainly the cost of maintaining the Friern buildings was becoming astronomical. There was a huge backlog of maintenance and I remember a chap from the Regional Health Authority coming down and saying that the cost of upgrading a ward was going to be huge and it would take 18 months to do it and I remembered from reading the history books that it only took 18 months to build the hospital in the first place. So that's progress for you! And I think it was at the time when the Health Service needed to look at what it was spending its money on and its priorities and couldn't really afford to keep upgrading old buildings. The main driving force though was the modernising of psychiatric services; unless you re-provided those services and took them away from places like that you were always going to perpetuate something that shouldn't really have taken us into the second half of the 20th century."

Geoff recalled how the transition worked:

> "When it was looked at initially it was wondered if these people would survive outside. Obviously some couldn't and they weren't transferred but lots could. One of the most satisfying involved a scheme somewhere in Hornsey Road. One patient I got to know really well was about fifty and had been at Friern since his teens or twenties and he was really apprehensive about moving in and he was one of six patients who were hand picked. They had had a lot of help from the nurses and therapists before they went in and there was follow up help afterwards. He said that he was not really sure that he could live on his own; I visited him about two months after and he said: "I never thought I could live a normal life." And it was things like that that made it really worthwhile. My take on all of this was that the re-provision schemes were really excellent and Friern was one of the first to be involved in a re-provision programme. There was money available because the Government and the Regional Health Authority at the time both wanted it to work. In subsequent years there hasn't been quite the same amount of money available because there are still some quite big psychiatric hospitals around, Goodmayes Hospital for example, in old buildings although it is about a third of

the size but it is still being used."

In the *Evening Standard* of 22 October 1990 Jerry Westall from the National Schizophrenic Fellowship made an interesting point. It was initially pressure from the Left which made people rethink the role of asylums ("mental illness was a form of distress and psychiatric hospitals were concentration camps for emotional dissidents") but it was the Right who actually saw the programme through, largely because of the money that could be made by the redevelopment of large asylums.

An organisation called Umbrella, comprising Bloomsbury Health Authority, the Departments of Housing and Social Services in Camden, three housing associations and the charity Mind was formed in 1989 and it produced a short report called *Care Based in the Community*. It stated that the closure of large psychiatric hospitals like Friern had been placed in jeopardy because of the failure to provide enough accommodation of the right design and type for people returning to the community. Umbrella had organised a scheme whereby for every bed closed down at Friern, a "dowry payment" equal to the cost of the bed was released to provide a network of alternative community care. The payments were made to the Bloomsbury Health Authority who passed on the money to the relevant community based services. When this money was added to grants from other organisations, Umbrella was able to manage three houses in the Camden area which catered for 27 former patients and provided them with daily visits from the Community Support Team. Residents attended regular meetings where their concerns could be aired and dealt with quickly.

Part of the support consisted of the running of the houses; a rota system for the cleaning and cooking and even watering the plants. Supervised outings were arranged, which helped to gradually get them used to shopping, using public transport, visiting theatres or other people's homes. For people who were very much used to their old lifestyle in Friern it required courage and bravery to leave and step into the unknown; even ordinary people would have found it disconcerting and challenging.

Had this level of support been more generally available, Care in the Community would have been an outstanding success. As it turned out, the general lack of funds meant that the support that was so vital could not continue to be provided and the problems that are so obvious today could have been avoided. When the closure of Friern was proposed in 1983 it was estimated that £72 million would be needed for capital projects for new facilities for Care in the Community – in fact only £50 million was available.[7]

In 1992 The North East Thames Regional Health Authority issued a booklet entitled *Leaving Friern, Coming Home* which gave details of projects that they had been developing since 1986. Once Friern had been closed, patients from health authorities in Bloomsbury and Islington, Haringey, Hampstead, Enfield and City and Hackney (the catchment areas for Friern) would be dealt with in a number of ways which could be tailored to their needs:

- Residential Homes that had been adapted or built for people with long-term mental health problems

- Day Centres would provide a welcoming place for people with long-term mental health problems. They would also have access to a mental health worker

- Mental Health Resource Teams would visit people in their own homes or provide supplementary care. They would be based in mental health resource centres

- Psychiatric Day Hospitals would provide a refuge where people could come for intensive care, whilst returning home in the evenings and at weekends

- Rehabilitation Units would enable people to either learn or regain their daily living skills

- Psychiatric departments at local hospitals for people who need to get away from their everyday environment for a period of rest and intensive treatment

- Community hospitals where elderly people with dementia could get continuous nursing care

- Medium secure units would offer a safe and secure environment for mentally ill offenders who had been referred by the courts

North East Thames had already spent £50 million on developing over 70 community homes and £21 million a year would be spent on providing support and care.

Because patients who had been released into the community lacked the kind of full time support and monitoring they would have received in a mental hospital, they often did not take their medication, often with disastrous consequences. One particularly horrible incident caused widespread public anger and brought into question the policy of releasing mental patients into the community. A musician, Jonathan Zito, was standing on a platform at Finsbury Park Underground station in December 1992 when he was stabbed in the eye and killed by a paranoid schizophrenic, Christopher Clunis, who had a long history of violent mental illness. Only in May that year he had stabbed a man in the neck but had been released when the victim failed to turn up at court. He had been in and out of hospital constantly for two months and on 28 September had been discharged by Guy's Hospital into the care of Friern. He failed to keep an appointment with a psychiatrist in October and his case notes did not arrive at Friern until 9 November. He was sentenced to be transferred to Rampton Hospital under the Mental Health Act without limit of time. Not surprisingly, Jonathan Zito's widow was extremely critical of the system: "Government policy for community care has failed in the extreme. They are closing down large institutions but not providing the resources for after-care. Someone has to tell me why Christopher Clunis was on the platform that day and murdered my husband."[8]

Dr Weller took the opportunity to restate his criticisms:

> "It gives me no comfort to know that we were right all along. I believed Friern should be reopened and the authorities should spend whatever is needed to bring it up to acceptable standards. But if it is not, an enormous amount of money will need to be poured into community care, otherwise there will be other catastrophes. They have spent £70 million decommissioning the finest hospital in Europe and I do not see how they can backtrack. But I fear we will see far more catastrophes unless more money is available."[9]

It is a sad fact that today some 2% of people will suffer from a severe psychotic illness – such as schizophrenia – in his or her lifetime and one in ten of all adults may suffer from anxiety or depression[10]. The GPs surgery is the first port of call for most people with mental health problems. Most NHS mental care and treatment is given by GPs, counsellors, pharmacists or community psychiatric nurses and most people make a full recovery. When people are in severe distress and do not recognise that they need help, they can be admitted to hospital under the Mental Health Act 1983 for a limited period of time without their consent; fortunately fewer than one in fifteen of all people admitted to psychiatric units are compulsorily detained under a 'section' of the Mental Health Act. Compulsory detention ('sectioning') cannot take place unless the criteria of the Act are met and there is no suitable alternative. Only a team of mental heath professionals can detain people for longer than 72 hours and only after a careful assessment and with compulsory detention as a last resort.[11]

Mrs Erna Karton was a Psychiatric Social Worker at St Ann's Hospital in Tottenham for nineteen years. When she started her career in 1968 it was in the Psychiatric Day Unit which had only just been created and was a new concept. Erna's job was to interview patients and their families and endeavour to ascertain the cause of their illness. A Psychiatric Team consisting of a Consultant, a Senior Registrar, and a Sister and a Psychologist would then assess the needs of patients and the kind of treatment they would need. Their progress would then be monitored on a weekly basis. Patients came from Friern and other mental hospitals such as Goodmayes.

Mrs Karton recalls one particularly disturbing interview she had with the wife of a patient:

> "He had been ill for some time and there was talk of him being discharged. I met his wife, an attractive lady, and before she left the room she said, rather like you would say "See you next week", "Well, of course, when he comes home I shall divorce him". I nearly fell off my chair. Sadly he committed suicide but, had we known earlier, we might have been able to help him to come to terms with the idea."

On another occasion a woman had been discharged from Friern and had been sent to the Psychiatric Day Centre for assessment:

> "I said "so they thought you were fine?" She said "Yes, but I don't really know as they found a knife under my mattress." And I was sitting there with her! And they had discharged her – that wasn't a good idea was it?"

Where suitable, patients would be moved into accommodation and they then came under the remit of the Psychiatric Health Visitor. The social workers in the community would come together with those in the hospitals to compare notes, although problems would sometimes arise because of the differences of opinion as to what constituted a mental problem Some of them for example reckoned there was no such a thing as schizophrenia.

CHAPTER TWENTY

Preparing for the end

As long ago as 1981, the Hospital Management Team was looking to a new future for Friern. They produced a paper called *Friern 2000* which called for a phased rebuilding programme and suggested that there would still be a requirement for about 750 inpatient places on the site by the end of the century. It was clear that there was a backlog of maintenance of the building and that this would remain for many years, but a ward improvement and upgrading programme should be embarked upon; a particular requirement was for the placement of elderly patients on the ground floor. Other things being looked at were the creation of new specialised units for adolescents, mothers and toddlers (especially for one-parent families) and alcoholics. In 1982, as part of the NHS restructuring, Friern became part of the newly created North Camden District Health Authority as part of North East Thames Regional Health Authority. Although there would be no change in the catchment area or its general role, greater operational and financial control would be given to local management.

Whilst changes were being considered at Friern, the national picture was one of a speeding up of closures of the large county lunatic asylums and the fate of Friern was already being decided. Around this time the annual cost of running Friern amounted to some £13,000,000, about 20% of the Health Authority's budget, although it was providing 950 beds and there were approximately 4000 out patient attendances and 20,000 day hospital patients were being seen.

When it was announced in 1983 that Friern would be closed within the next ten years, the problem of long stay patients was one that concerned many of the doctors and nursing staff. Dr Stephanie Westfield highlighted the problem[1]:

> "Amongst the patients on the two rehabilitation wards where I work, probably half consider Friern their home, and view with dismay suggestions that they go out again into the community accommodation. These people should not be considered simply institutionalised; many of them are tormented daily by frightening auditory hallucinations, or hold so firmly to, and act on, delusional beliefs, that it is impossible for them to cope without high levels of support. Friern used to house 3000 people, now 800: those people who can survive with the present type of community facilities have long departed. Many people with chronic disability are now ageing, but a significant number of disabled young people will continue to need specialised care.
>
> So where is the master plan that will emerge and make more supportive present community services? Where are the hostels, the community nurses, the industrial workshops, the day centres? Where is there special note taken of the itinerant, often homeless population, the hospital services, containing as it does in its catchment area three major mainline stations (Euston, King's Cross, St Pancras)?
>
> There is no plan. There is inadequate money to fund any reasonable plan."

It was not just doctors who opposed the closure of Friern; the trade unions were vocal in their criticism and when Margaret Thatcher visited the hospital in April 1985 trade union representatives refused to attend a briefing session.

Vernon Muller, the chaplain of the hospital was also against the closure:

> "I think my main opposition to the closure of Friern was twofold. One, there were a number of patients in Friern who needed asylum, and turfing these patients out

into the community without almost 24 hour support was madness, so when patients started to be moved out I went to visit them and I saw flats with brand new furniture and within weeks they were an absolute tip, because the patients weren't able to care for themselves. The other side, in Friern there was excellent work going on which a lot of people never saw. "

With the announcement that the hospital would be closing, problems arose with the recruitment of new staff and, more importantly, the retention of existing staff. In 1986 the Hampstead Health Authority employed the services of a Public Relations company to try and prevent nurses leaving Friern and 'agony aunt' Claire Rayner was hired to chair a meeting for nursing staff.[2]

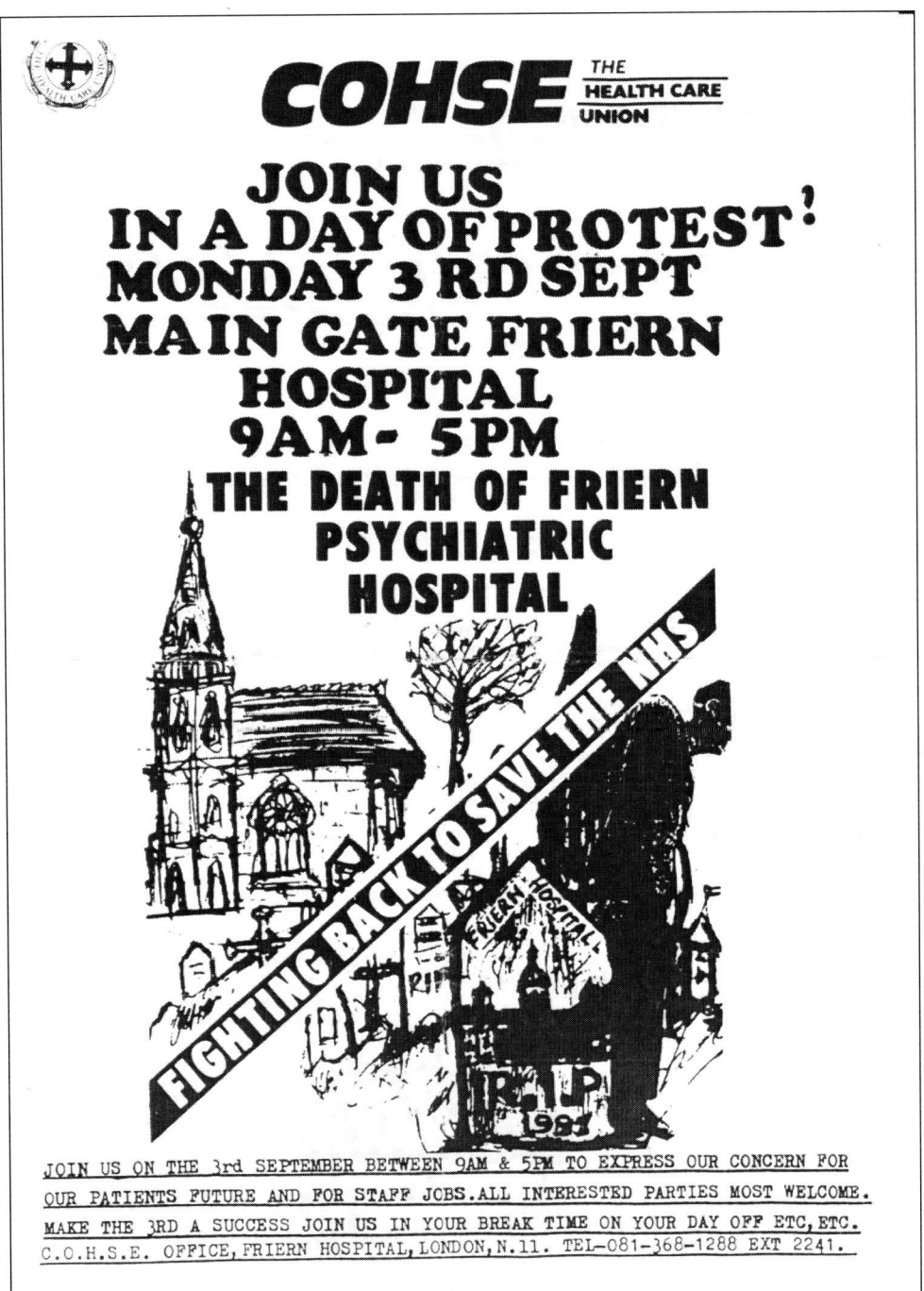

Needless to say, the trade unions were against any loss of jobs.
(FB&DLHS Archive)

The inevitable happened, however, and a Service of Thanksgiving was held at 4.40pm in the Main Hall of the hospital on Wednesday 17 February 1993 with the officiating guests being The Right Reverend J Klyberg, Church of England Bishop of Fulham; The Right Reverend Vincent Nicholas, Roman Catholic Bishop in North London; Rabbi Alan Plancey, of the United Synagogue in London and The Reverend David Staple, General Secretary of the Free Church Federal Council. The history of the hospital was covered by three presentations at the service. Dr Patrick Campbell, former Chairman of Friern Hospital Medical Committee, covered the period up to the Second World war; Mrs Zeba Ariff, Staff Nurse on Ward 36, covered the period from the Second World War to 1993 and Ms Clare Murdoch, Assistant General Manager, Mental Health Services, Bloomsbury and Islington Health Authority, outlined the future hope and provision for those who had previously been admitted to Friern.

In March 1993 the North East Thames Regional Health Authority produced a booklet in conjunction with the WVRS, the League of Jewish Friends, Friends of Friern and Friern Radio. *142 Years of Caring* was clearly meant to prepare people for the eventual closure and to reassure patients that things would only be better with treatment in the community as some of the quotations in the book show:

> "I think a lot of patients have been happy to be here. But a lot of patients I've spoken to recently have told me how happy they are to have moved back into the world"

> "There have been some very careful plans made to look after the patients when they go back into the outside world – some nice places, some beautiful homes"

> "Patients are cared for here in a very good way. They're given a lot of help"

The decommissioning of the hospital was a monumental task. An inventory of every item was made, ranging from a giant washing machine in the laundry down to a picture on a wall. Hampstead NHS Trust had first choice of equipment that could be useful to them

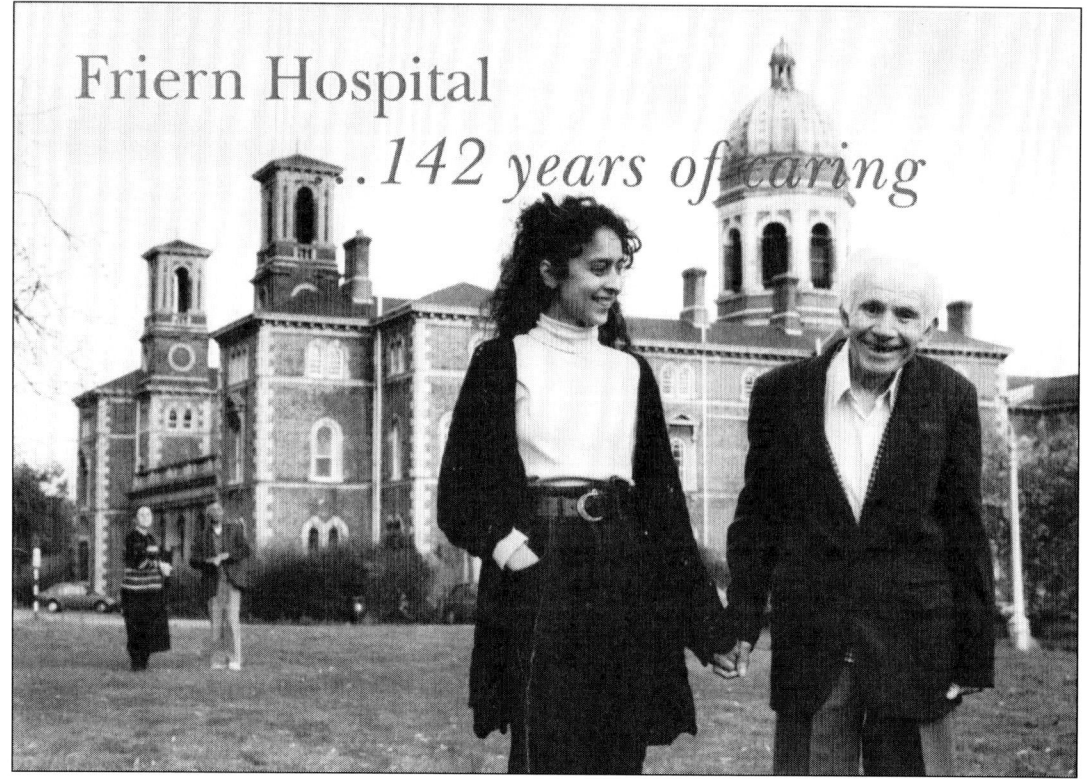

(FB&DLHS Archive)

elsewhere. The remaining items were sold at public auction and, for those still unsold, at private auctions. A deal even was struck with the Sudanese government for the sale of 400 beds and mattresses for £3720.[3] One unforeseen problem with the building was the presence of asbestos in various locations. This was eventually removed at a cost of £537,451.[4]

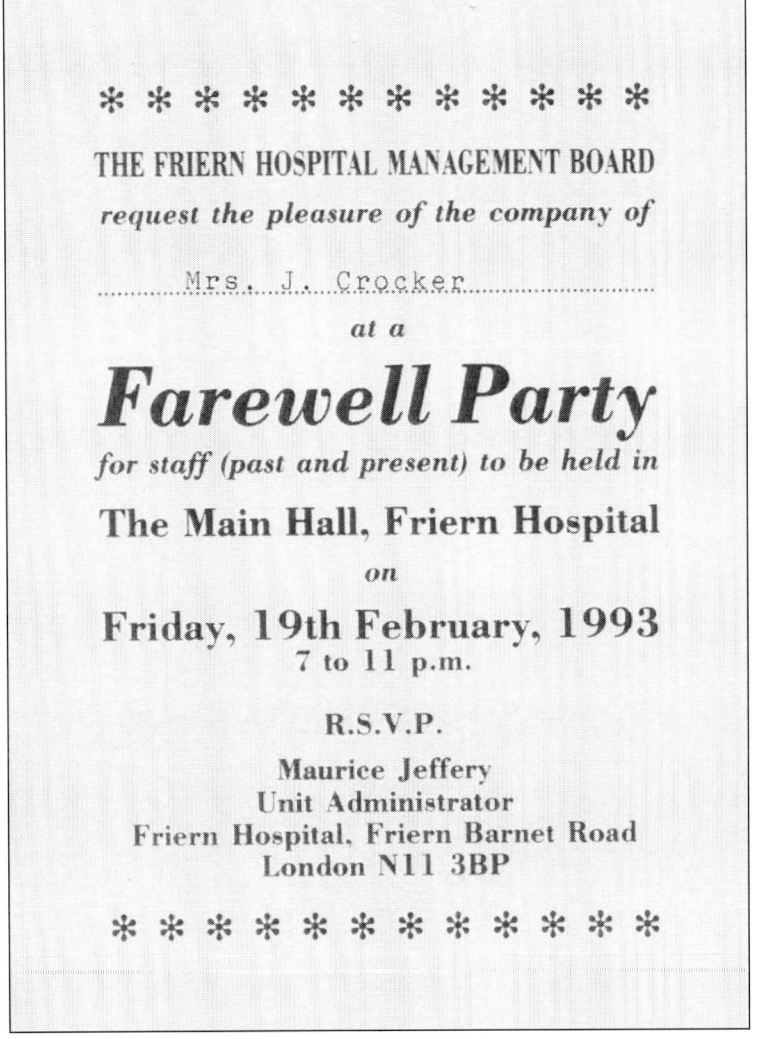

All good things come to an end.......
(Jean Crocker Collection)

Once the contents of the building were disposed of, services were cut off, except for water supplies to the fire hydrants and electricity to supply the fire alarms. A decommissioning team was on the site until July 1993, after which time only security personnel were present. To the rear of the building several wings had been empty for some time following the gradual running down of the hospital and these were demolished and the site was secured. Three buildings were, however, operational for some time after the closure – the Haringey Day Unit; the Regional Computer Centre and the Sterile Supplies Unit. The SSD Unit remained open until 1996 but lost the use of water from the well and had to get its supply from Lea Valley Water. Apparently the hospitals it supplied were not told in advance that it was closing, which caused some inconvenience as they had closed their own departments when the service was centralised at Friern.

The security personnel were briefed that any patients turning up after the closure were to be referred to the Haringey Day Unit where advice would be given. Those turning up after dark were to be referred to local general hospitals; in the case of difficult patients the police were to be called in to deal with them.

The cost of decommissioning was in the region of £990,000. A further £500,000 was earmarked for the reclamation of the land to the south of the site that had been used for tipping and waste disposal in the 1970s. This was necessary before the site could be sold for redevelopment as a retail park.[5]

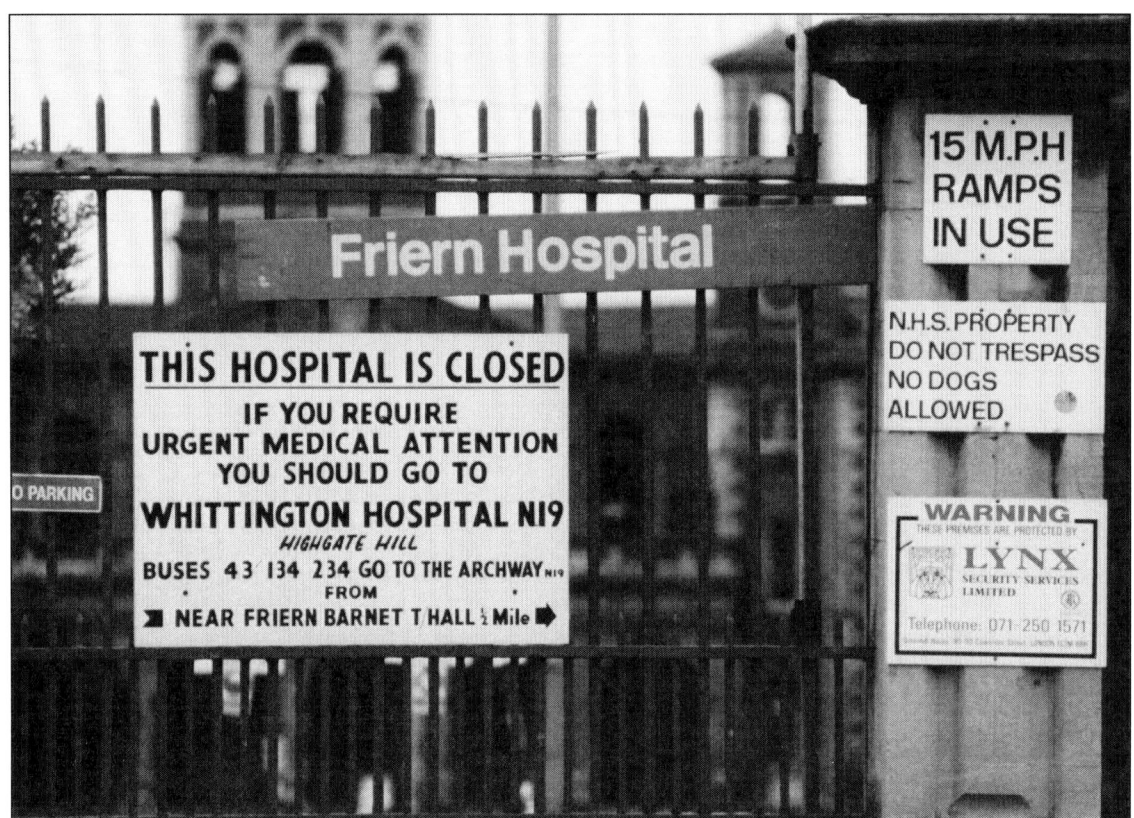

(John Donovan)

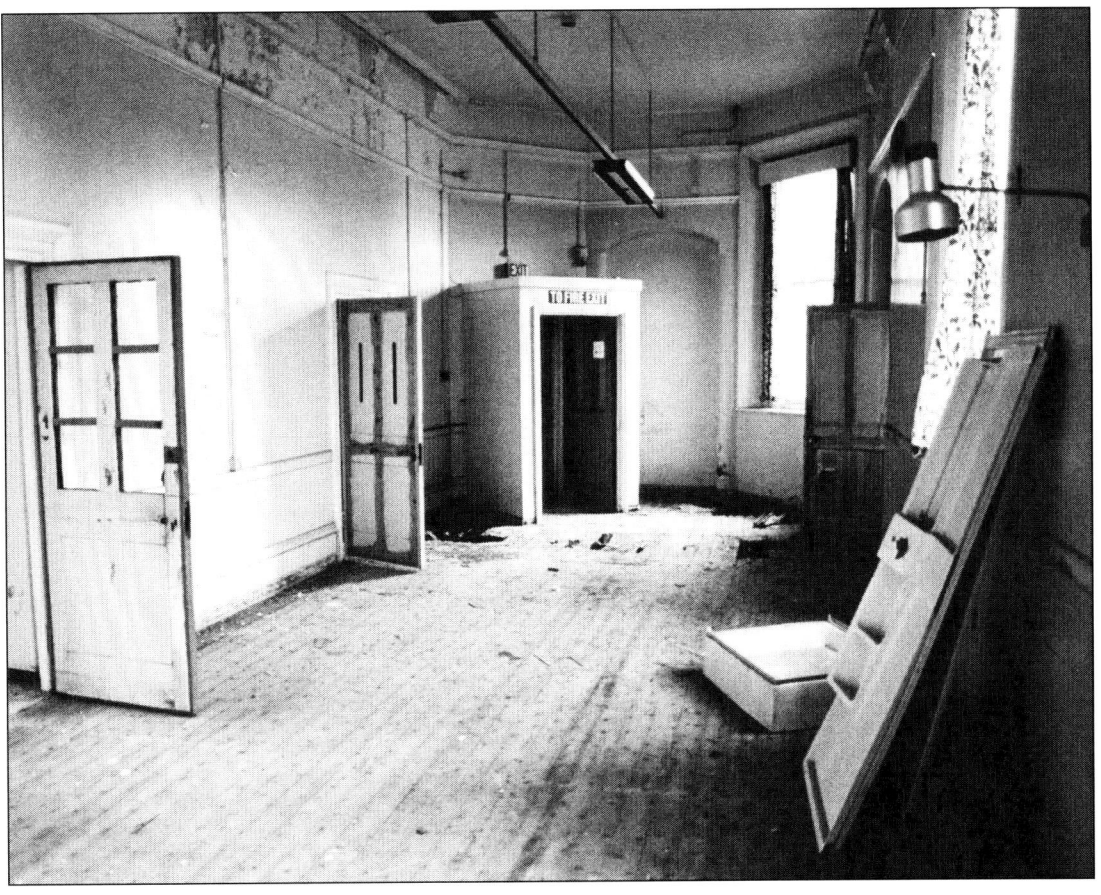

A sad end. (Mark Wickwar)

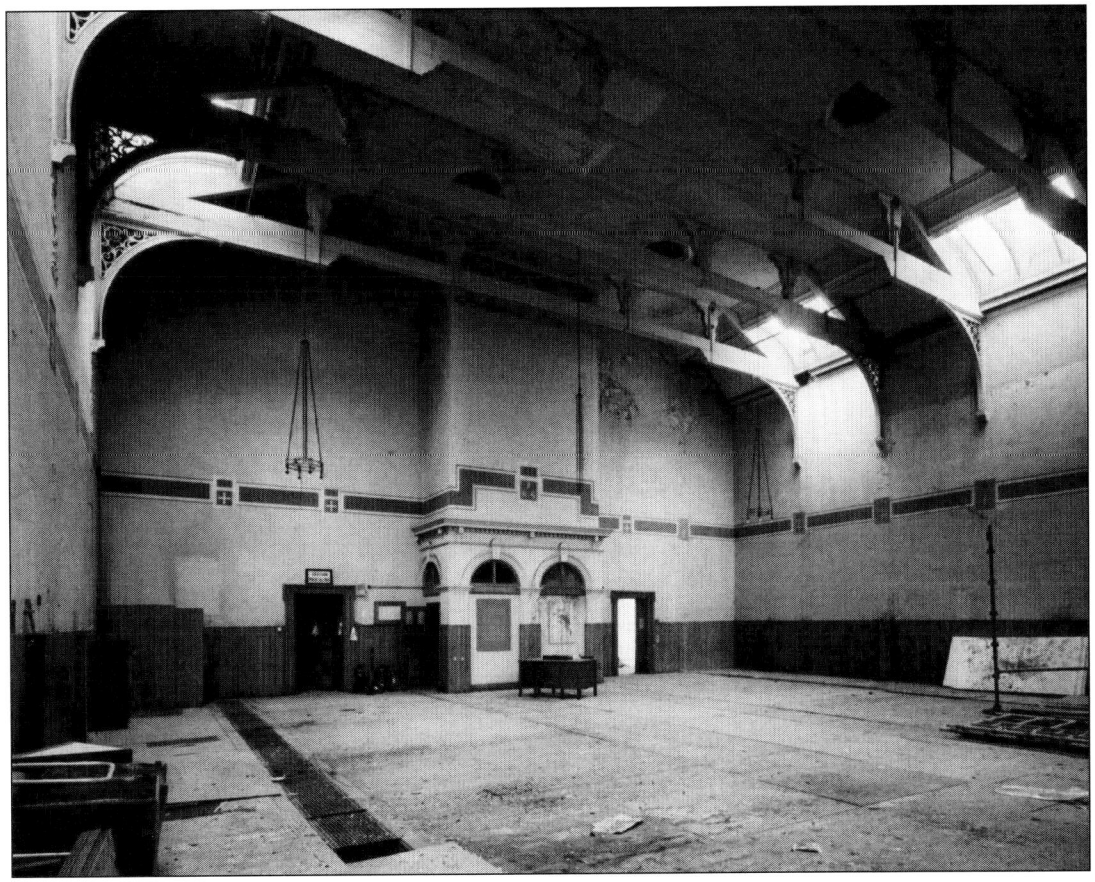

The main hall lies empty. (©Crown Copyright.EH)

CHAPTER TWENTY ONE

Development of the site

Parts of the Friern Hospital site had been sold off some years before the actual closure of the hospital. The extreme south western corner, where it abutted Colney Hatch Lane and the North Circular Road, was the first to be sold off for development. In 1982 an estate was created by Fairview Estates which consisted of a central road, Poplar Grove, off which ran Elm Way, Greenway Close, Hornbeams Rise, Laburnum Close, Larch Close, Silver Birch Close, and Sycamore Hill. Altogether there were 200 houses and 349 apartments and many of the properties were part of a shared housing scheme. For some years prior to this, this low lying site alongside Bounds Green Brook had been subject to flooding, although this problem seems to have been solved.

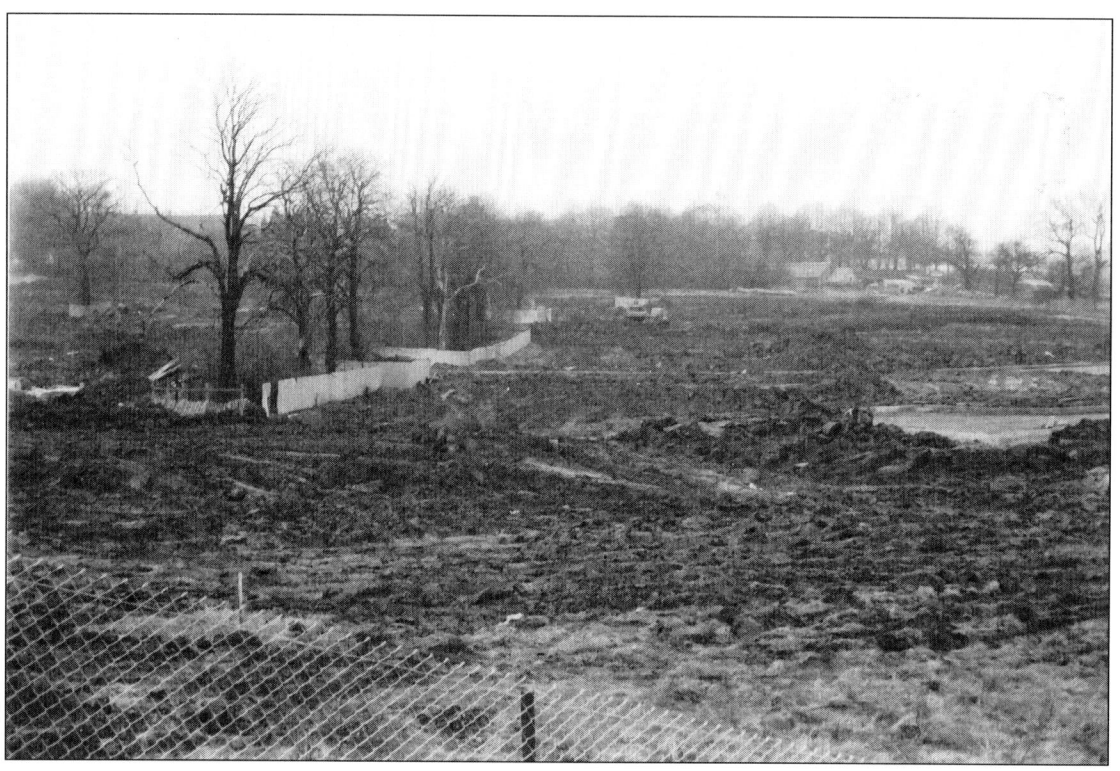

Work has just started on the building of Poplar Grove in this view from March 1982.
(John Donovan)

In 1986 a new road Firs Avenue, was built to the north of the Fairview Estate. The associated development comprised 170 houses. The road was notable for being sinuous and rather narrow, which was to cause problems later on as the number of vehicles increased and parked cars made access difficult, particularly for council refuse lorries.

In 1992 four acres to the rear of Halliwick Hospital were sold to Jewish Care, a charity caring for the aged which in 1997 opened a three storey home for the elderly and those suffering from dementia. The scheme cost £10.5 million and as well as 120 bedrooms it has a hydrotherapy pool, therapy rooms and its own synagogue. A new road, Asher Loftus Way, was built to link the home to Colney Hatch Lane.

In 1988 outline plans were submitted to Barnet Council for a retail park consisting of 13 retail units, a public park and space for the possible provision for a one form entry primary school for 210 children, which would have been up to Barnet Council to provide. The school was never built.

Objectors from over twenty local voluntary and conservation groups felt that the scheme was too large and would threaten the livelihood of local shops in North Finchley and Wood Green and would also lead to a large increase in traffic in local roads. The Secretary of State for the Environment, Nicholas Ridley, rejected calls for a public inquiry into the plans on the grounds that it was a local, not a national, issue and could therefore be dealt with by the local council. At a public inquiry in September 1988 Hampstead Health Authority said that the land near Pinkham Way was not the fine landscape that some had described it and would not suffer severe visual damage if a slip road with a roundabout at each end was constructed. It was "a wasted asset and a dump".[1]

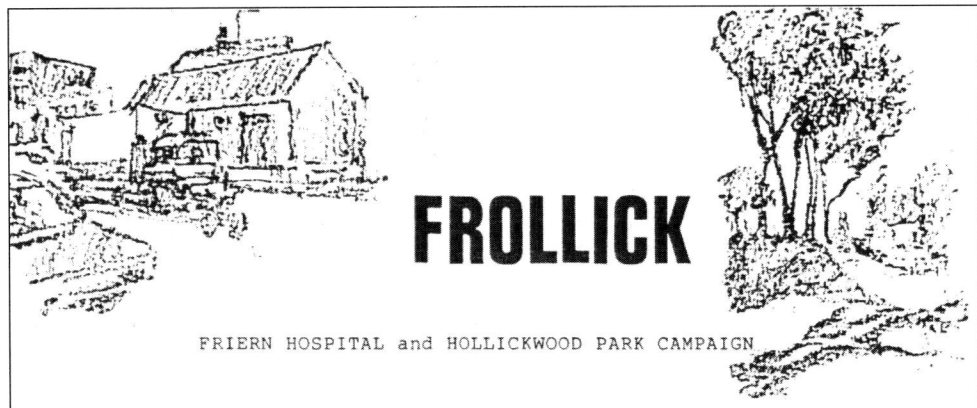

(FB&DLHS Archive)

The inspector found in favour of the development and the plan for the retail park was eventually scaled back to 10 retail units plus a McDonald's restaurant. The units were reconfigured into two sides of a rectangle which enclosed a car park. The developers argued that since the land that the main hospital building stood on was some 5 metres higher than the proposed retail park, there was no question of the latter dominating the site. Barnet Council approved the scheme by a narrow majority (nine votes for, 8 against) on 27 April 1994.

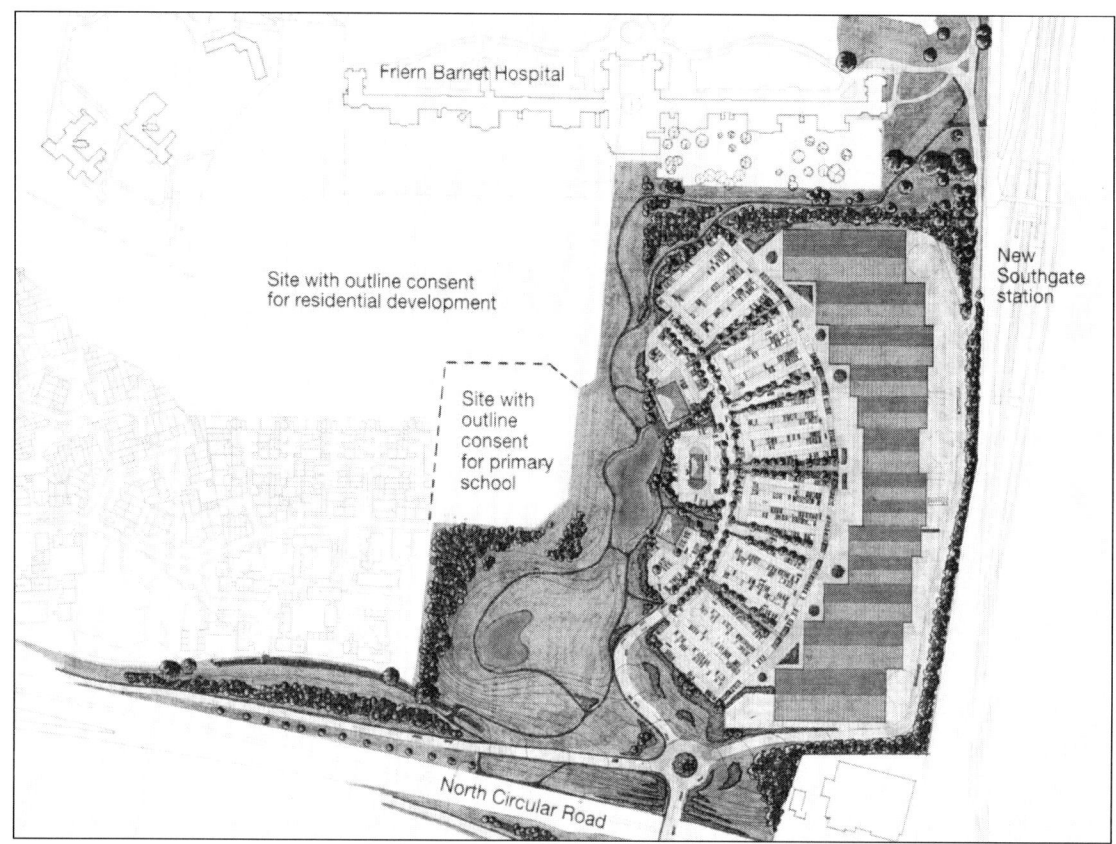

The initial plan was for thirteen retail units set out in a semi-circle.
(FB&DLHS Archive)

Agreement was reached between the Regional Health Authority and Haslemere Estates, a subsidiary of Rodamco, a Dutch investment group[2] for the sale of 31 acres for £4,000,000 A consortium of Try Construction Ltd and Tarmac Construction Ltd were responsible for the construction. Work started in July 1996 and the first task was to clear the land which was overgrown with low-value scrub, particularly bramble, goat willow and the invasive Japanese Knotweed. Access to the retail park was via a new slip road (Atlas Road) on the northern side of the A406 and egress was via a newly constructed bridge over the North Circular and thence via a slip road (Orion Road) to the south.

The work was completed in March 1998 and the first occupants moved in soon after. The retailers were Tempo electrical store, Carpet Right, Curry's electrical store, Allied Carpets, Furniture Village, Halfords, JJB Sports, Harveys Linens, Comet electrical and MFI furniture.

Because the retail park was specifically excluded from containing any food retailers such as supermarkets, the effects on local traders turned out to be negligible and the fears of huge volumes of traffic clogging up local roads also proved unfounded, manly because the access to the site was restricted to slip roads to and from the North Circular Road.

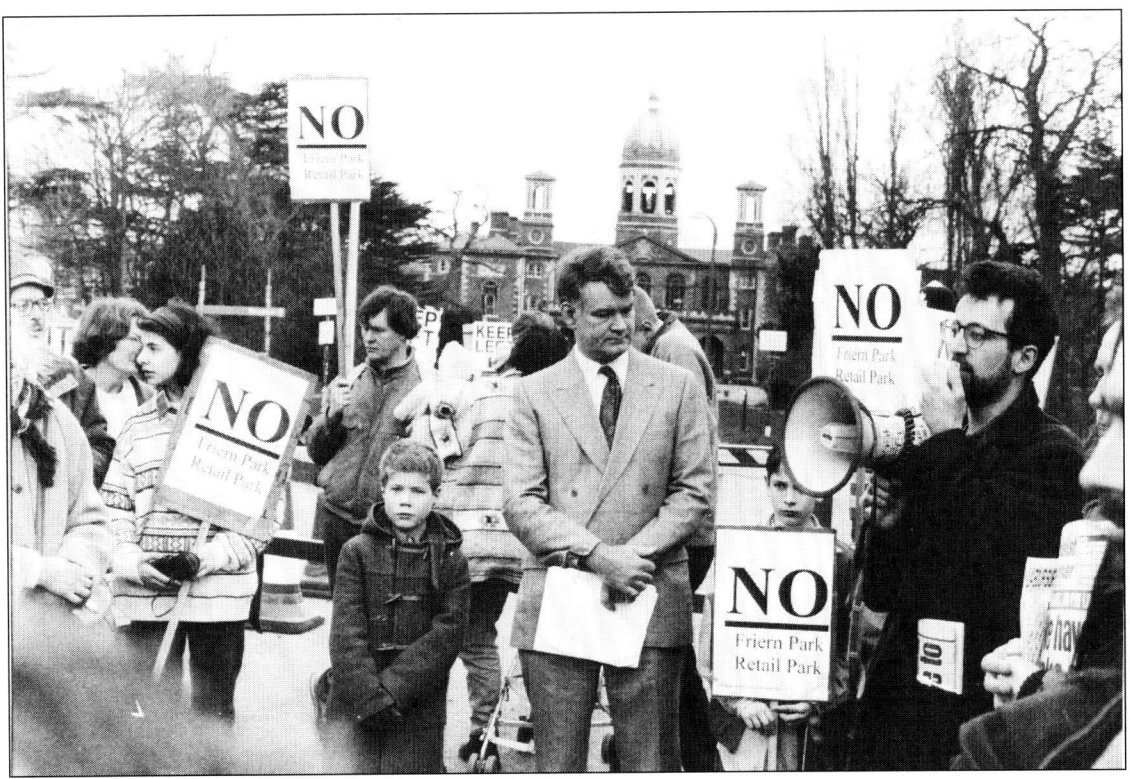

Objectors gather outside the gates of the Hospital. (John Donovan)

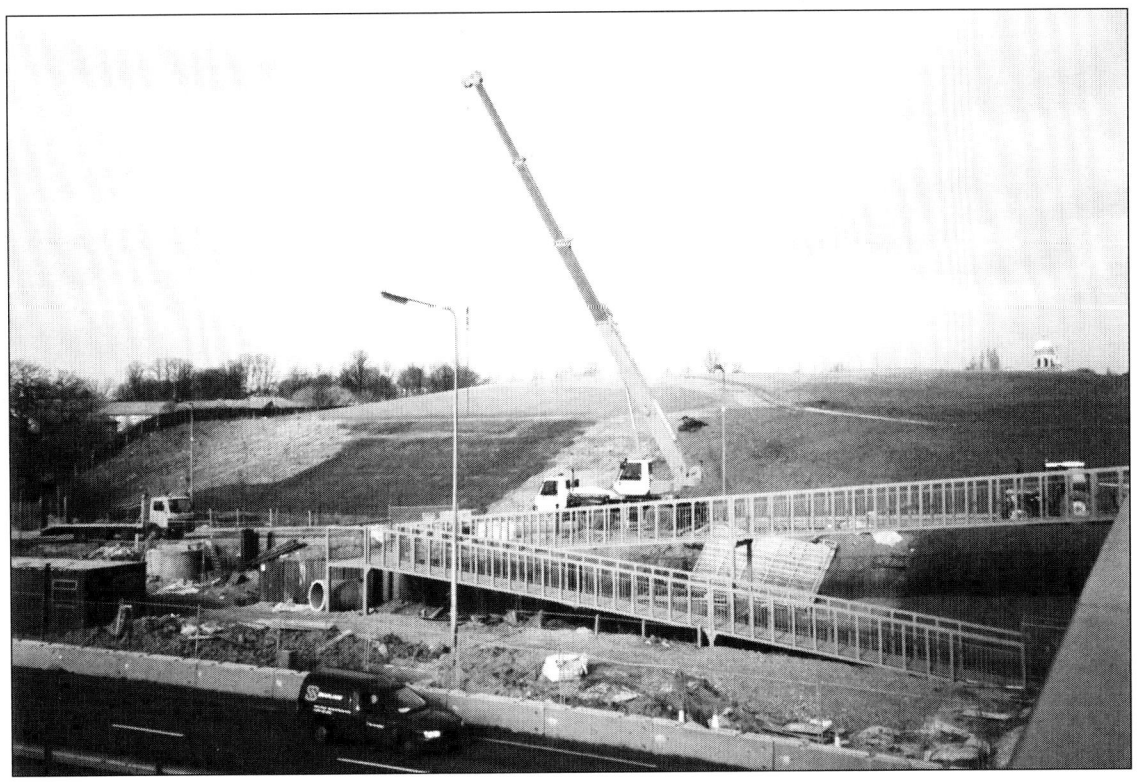

Landscaping work on the slip road to the North Circular nears completion
in February 1998. (John Donovan)

In 1997 a new access road, Regal Drive, was created at the eastern end of the site running parallel to the line path. Eight new roads were built off it, all with a royal connotation. Balmoral Avenue, Baron Close, Duchess Close, Earl Close, Hampton Close, Highgrove Close and Kensington Close were built by Try Construction and marketed by Bellway Homes under the name Princes Gate. The estate numbered 144 houses, with the largest road, Balmoral Avenue, having 36. A 2-bedroom house sold for £105,995, a 3-bedroom for £141,995 and a 4-bedroom for £178,950.

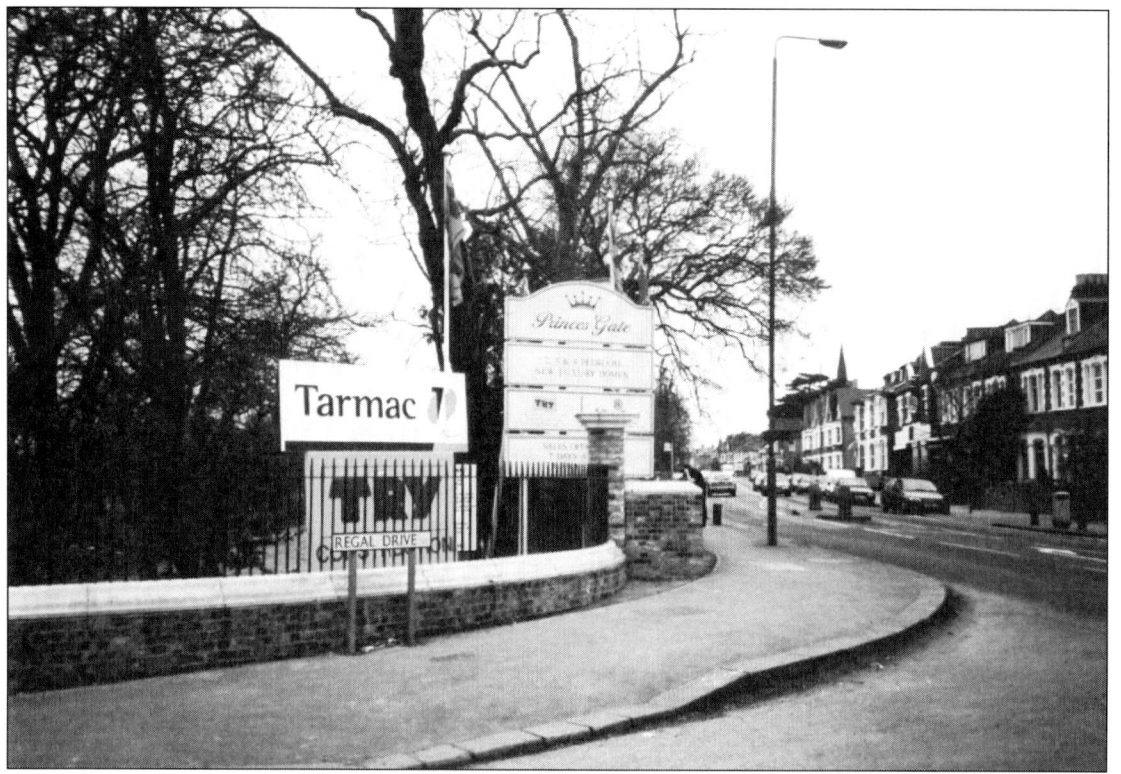

Princes Gate, off Friern Barnet Road, under development. (John Donovan)

At the other end of the site, north of Firs Avenue, on the western side and adjoining Colney Hatch Lane, the biggest development was being created. The name given by the developers, Bryant Homes, was Halliwick Park. The first show house opened in December 1998. The estate comprised fourteen new roads, all named after places in Yorkshire: Arncliffe Close, Catterick Close, Coverdale Close, Deepdale Close, Garsdale Close, Grassington Close, Pickering Gardens, Skipton Close, Wensleydale Close, Wharfedale Close and Winterburn Close all ran off the main road, Ribblesdale Avenue. Work started in 1999 and was completed in 2001. The development totalled 224 houses and 4 blocks of flats. The first phase of 32 houses included detached houses at prices ranging from £184,995 to £214,995

In 1972 land to the extreme west, fronting onto Colney Hatch Lane had been used to build a computer centre for North West Thames Regional Health Authority. This was demolished in 1998 and Halton Close, a development of 39 houses, was built on the site and completed in 1999.

On the north west of the site, where the former Hallwick Hospital had stood, five new roads were built - Martock Gardens, Cheddar Close, Shapwick Close and Radstock Close had 63 houses plus three blocks of flats (Harrogate Court, Wincanton Court and Battleton Court) and Sparkford Gardens had 28 houses and one block of flats (Yarlington Court).

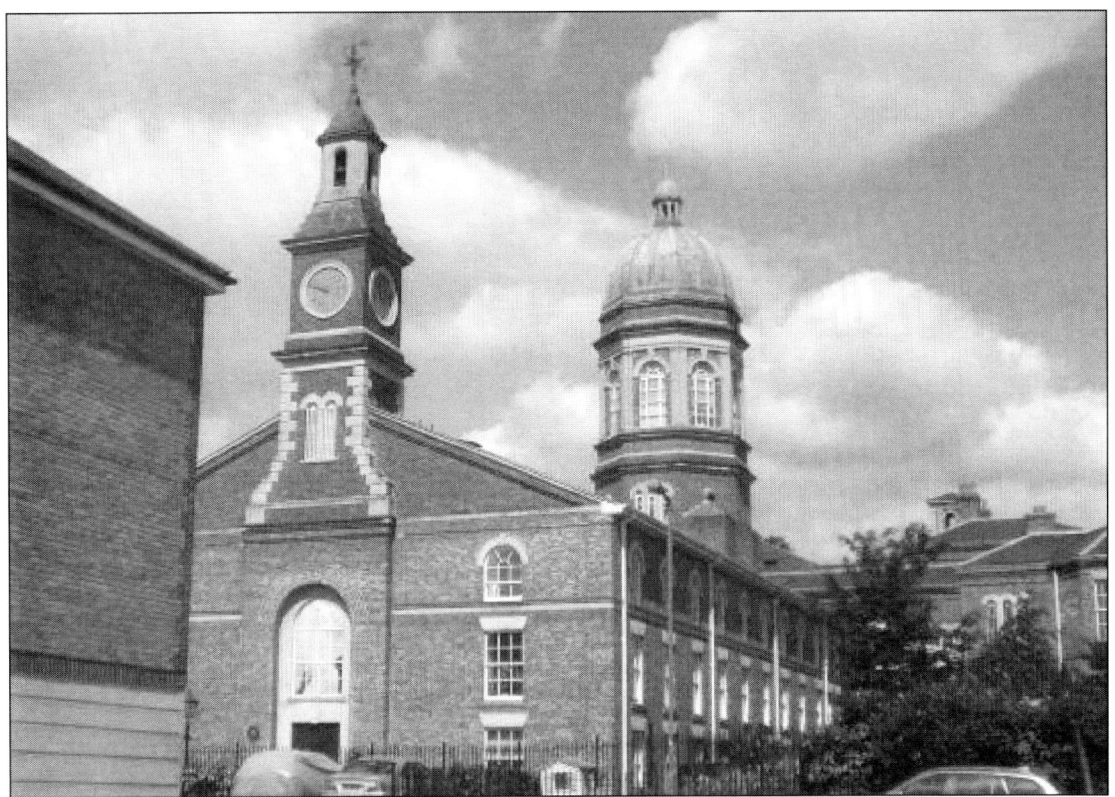

View northwards from Hampton Close (Author)

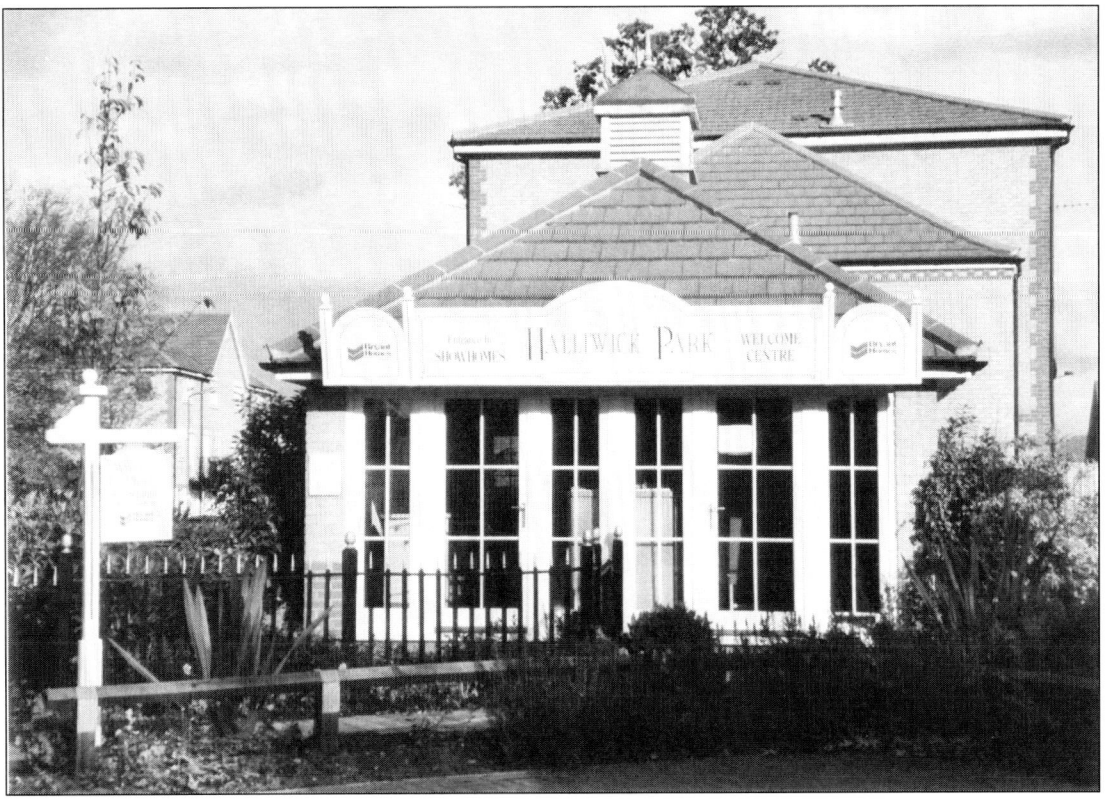

The Halliwick Park Sales Office. (Author)

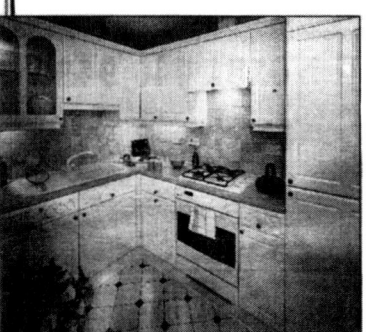
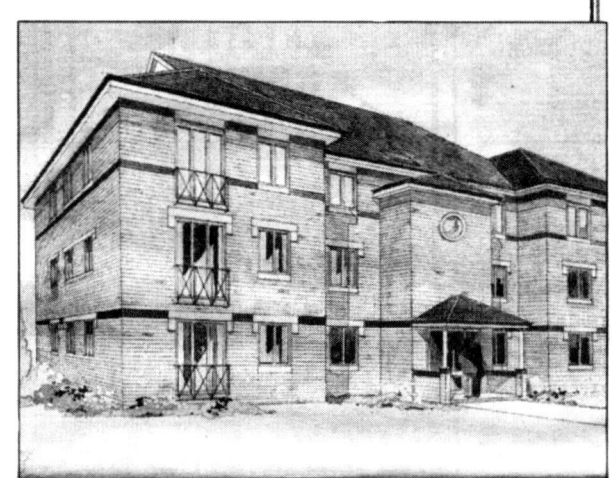
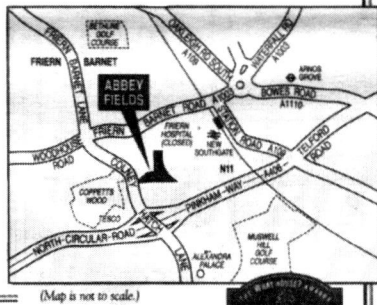

Abbey Fields, in Ribblesdale Avenue, was later renamed
Ripon Court and comprises 32 apartments.
(FB&DLHS Archive)

CHAPTER TWENTY TWO

Princess Park Manor

An application was made in 1986 to demolish Friern Hospital[1] but, not surprisingly, this was turned down since it had been granted a Grade II listing in September 1982.

Since its closure in 1993, the building had been allowed to deteriorate, resulting in a scene of complete desolation. An article in a local newspaper[2] described the scene:

> "Nature and neglect have taken the greatest toll on the floorboards. Dry rot has turned a great expanse of floor to powder and gaping holes leave beams exposed. The cornices trimming the high ceilings are dotted with colourful fungi and the most spectacular cobwebs I have ever seen. The longest corridor in Europe is strewn with rubble and the back of the building, where hospital wings have been demolished, looks as if a small Spanish town has been razed to the ground."

In October 1995 the hospital buildings and the remaining land were bought by Brookstream Corporation, a subsidiary of Finchley based Opec Prime Properties Ltd, whose owner was Luke Comer. The exact purchase price was not disclosed, but it had been described in the press as 'a nominal sum'.[3] In 1994 Debenham Thorpe Zadelhoff had advised the Royal Free Hospital to expect around £14,000,000 for the sale of land for residential use[4]. Surprisingly, the North West Thames Regional Health Authority claimed that they had not received many offers to buy the site. Several plans for the redevelopment of the Friern Hospital site were submitted to Barnet Council and there then followed lengthy discussions involving Barnet Council, English Heritage and local residents. English Heritage's main concern was, of course, that the hospital building should not be dramatically altered externally but they withdrew their opposition to the scheme and in June 1996 Barnet Council granted planning permission for the scheme so the green light was given for work to start in July 1996.

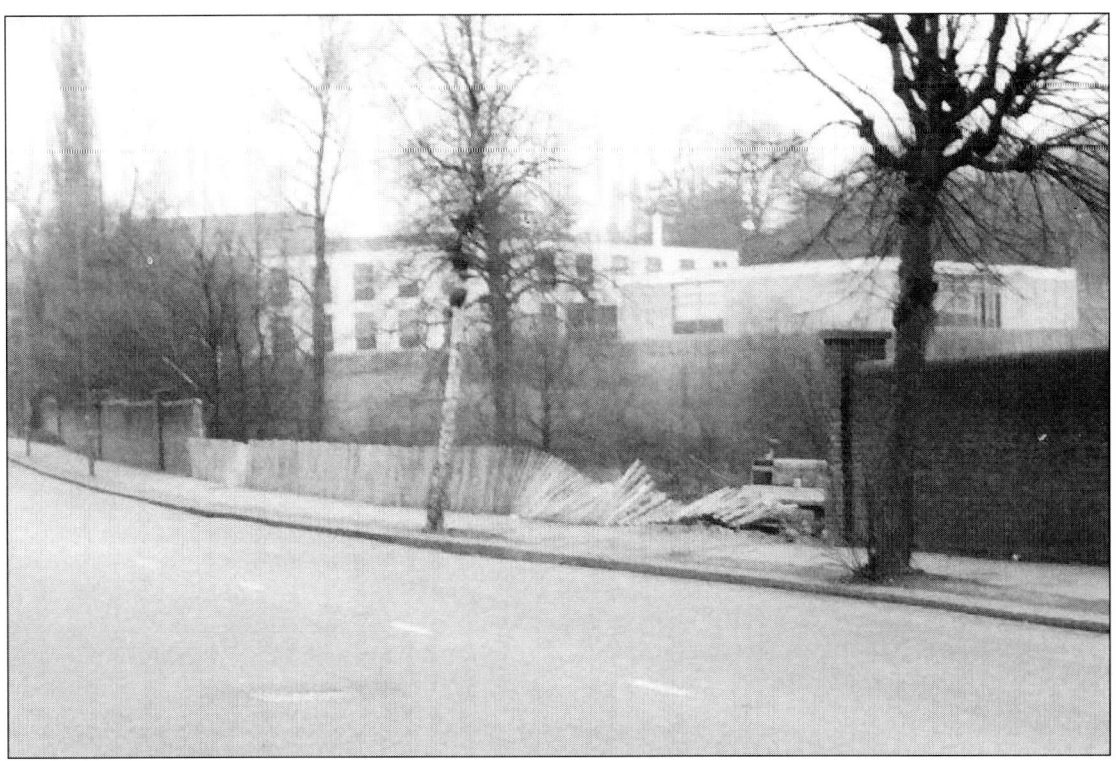

The computer centre photographed in 1982. (John Donovan)

The architect for the project was Peter Smith who had been responsible for the successful restoration of Alexandra Palace, another large Victorian building in North London, and his design called for the demolition of some of the wings to the rear of the building. Although these were listed, English Heritage did not object as the bulk of the building was being retained and renovated and any new parts had to be built in the same style as the original. Most of the interior of the hospital was gutted and two floors were replaced by three which, since the old ceilings were high, meant that in some apartments the new ceiling heights did not match up with the windows. It was hoped that, wherever possible, features such as original windows, door openings, chimney breasts and decorative plasterwork could be retained, however it was not possible, or even desirable, to retain the long corridor to the north of the building and this was divided up into various rooms and incorporated into apartments. Prospective buyers who were in at the early stages, when the building was still a shell, had the opportunity to get involved with the planning of their new apartments.

Altogether there were over 70 different types of apartments, ranging from one-bedroom flats at £169,000 to a 3-bedroom, 2-bathroom penthouse within the dome at £1,000,000. Service charges ranged from £895 to £1100.

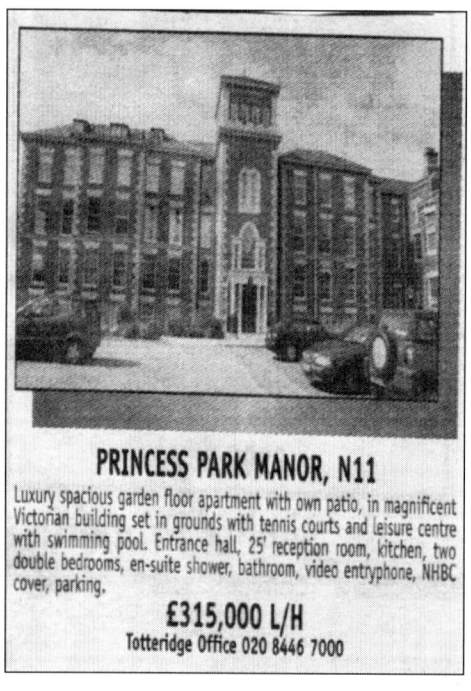

May 2002

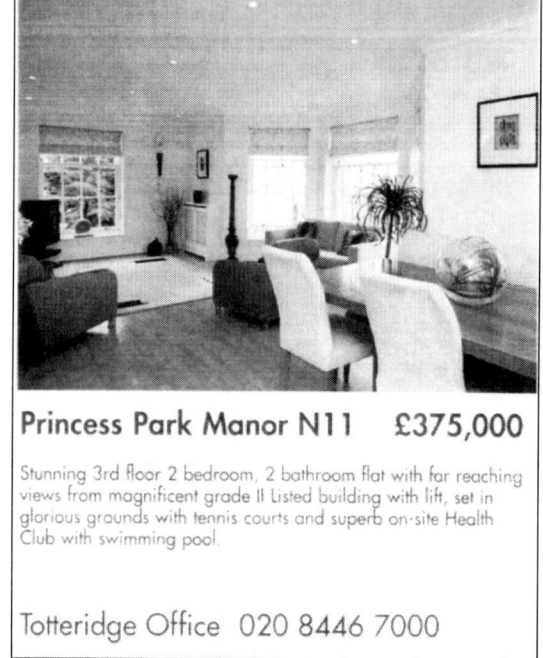

July 2004

The conversion of the building was done in five phases and in order to raise the revenue necessary for the completion of the scheme, as each phase was completed it was immediately put on the market; thus purchasers of apartments in Phase One lived in what was a building site for some time until the last phase was completed in 2009. All 366 apartments had leases running for 125 years from 25 March 1998 and the lease for the first apartment to be sold (number 192) was signed on 20 October 1998[4].

Part of the conversion included the replacement of the former chapel by a sporting club with its own 20 metre swimming pool, a bar and restaurant, solariums, dance and aerobic studios and outdoor tennis courts, the complex being run by Esporta. Phase six of the development consisted of brand new buildings attached to the existing eastern wing. The original planning application in January 2004 was for 64 flats, but when finished, the size had been increased to 83 and unauthorised alterations had been made to the building. In June 2009 Barnet Council served the group with enforcement notices which it appealed against. A public inquiry into the case was held over several days in May and June but, during adjournments, the council and the developer came to a mutual agreement. The planning inspector granted permission for 82 of the flats – one has been deemed not fit for residential purposes – subject to the group making some alterations to keep it in line with the building's Grade II listing. In addition, the firm was instructed to

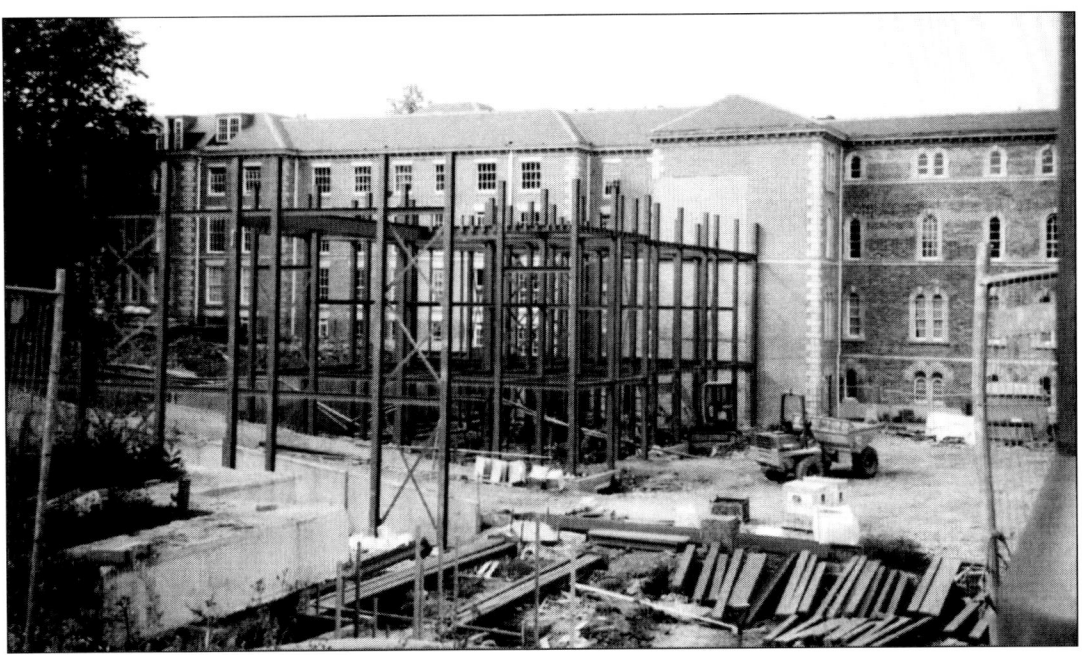

In August 2004 the steelwork goes up for the new extension on the eastern end. (Author)

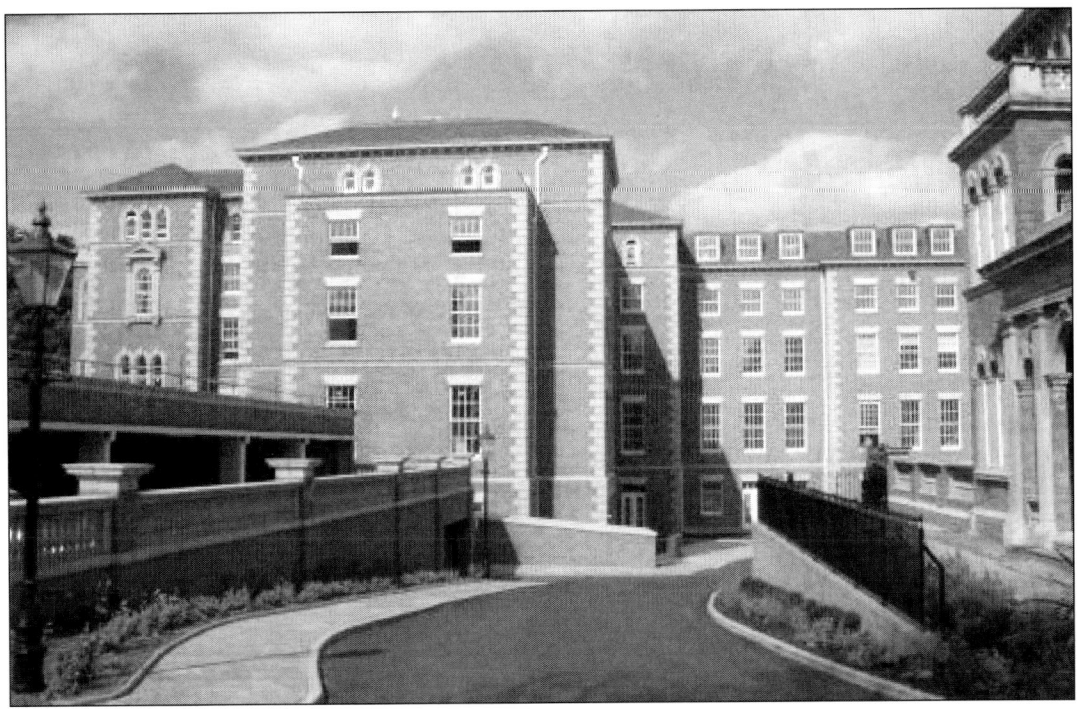

The newly built extension to the east wing in the same style as
the main building, but with four floors (Author)

pay the council's legal costs. The group were also told to make contributions to the council, of which £3.4 million would go towards the building of affordable homes in the area and almost £250,000 towards education provisions.

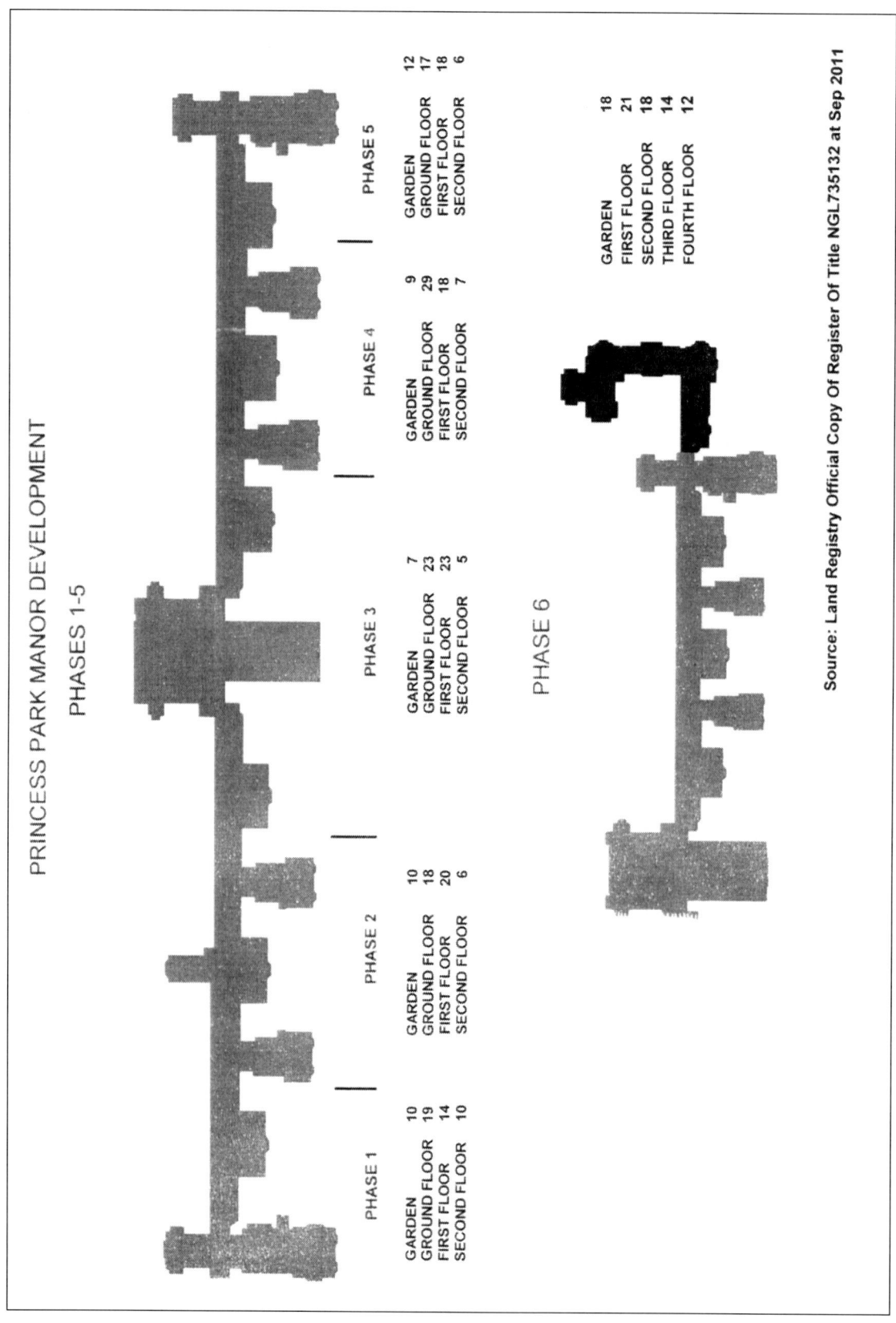

The refurbishment was done in phases. A comparison with the plan on page 111 will show how much of the original building was demolished in the refurbishment.

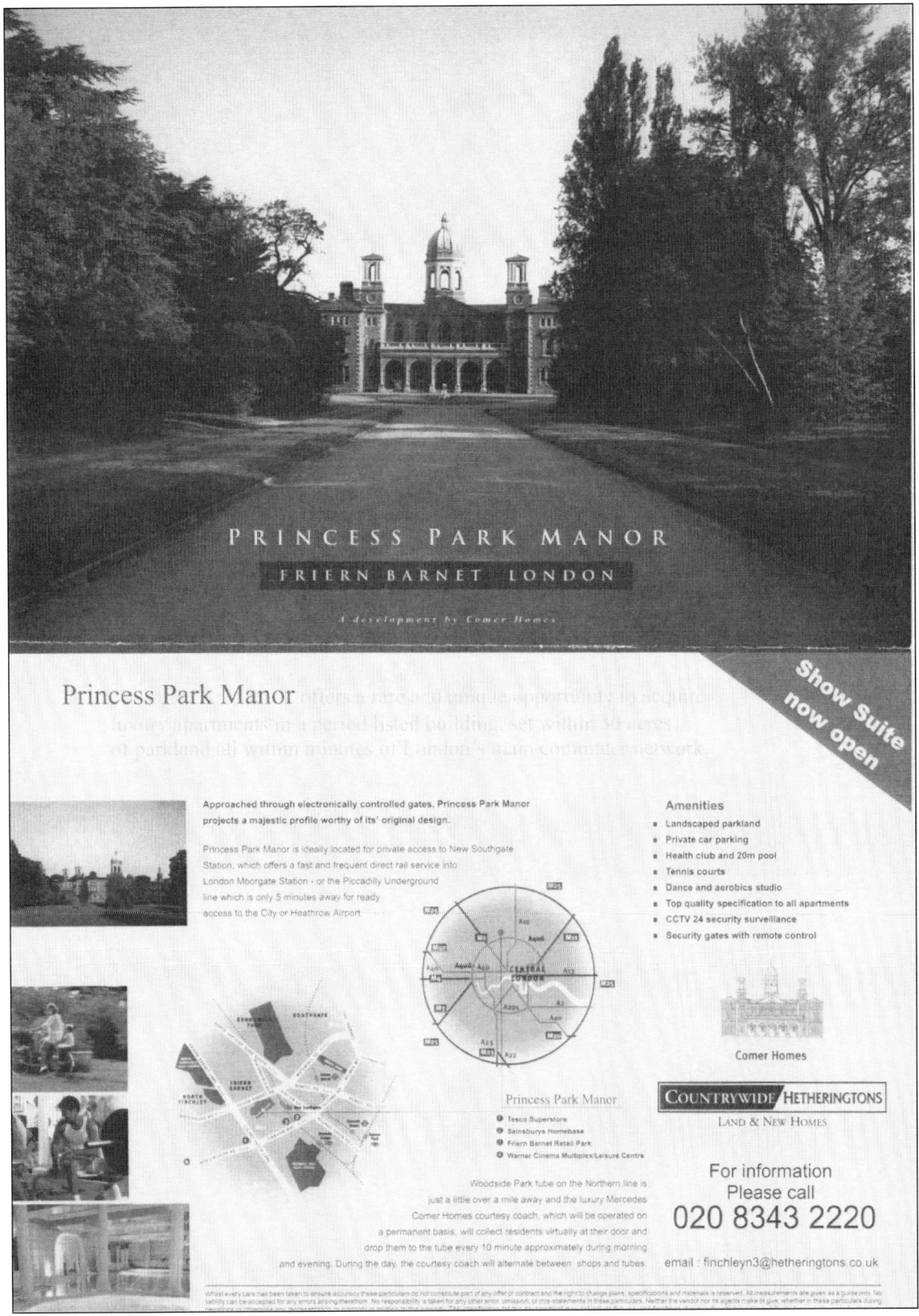

(FB&DLHS Archive)

Barnet's cabinet member for housing, Richard Cornelius said[5]:

> "This was a difficult and unprecedented case, involving a huge amount of hard work by the council, which will see a significant benefit to the community. I am delighted we stood firm and have finally reached a resolution which benefits the

Borough and the flat owners themselves who were in a difficult position living in properties without planning permission." Luke Comer from Comer Homes Group told *The Press* the issue had occurred after an "oversight" by the group's architects. He said: "We decided smaller flats would be better to sell and submitted planning permission, which was never dealt with properly. We tried to put the mistake right as soon as we knew about it. We advised residents not to sell at this time, but if they had to, we would buy the flat and cover their costs – but nobody did sell."

Another bone of contention was the status of the area of parkland to the north west of the site. One of the terms of the granting of the original planning application was that this area would be open to the public as a park, although this may not have been communicated to the purchasers of apartments in the renovated building; consequently there was opposition by them to the scheme. Amongst the objections was that the park had been opened prematurely and without consultation with the residents; that the grounds belonged to the estate and were not for the use of the public and that the park had been opened even though part of the site was still undergoing building work.

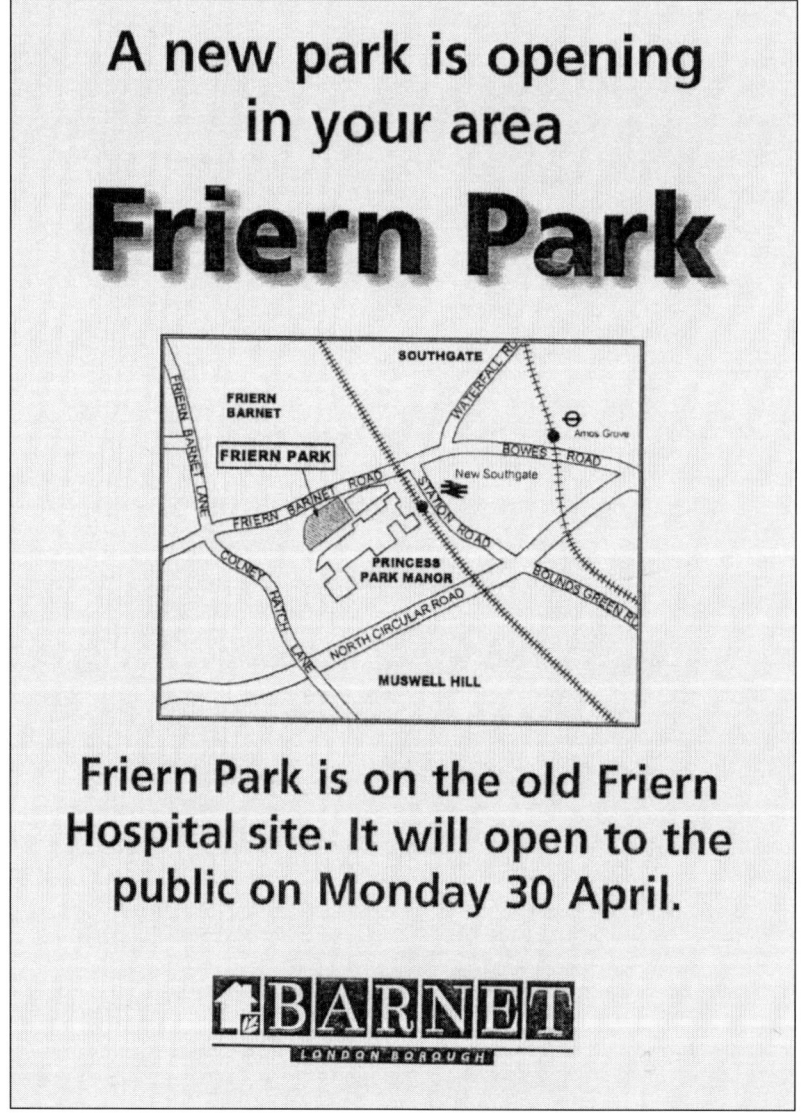

The leaflet was distributed in 2011
(FB&DLHS Archive)

PRINCESS PARK MANOR

improving quality of life

Barnet Council

Welcome to Friern Park

Set in the grounds of the former Friern Hospital, Friern Park offers extensive grassland and mature parkland trees. The character of the open space is dominated by the former hospital which has been extensively refurbished to provide luxury accommodation.

The open space is laid out in two distinct and separate areas. The landscaped open space will be maintained by Barnet Council, in keeping with its function as the setting of a listed frontage. The style of park furniture such as seats, litter bins and dog waste disposal bins have been approved by English Heritage. Furniture will be installed in early June.

Access to Friern Park
- The park can be entered through the pedestrian gates on the Friern Barnet Road entrance.
- The park is open to the public daily dawn till dusk.
- The areas shown with the solid line on the plan are available to the public. The remaining shaded areas including the perimeter access road are private property. Visitors to Friern Park are not permitted access to the private areas.
- Users of the open space are not permitted to bring vehicles beyond the main entrance gate.

Facilities at Friern Park
- Due to the character of Friern Park, it is ideally suited for passive recreation such as walking, sitting, sunbathing and dog walking.
- There is no play area or organised sport facilities within the park. The nearest children's play area to this site is Friary Park, Friern Barnet Lane.

Use of Friern Park
- When in the park please be considerate of other users and local residents.
- Please take your litter home.
- Please keep dogs under control and clear up if they foul in the park. Failure to clean up after your dog can result in an instant fine of £25. Council officers patrol this park.
- Organised team ball games are not permitted in the park.
- Due to construction works that are taking place at the eastern end of the former hospital building, the open space which fronts the building will not be available to the public until the construction work is complete. It is anticipated that this addition to Friern Park will be accessible to the public around December 2002.

We hope you enjoy your visits to Friern Park

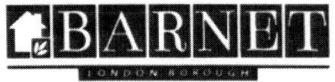

(FB&DLHS Archive)

After the new park had opened, Barnet Council asked for suggested names for it and among those offered by Friern Village Residents' Association, Princess Park Manor Residents' Association and Holly Park School were Asylum Park; Colney Hatch Park;

Curtis Park; Friern Village Gardens; Friern Village Park; Hawkins Park; Holly Bush Park; Holly Green; Prince Albert Park; Princess Gardens; Princess Park Gardens and Sparrows Acres. Surprisingly, the long established local organisations that were aware of the historical significance of the area (Arnos West Community Association; The Finchley Society; Friern Barnet & Whetstone Residents' Association and the Whetstone Society) were not consulted.

The eventual choice of the name "Friern Park" was confusing since there is a street nearby called Friern Park, and Friary Park was just up the road in Friern Barnet Lane and had been there since 1910. Some time later "Friern Park" was amended to "Friern Village Park" and a signboard carrying this name was erected outside the railings. The name "Friern Village" has no historical significance but was concocted by estate agents anxious to brand the estate of new houses in and around Ribblesdale Avenue.

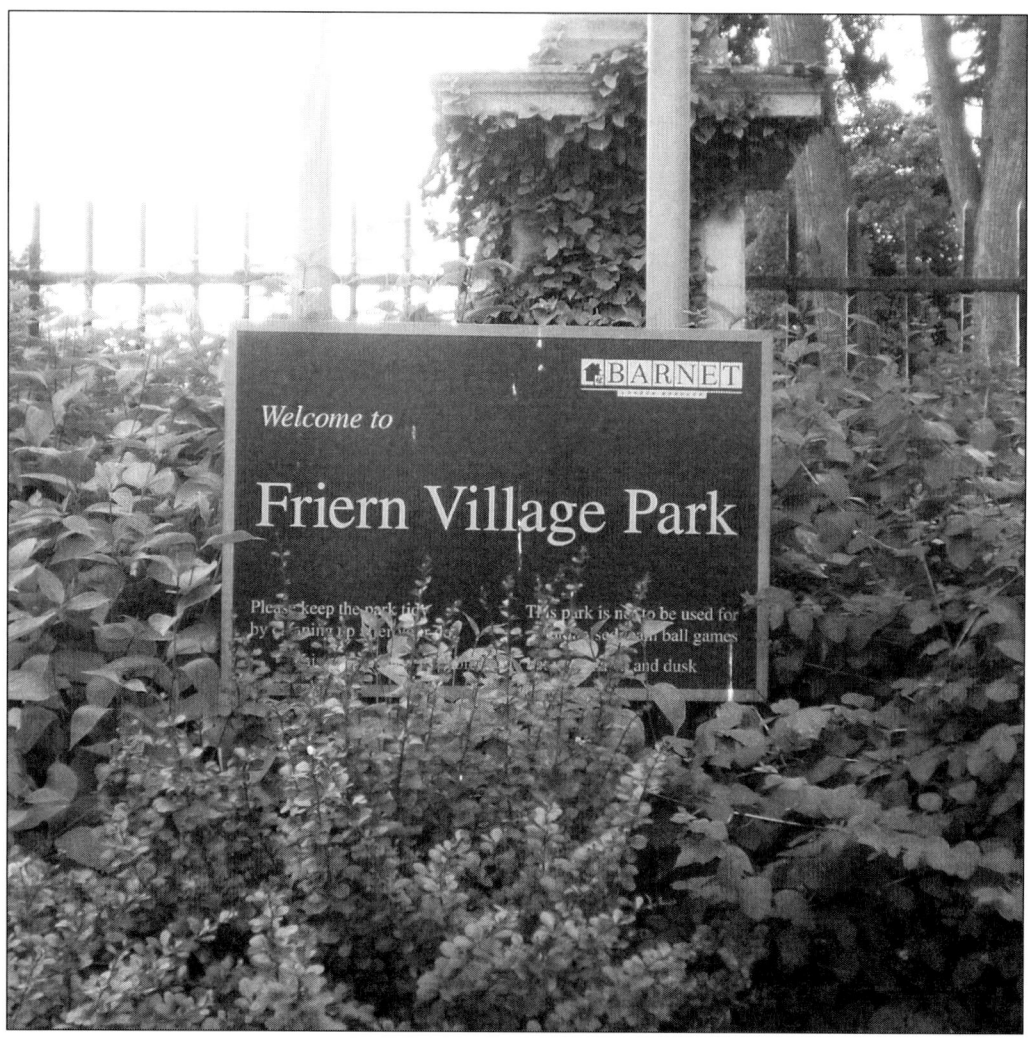

The sign alongside the entrance in Friern Barnet Road.
(Author)

CHAPTER TWENTY THREE

See You in Court

The administrators of hospitals do not usually end up in the courtroom, however Friern was involved in two court cases, one where it was the plaintiff, the other the defendant.

In November 1855 it was decided that the asylum was in need of enlargement and a plan was prepared by the Asylum Steward for extra accommodation for 593 patients at an estimated cost of some £39,000. It would have seemed natural for Daukes to have been chosen for this work, but the work was given to a James Harris. In February 1856 the Clerk of Works reported to the Committee that he had discovered some cracking in the plaster of the inner walls and one ward in particular was in a very dangerous state. Daukes was asked to comment on this and after inspection he assured the Committee that there as no danger to the patients and that he would repair the damage at his own expense.

In the meantime, another architect, Andrew Timen, had visited the asylum and had also noted cracks in the building which he reported to the Committee. The Committee were clearly alarmed at this and they contacted Lewis Cubitt, the designer of the iconic King's Cross Station, and asked him to prepare a report which he did in September 1856. He recommended that the foundations be underpinned, that the roof should be redone, that ceiling arches be removed and that the fireproofing of the ceiling should be discontinued. Cubitt estimated that the improvements would cost in the region of £40,000. Daukes offered to meet Cubitt to discuss the situation but Cubitt declined.

In January 1857 Cubitt was appointed to carry out the necessary work which cost £67,000. The drama continued when Daukes visited the asylum in July 1867 with two other architects and was of the opinion that the work taking place was unnecessary as the defects were not of a structural nature.

The sorry affair continued and ended with Daukes being prosecuted by the Committee for breach of duty in not constructing the asylum in accordance with his specifications but, after three days of the trial, and before several architects were due to give their opinions in favour of Daukes, the case was withdrawn. The judge was of the opinion that Daukes had been victimised by other architects who had influenced the Middlesex magistrates into bringing the case.

The second case occurred almost exactly one hundred years later, in 1957, and was to become a classic example of tort law. On 23 August 1954, a voluntary patient at Friern, a John Bolam, who was a manic-depressive, agreed to undergo electro-convulsive therapy (ECT) at the hospital. In some cases ECT involves the use of relaxant drugs, to minimise the harm to patients when they involuntarily thrash about when the electric shock is given to their brain. However, in Mr Bolam's case he was not given a relaxant and furthermore he was not restrained while the treatment was going on. As a result, he suffered several severe injuries including fracture to his hip bone. He sued the Friern Hospital Management Committee and claimed compensation for negligence, claiming that the doctors had not issued relaxants, had not restrained him and had not warned him of the risks involved in the treatment. The case was heard in the High Court and several expert medical witnesses were called upon to give their opinion. Some used relaxants and restraints in the course of ECT while others did not. In his summing up the judge said:

> "In the realm of diagnosis and treatment there is ample scope for genuine difference of opinion and one man clearly is not negligent merely because his conclusion differs from that of another professional man, nor because he has

displayed less skill or knowledge than other would have shown. The true test of establishing negligence in diagnosis or treatment on the part of the doctor is whether he has proved to be guilty of such failure as no doctor of ordinary skill would be of if acting with ordinary care…..We should be doing a disservice to the community at large if we were to impose liability on hospitals or doctors for everything that happens to go wrong. Doctors would be led to think of their own safety than of the good of the patients. Initiative would be stifled and confidence shaken. A proper sense of proportion requires us to have regard to the conditions in hospitals and doctors have to work. We must insist on due care for the patient at every point, but we must not condemn as negligence that which is only a misadventure."

The jury found in favour of Friern Hospital and the Bolam case became an important part of English law when dealing with claims of professional negligence.

In 1997 the *Daily Telegraph* published an article criticising the standards of psychiatric care and treatment at Friern. Six years later, in July 1983, the paper agreed to pay what were described as "substantial damages" to 17 consultant psychiatrists at Friern for their libel. The paper admitted that they had made "what are now recognised to have been completely unfounded allegations". They went on to say "the allegations were wholly without justification, and are pleased to pay tribute to the high standards of skill and care which are provided at Friern Hospital".

CHAPTER TWENTY FOUR

Friern in the media

The name Colney Hatch became synonymous with mental illness in much the same way as Bethlem (or "Bedlam") had in earlier times. In 1890 there was even a comic song published entitled *Here's Another One Off to Colney Hatch*.

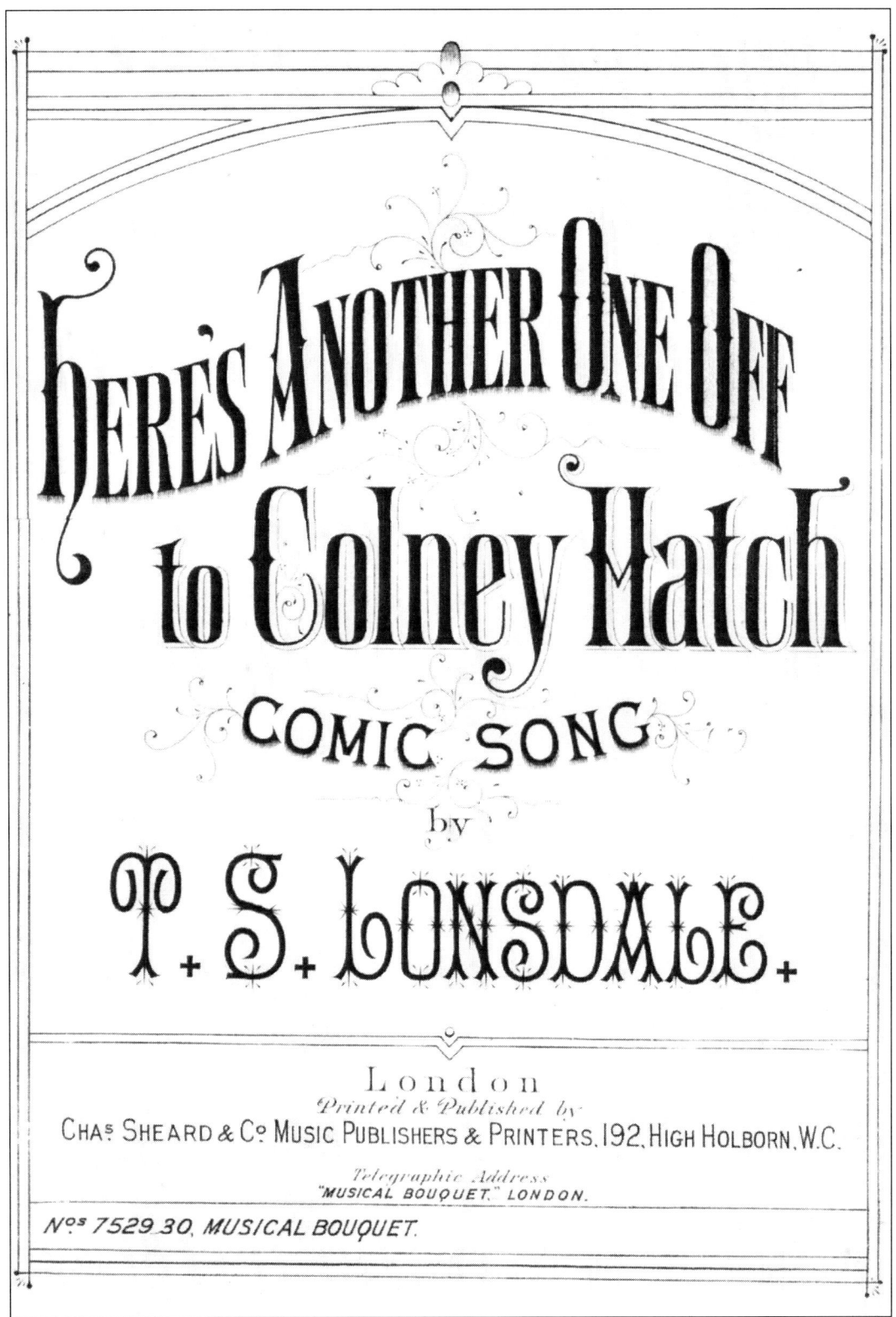

(FB&DLHS Archive)

For good measure, the chorus even managed to incorporate three other asylums:

> "There's another one off to Colney Hatch,
> Another one right for Bedlam,
> Another one off to join the batch,
> And poor Missis Wedlam.
> As a member now for Earlswood,
> I'm sure that you would stand well!
> Anyone now going on,
> Anymore for Hanwell?"

For people in North London the name was commonly used when referring to anyone slightly out of the ordinary: "He'll end up in Colney Hatch."

In 1950 a short promotional film was made entitled *Time Marches on at Friern,* presumably to mark the centenary. The director was D C Kessock Philip who was a doctor at the hospital and the editor and technical advisor was Dr A C Dalzell. The only surviving copy is a silent version and because of this it is difficult to ascertain the purpose of the film – it appears to have been made as a promotional tool to encourage nurses to join the hospital. Although of very poor quality technically, the film does contain some interesting views of the staff and the buildings and grounds.

In 1981 Friern was used as the setting for a movie called *Britannia Hospital,* starring Leonard Rossiter, Malcolm McDowell, Peter Jeffries, Joan Plowright and Graham Crowden and directed by Lindsay Anderson. The satire is based on an NHS hospital celebrating its five hundredth anniversary which is expecting the arrival of the Queen Mother who is coming to open a Centre for Advanced Science which is run by a crazed surgeon who creates people using parts from dead patients. In tune with the times, it also features militant striking workers who refuse to admit anybody to the hospital unless they are actually dying. The film was generally assumed to be an allegory for the state of Britain at the time. The exteriors were filmed at Friern and the hospital was paid £500 a day by the film company. The Manager of Friern at the time, Geoff Smith, describes how it all came about:

> "I was sitting in my office one Friday evening and a chap suddenly appeared and said he was a Location Manager and he explained that he was looking for a location for a film on a hospital. He said that he had just been driving by and had spotted the hospital and thought it was ideal. The reason I agreed to the film *Britannia Hospital* being made at Friern was that it was about a general hospital, not a psychiatric one. I met the producer, and Lindsay Anderson came up for a meeting and we got approval for about two or three weeks but it overran and we negotiated a fee of so much per day. They wanted something that looked something like a private patients' wing and one of the things that we had wanted to do was upgrade the doctors' bedrooms in the main block so they upgraded those free of charge, then they wanted to use the kitchen and my deputy suggested that it needed painting and they did that as well; we got all sorts of things done. And the patients loved it – it was activity on the site for the best part of six weeks. Leonard Rossiter was fantastic and there is so much time when they are not actually filming so they are at a loose end and he went to the Art Therapy Department and saw Mrs Reddy and he judged a patients' competition which the patients did once a year. He played the Administrator and I tried to explain how I worked. When it got near the end of the filming the producer asked us if we would like to go to the premiere and Sandra and I went to a little cinema off

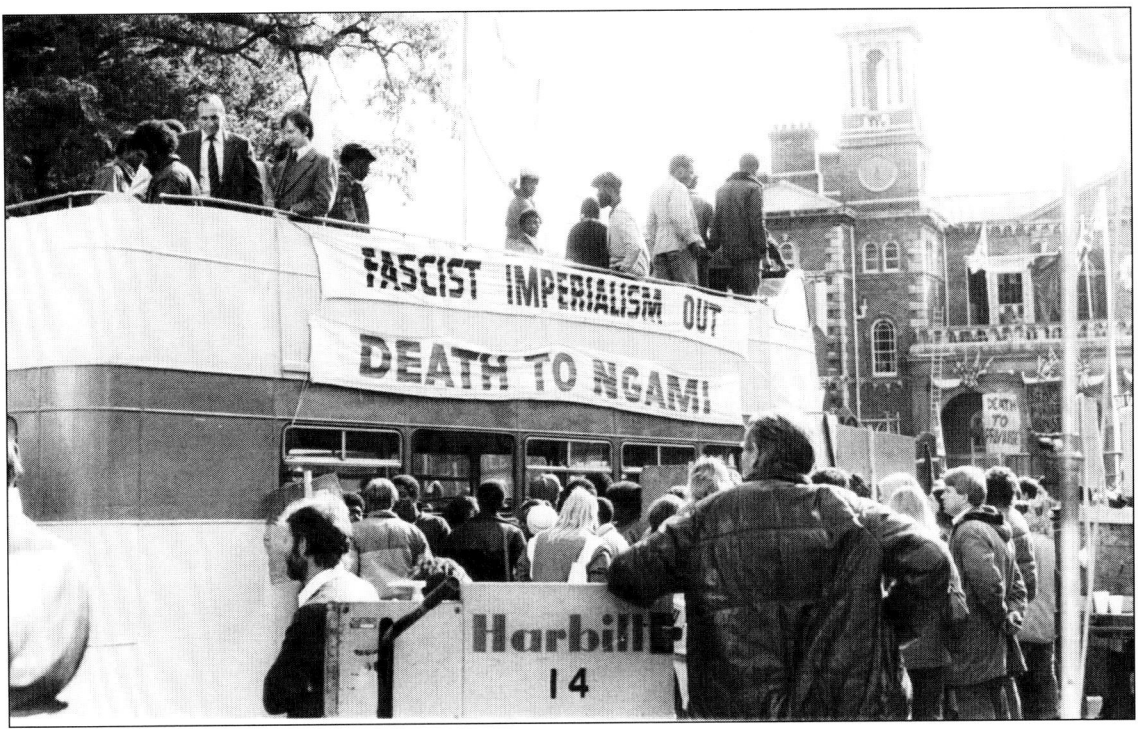

Filming Britannia Hospital. (Geoff Smith Collection)

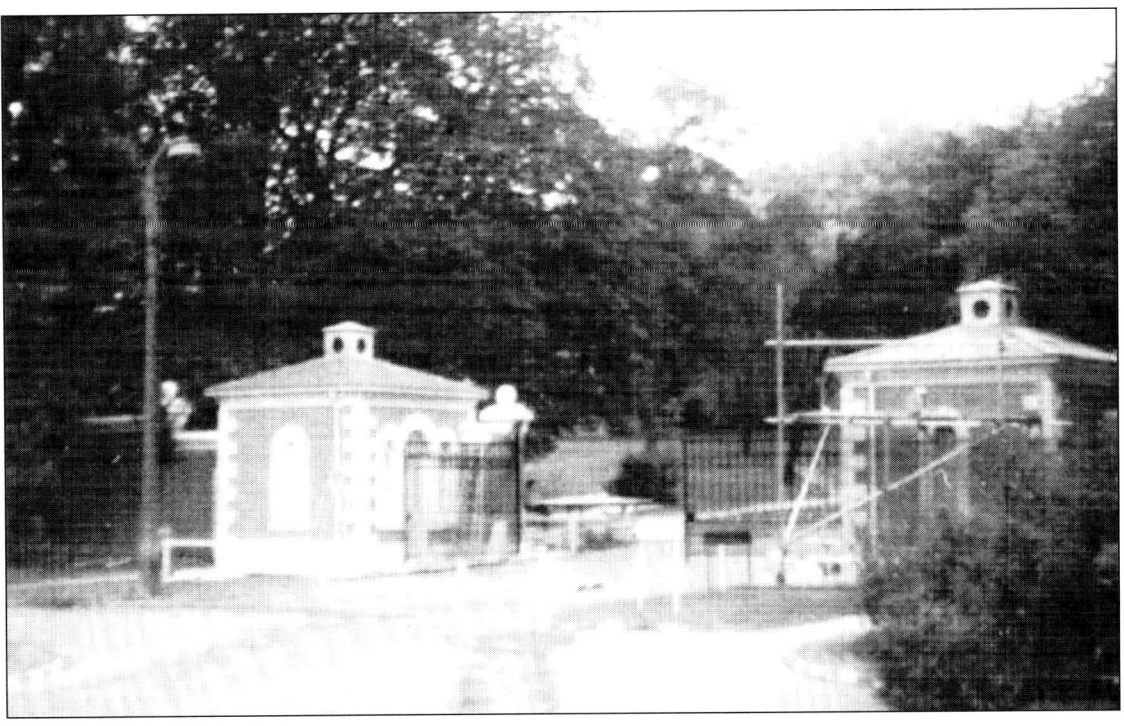

The film company even built two fake buildings at the bottom of the main drive.
(Vernon Muller)

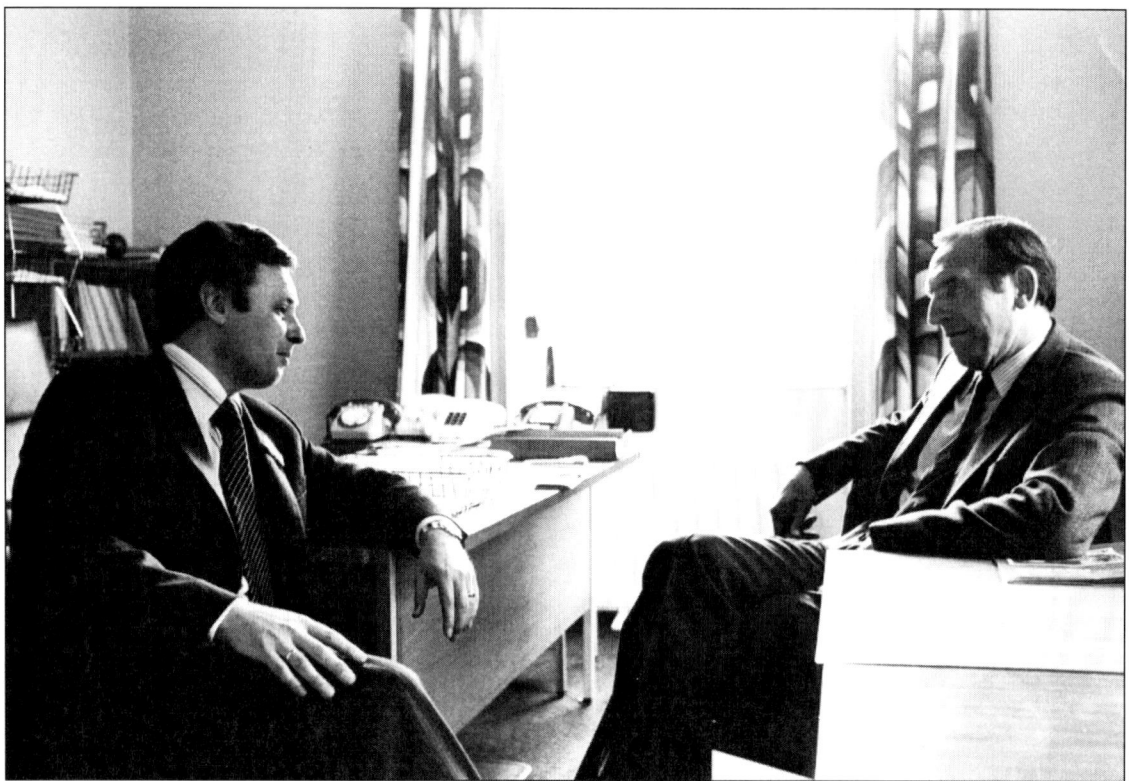

Geoff Smith (left) chatting to Leonard Rossiter in his office. (Geoff Smith Collection)

Tottenham Court Road on a Sunday morning and some of the cast were there, but it wasn't like the film premieres you see, with red carpet and everything."

Betty Inman was a secretary to the Consultant Psychiatrist at the time and she recalled that the making of *Britannia Hospital* caused a lot of excitement among the staff, some of whom had been promised parts in the crowd scenes. This never transpired as they were later told that they needed an Equity card!

In 1985 a BBC2 documentary programme in the Horizon series entitled *A World of Their Own* featured patients and staff at Friern and a documentary was broadcast on BBC Radio 4 on 28 June 1990 entitled *Up the Road to Colney Hatch*.

In 1993 the derelict asylum was used for location shooting of a British film entitled *Beyond Bedlam,* starring Craig Fairbrass, Elizabeth Hurley, Keith Allen and Anita Dobson and directed by Vadim Jean. The story is based on a novel by Harry Adam Knight and tells of policeman and a doctor struggling to defeat a serial killer. The executive producer Alan Martin described the location[1]:

"As we're filming there are guys wandering around with spanners and carrying out giant spin dryers. Once we had an option on the book we were always going to use Friern. It's the most wonderful place to film a psychological thriller."

In the same year an episode in the BBCTV series *Love Hurts III* was filmed in the hospital laundry. The programme was broadcast in the first week of January 1994.

In October 1994 a 14 minute 16mm colour film was shot at Friern. *The Holy Time* told the story of Paul Schreber, an eminent judge who was plagued in his later life by attacks of insanity. The film told of his visions, his hallucinations, and his subsequent recovery. It was directed by Ben Hopkins, produced by Tony Emsley and was entered in the British Short Film Festival in September 1994.

In March 1999 a Channel 4 programme in the Cutting Edge series directed by Rebecca Frayn and entitled *Asylum,* featured interviews with future residents of Princess Park Manor and three former patients of the hospital. The patients had conflicting views – one said it did him good to chat to someone every day, especially doctors, and there was no pressure, which gave him a chance to unwind and recuperate; another felt that as there was no decision making, he found it difficult to cope when he was discharged and he was later readmitted "back into the womb again". The third man found it difficult and lonely being left to his own devices in the outside world.

In 2006 Friern was the subject of a programme in the *Hidden House Histories* series on The History Channel which traced the story of the hospital and its subsequent conversion to apartments. The Chairman of Friern Barnet & District Local History Society, David Berguer, and the architect in charge of the conversion, Peter Smith, were interviewed by Nick Barratt who hosted the programme.

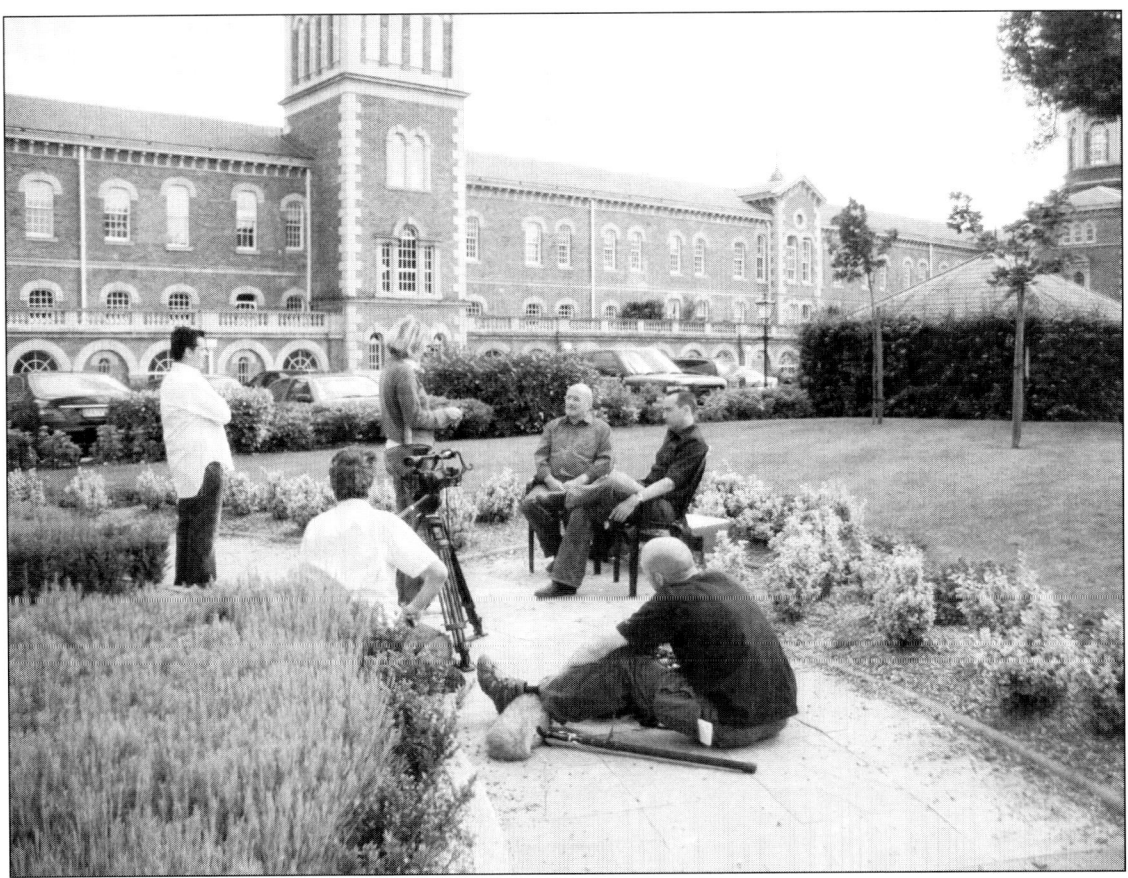

Nick Barratt and the author being filmed in front of Princess Park Manor on 11 June 2006.
(Patricia Berguer)

CHAPTER TWENTY FIVE
Reminiscences

A number of local residents and former staff have kindly given their recollections of Friern.

"It was about 1966 when I was asked by my then music teacher if I would help him give out Christmas presents to the patients. What he did not tell me was that we would be going into the locked wards. It was quite frightening to have the doors locked behind you as you went from one ward to another. Nothing happened although some of the patients' approach was rather frightening. Although it happened a long time ago it is something I have always remembered."
Margaret Price

"I have memories of problems at Friern Barnet Library and the things the staff had to put up with from inmates allowed out. There was one chap called Stavros (nothing to do with Harry Enfield!) who had learnt that if he stood on the table in the reference area and dropped his trousers there was a good chance that he would get a lift back to the hospital in a police car. It got to the stage that when Frances or one of the staff rang the police they would say: "Oh, not Stavros again!" I went and paid a visit to the boss of the hospital about it and he turned out to be the son in law of, I think it was, one of my own staff. He listened sympathetically but said there was precious little he could do about it. I reckon it's much quieter nowadays in Friern Barnet Library."
David Ruddom

"There was also a patient on the 221 bus and she took all her clothes off. She was a big woman and they had to get all the passengers off and take the bus out of service. Eventually the police came, but they couldn't get her off. The police then asked the driver to drive into Friern!"
Vernon Muller

"One of my mother's sisters, born about 1898, was playing in Colney Hatch Lane one day when she was about six and a long crocodile of patients walked past two-by-two with a member of hospital staff at the front and another at the back – apparently they were often taken for a walk like this. What neither member of staff initially noticed was that one of the patients picked up a little girl and carried her along very gently for some distance. When it was realised what had happened one of the staff carried her back to the place where she had been picked up."
Eileen Bostle

"For twenty three years I was a BBC secretary and in middle age I left and became a temporary secretary at Friern Hospital for two months in 1969. It was a large office holding four secretaries, all working for psychiatrists. I worked for the consultant Dr Hunter, and occasionally for his mother, Dr Ida McAlpine, who was a member of the construction family. Dr McAlpine was very kind to me, instructing me in the basics of psychiatry from a phrenology model! I remember that the office stationery was of very poor quality and the copying machine was a museum piece – it was literally like the first ever attempts at photography. I was offered a permanent secretarial job there, but they were only able to offer me £14 a week – basic rates, I think. I had matric, intermediate BA and BA to offer, but their scales paid for Higher Schools (now A levels), which I had skipped."
Mary Beagles, nee Comyns

"I started my career with the Prudential Assurance Company in 1968 and to facilitate the payment of claims (death, surrender or maturity) part of my duties as District Agent would be to obtain the signature of persons who were named as "Proposers" or "Life Assureds" on "Own Life" or "Life of Another" Industrial Branch Policies. This did, on occasion, require me to visit the hospital to complete the task. I would report to the office and then be taken to the relevant ward where I would talk to the patient concerned; Unfortunately, not all of them were able to give me relevant answers As a personal observation, I found that the place was a bit intimidating and sad but, having said that, I also felt it represented a place of refuge for the patients" *Dave Gladding*

"I have some memories of Friern Hospital, from the 1980's until its closure, from the links between St John's Church, Friern Barnet and the hospital chapel. We had a rota - about 5 or 6 members of the congregation - on which we would go in turn on Sunday mornings to help the chaplain at the hospital service - e.g. getting patients who needed escorting from their wards. I particularly remember, Queenie, who was brought in a wheelchair. She had lived in North Finchley as a child, above a shop in the High Road, a newsagent in the parade near Britannia Road (still a newsagent and food shop, I think) and went to St John's School, Whetstone. She had clear memories of those days, some of which were shared by my mother, who also lived above a High Road shop (the one that for many years was Harris's, the shoe repairer). Sadly, Queenie's problem was with the present; it was often difficult to get her into the chair to go back to her ward as, she would say, she had no body, so they wouldn't want her. There were many others who were very regular, and I wondered whether they would feel a loss when they were dispersed as the hospital closed. At the time I was involved, the old chapel was no longer in use - I think it needed restoration and was considered dangerous. Instead, there was a multi-faith room used for Jewish, Roman Catholic (they had their mass on Saturday evening, with priest and people coming from Our Lady of Lourdes, Arnos Grove) and Anglican. The room was furnished appropriately for each. On Remembrance Sunday, following the service, we would process to the war memorial, the fountain in front of the main doorway. It was my job to lead with the processional cross, trying to judge the pace so that the tail wasn't left too far behind and that I wasn't overtaken by the more impatient, and taking care to avoid catching the cross on the corridor ceiling, which varied in height. As well as the link with the hospital service, some patients, able to leave the hospital, would come regularly to the service in St John's." *John Philpott*

"As a qualified Engineer I was often involved with major problems on the electricity network, being called out at all hours of the night and day. On one occasion I was called out to Colney Hatch Hospital, one dark winter's night when the electricity had gone off in a section of one of the very long corridors. If I remember rightly, the doors in the corridors didn't have exterior handles; staff used to get in and out with a special type of T key that used to turn the lock. I went to the switch room with their Chief Engineer and we worked on this piece of switchgear for some time, finally restoring the supply. As I left and started walking down the corridor, the switch tripped out again and all the lights went out. By this time quite a number of patients were promenading up and down and immediately the lights went out they started to scream and shout. My heart was in my mouth and I quickly moved to the side wall, backtracking quite a way to where I thought the door had been and that I had not long come out of. I luckily banged on the right door and was greeted by the Engineer who had a wry smile on his face. "Worried were we?" he said. I just looked back at him and tried to stop shaking, thinking in my vivid imagination about what might have happened. We finally fixed the problem after another session and I got home late that evening." *Ray Lewis*

"An ancestor of mine, Abie Butfoy, was admitted in 1851. He had been a serving Police Officer in Dagenham before being implicated as one of the suspects in PC Clark's murder in what became known as 'The Dagenham Murder' in 1846. No charges were

pressed but he was a prime suspect. After the murder he returned to Bethnal Green and returned to his previous employment as a silk weaver. On 17 January 1851 Butfoy was taken from home and admitted to Bethnal Green Workhouse as a lunatic, then some months later to Colney Hatch where he was the second patient to be admitted. On 7 July 1853 he died, aged 43, the cause of death being given as 'Chronic changes of brain'. He was laid to rest in the asylum burial ground four days later, the service being carried out by the Chaplain Henry Murray."
Sara Brooks

"When I was in my early twenties I used to sing in a very amateur old-time Music Hall. The troupe was run by a man called Jo Blake who was dedicated to Music Hall, and organised local shows. One booking was on a Saturday evening at Friern Hospital, round about 1964. There was, as I recall, a reasonably sized theatre with a stage and changing rooms. I arrived early and asked someone (who I imagined was a member of staff) where the theatre was. After following his directions I found myself outside the operating theatre! I have no idea what sort of operations they performed there. I can recall standing on the stage dressed up as Al Jolson, and doing my best to entertain the audience. As you can imagine, there was quite a mixed reaction. Some were asleep, others were wandering about the theatre, and others were not able to enter into the spirit of the show to any extent. But I do remember that there was a general air of enjoyment, although many of the patients didn't really have the ability to show their feelings. I can recall, however, being made very welcome and I did feel at the end of the evening some pleasure had been brought to the patients and staff."
Richard Testar

"At school, Woodhouse Grammar, it was quite common for a schoolchild to ask if another had a "green card", meaning for the lunatic asylum, if something stupid had been committed. Fortunately, they didn't know that I had been born there even if it was part of an emergency hospital during World War II. I never heard anyone else mention that they had been born there, but then it would have been considered a stigma. Strangely enough ten years ago I met someone, now living in Bognor Regis, whose brother was also born at the EMH."
Elizabeth Carter

"There was a cashier and the patients would get their weekly allowances and there was a Pope who had died and another Pope was appointed and he died shortly afterwards. When the second Pope died, one of the patients, who was a Roman Catholic said: "Have you heard the Pope has died? and the lady said: "Oh, yes we know the Pope died" and he said "No, the new Pope" and she said "Yes, we know the Pope died!" and they didn't believe him. The patients used to watch the television and read the newspapers."
Vernon Muller

"I worked at Friern as a secretary to three psychiatrists for ten years. During that time I only used the dentist and the hairdresser at the hospital once. I remember sitting in the hairdressing salon at the back of the building having my hair done and watching the fire at Alexandra Palace. It was on Thursday 10 July 1980."
Betty Inman

"In the early seventies I was a young black cab driver. One day I picked up a woman outside Friern Barnet Town Hall and at her request took her to an address in Finsbury Park. She asked me to wait while she went up to a house and rang the doorbell. There was no reply, so she then asked to be taken to Golders Green where the same thing happened. I should have realised early on that something was not quite right, but I was young and inexperienced. She then asked me to take her back to Friern Barnet and once there to go on to Friern Hospital. When I told her the fare she said she had no money.

Two nurses came out to escort her into the building and I explained what had happened. Fortunately, they paid for her fare and told me that the money would come out of the Sunday Fund. Apparently this was not an uncommon occurrence, but from then on I was a bit wiser. I later learned that it was not unknown for some black cab drivers to switch off their 'For Hire' signs as they drove past the Hospital!"
Gordon Brown

"One thing I remember about the place is the smell of it. It had a completely unique smell that I have never smelled since, even in hospital. It was a combination of bleach, that kind of sanitised smell that you get in hospitals, but with a strong undertone of food. The two mixed together made this very odd and although I was there four or five years it was the first thing that hit you and I never got used to it. Another thing I remember was that the place was very shiny: the interior was that shiny paint that was on everything, ceilings, walls, floors. The other thing was the shops on the other side of the road, the little newsagent used to sell single cigarettes 2p each."
Pete Abbott

"Whilst working in Friern Barnet Town Hall we would be visited by some of the patients from the hospital. One man would come and stand in the car park and salute the flag then happily go on his way. Another would come in to our receptionist and hand her a letter. This would be lines of scribble, but she would go and get a member of staff and who would pretend to read the letter and then tell the man that we would take it to a senior officer. This would satisfy him, and off he would go until the next time when the whole scenario would be repeated again. There were also two sisters who pushed a large coach-built pram around the area – they must have walked for miles. I remember this going back to my childhood and it went on for a good number of years but I can't remember if there was anything in the pram. It was so sad when the hospital eventually closed as the patients seemed totally lost and wandered around having lost the only way of life that they had ever known. I am told that both my paternal grandfather, with the surname of Martin, and my stepmother's father, surname Wakenell, both worked at the hospital, one as a nurse and the other as mortician, but I have nothing to substantiate this and nobody who would be likely to know left to ask."
Doreen Holmes

"An uncle of mine, by marriage, was a male nurse at the hospital and I remember that he used to play football for the hospital team. On one occasion he asked me to come along when they played a visiting team from Poland - a very rough side – and my uncle ended up having his leg broken. I am not sure that he ever played again, but I got a nice football shirt out of it (blue and white squares) and I wore it during my sports lessons at school."
Derek Spurgeon

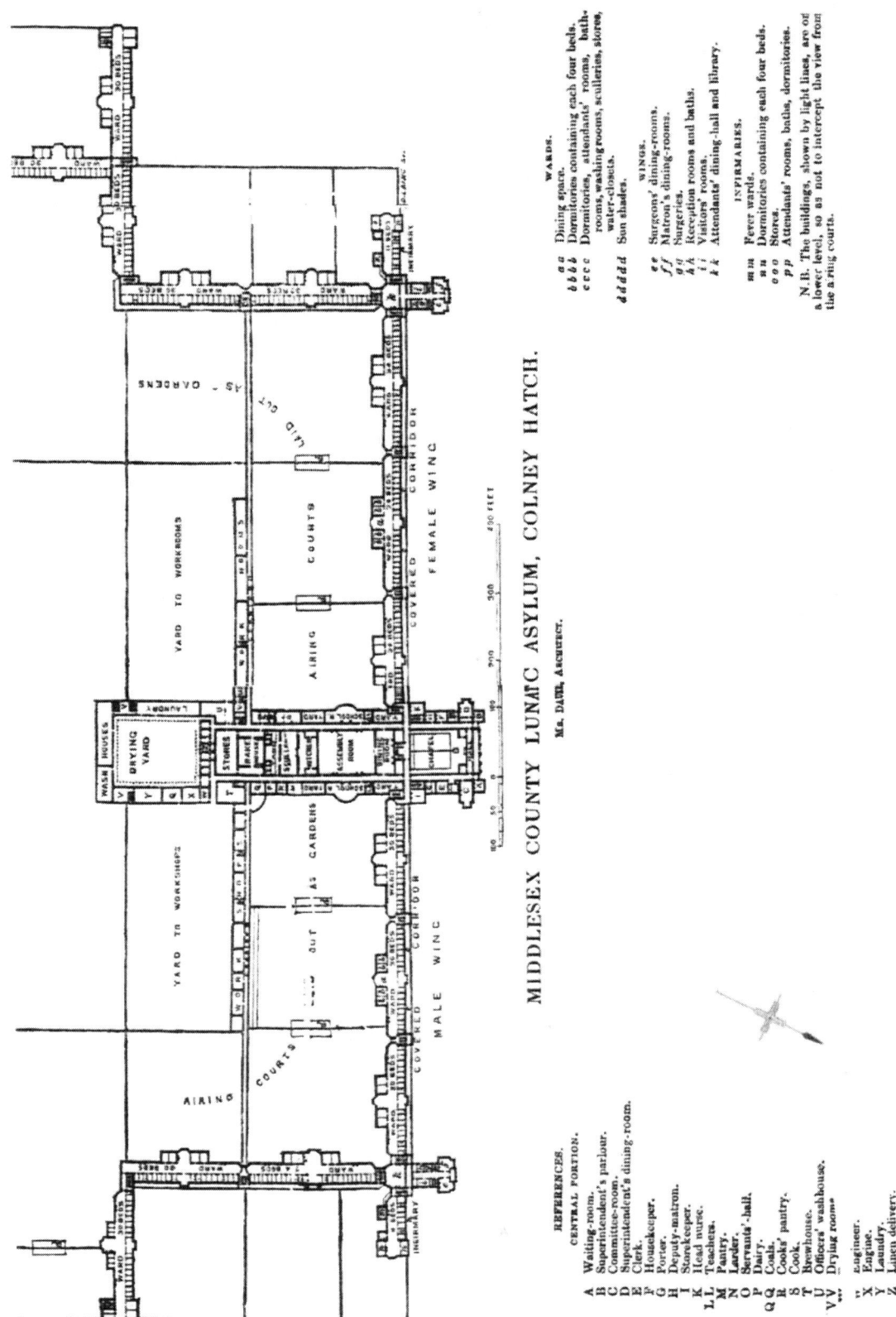

How it all started. The original plan of the asylum
(The Builder)

NOTES

CHAPTER 1 MENTAL ILLNESS AND POVERTY
1 Kathryn Morrison. *The Workhouse.* (English Heritage 1999). Page 156
2 *The Builder.* 5 November 1859. Page 722
3 Barnet Local Studies and Archives. MS 9380/1
4 *The Times* 13 June 1851. Page 6
5 *The Times.* 2 July 1851. Page 8

CHAPTER 2 CHOOSING THE SITE AT COLNEY HATCH
1 London Metropolitan Archives H12/CH/A/01/001/001
2 London Metropolitan Archives H12/CH/A/01/001/001
3 London Metropolitan Archives MF/A/004
4 *Victoria History of the County of Middlesex.* Constable & Co. 1911

CHAPTER 3 DESIGN
1 *The Builder.* 16 October 1847
2 *The Pictorial Handbook of London.* 1854
3 *The Pictorial Handbook of London.* 1854

CHAPTER 4 BUILDING THE ASYLUM
1 London Metropolitan Archives H12/CH/A/01/002/001
2 London Metropolitan Archives
3 Richard Hunter and Ida Macalpine. *Psychiatry for the Poor* (Dawsons of Pall Mall) 1974. Page 146
4 www.moneysorter.co.uk/calculator_inflation

CHAPTER 5 PROBLEMS WITH SEWAGE
1 London Metropolitan Archives H12/CH/A/01/006
2 *Barnet Press* 13 February 1869

CHAPTER 6 GAS AND WATER
1 London Metropolitan Archives H12/CH/A/01/002/004
2 *New Southgate Gas Works*: A Brief History (Friern Barnet & District Local History Society) 2007
3 *Friern Hospital Magazine.* October-November 1950. Page 17
4 London Metropolitan Archives MJ/SP/1885/04/019

CHAPTER 7 THE EARLY DAYS
1 Burnt Oak Register Office
2 *Chapters on Mental Physiology* (Longman, Brown Green and Longmans) 1852 page 113
3 *New Southgate: A Brief History* (Friern Barnet & District Local History Society) 2007
4 London Metropolitan Archives H12/CH/1/10/007

CHAPTER 8 HOUSEKEEPING
1 London Metropolitan Archives H12/CH/A/01/007
2 Richard Hunter and Ida Macalpine. *Psychiatry for the Poor* (Dawsons of Pall Mall) 1974. Page 115
3 *The Builder* 5 July 1851. Page 415
4 London Metropolitan Archives H12/CH/A/02/005
5 London Metropolitan Archives H12/CH/A/02/005

6 London Metropolitan Archives LCC/MIN/009/76
7 *Friern Hospital Magazine* October-November 1950. Page 38
8 *Friern Hospital Magazine* October-November 1950. Page 35
9 Richard Hunter and Ida Macalpine. *Psychiatry for the Poor* (Dawsons of Pall Mall) 1974. Page 119-121
10 *Friern Hospital Magazine* October-November 1950. Page 36

CHAPTER 9 PATIENTS
1 *The Times* 21 January 1852
2 Committee Report Number 4 London Metropolitan Archives H12/CH/A/08/001
3 Shifrin, Malcolm R *Victorian Turkish Baths* –encephalograph from a group of schizophrenics in a catatonic stupor. March 2011
4 London Metropolitan Archives H12/CH/A/01/010
5 *Express & News.* 5 August 1977. Page 10
6 *The Times.* 13 September 1977. Page 2

CHAPTER 10 TREATMENT
1 *Illustrated London News*
2 Wilkie Collins. *The Woman in White.* (Penguin Books) 1999. Introduction by Matthew Sweet. Page xviii
3 Shifrin, Malcolm R. *Victorian Turkish Baths* www.victorianturkishbath.org. March 2011
4 *Everyday Life Through the Ages.* Reader's Digest Association 1992
5 London Metropolitan Archives H/12/CH/A/004
6. London Metropolitan Archives H/12/CH/A/7/10/1-6
7 *Mental Health Guide.* Mind in Barnet. 2007. Page 2
8 *British Medical Journal.* 14 December 1974. Page 637
9 Roy Porter. *Madness* (Oxford University Press) 2002. Page 205
10 Roy Porter. *Madness* (Oxford University Press) 2002. Page 206
11 Mental Health Guide. Mind in Barnet. 2007. Page 6
12 London Metropolitan Archives H/12/CH/A/07/011
13 Jo Brand.. *Look Back in Hunger.* Headline Publishing Group 2009

CHAPTER 11 WORK AND THERAPY
1 London Metropolitan Archives H/12/CH/A/07/011
2 Mental Health Network Journal. January 1985. Page 1
3 *The Times.* 28 Dec 1974. Page 12

CHAPTER 12 TAKING CARE OF THE SOUL
1 *Friern Hospital Magazine.* October-November 1950. Page 27
2 *Friern Hospital Magazine.* October-November 1950. Page 28
3 www.together-uk.org/about-us/our-history/henry-hawkins. December 2011
4 London Metropolitan Archives H12/CH/Y/03/022

CHAPTER 13 ENTERTAINMENT
1 *Hendon & Finchley Times.* 18 March 1993. Page 17

CHAPTER 14 STAFF
1 Richard Hunter and Ida Macalpine. *Psychiatry for the Poor* (Dawsons of Pall Mall) 1974. Page 89

2 *Supplement to the London Gazette*, May 21, 1884
3 London Metropolitan Archives H12/CH/A/07/004
4 *Barnet Press* 7 August 1981
5 Friern Hospital Magazine. October-November 1950. Page 21

CHAPTER 15 FIRE!
1 Jack While. *Fifty Years of Fire Fighting in London* (Hutchinson & Co) 1931
2 Royal Free Hospital Archives ACC 4/99

CHAPTER 16 WARTIME
1 Maggie Butt. *Ally Pally Prison Camp* (Overstep Books) 2011. Page 54
2 London Metropolitan Archives H12/CH/A/08/001
3 Percy Reboul and John Heathfield. *Days of Darkness* (Sutton Publishing) 1995
4 London Metropolitan Archives H12/CH/A/7/9
5 London Metropolitan Archives H12/CH/A/79

CHAPTER 17 CHANGES & IMPROVEMNETS
1 London Metropolitan Archives. MCC/CL/L/CC/02/021
2 The Builder 5 November 1859. Page 723
3 London Metropolitan Archives MCC/CL/CC/2/21
4 London Metropolitan Archives A/KE/736/24
5 London Metropolitan Archives H/12/CH/A/07/011
6 Richard Hunter and Ida Macalpine. *Psychiatry for the Poor* (Dawsons of Pall Mall) 1974. Page 144

CHAPTER 18. SANS EVERYTHING
1 *Findings and Recommendations Following Enquiries into Allegations Concerning the Care of Elderly Patients in Certain Hospitals.* HMSO 1968
2 *Daily Mail* 10 Sept 1965

CHAPTER 19 CARE IN THE COMMUNITY
1 *Richard Hunter and Ida Macapline.* Psychiatry for the Poor (Dawsons of Pall Mall) 1974. Page 155
2 Royal Free Hospital Archives
3 *The Guardian.* 15 November 1977
4 London Metropolitan Archives H12/CH/Y/03/011 *Neurone* Magazine
5 *Evening Standard.* 22 November 1984. Page 7
6 *The Friern Report: An experiment in resettlement.* 1990
7 *Openmind.* October/November 1983. Page 7
8 *Hendon & Finchley Times* 1 July 1993. Page 5
9 *Hendon & Finchley Times* 8 July 1993. Page 1
10 *The Mental Health Guide.* Sixth edition. Mind in Barnet 2007. Page 2
11 *The Mental Health Guide.* Sixth edition. Mind in Barnet 2007. Page 20

CHAPTER 20 PREPARING FOR THE END
1 *Openmind*, October/November 1983. Page 7
2 *Health and Social Service Journal,* 23 January 1986. Page 97
3 *Finchley Press.* 10 June 1993
4 Royal Free Hospital Archives ACC 4/99
5 Royal Free Hospital Archives ACC 4/99

CHAPTER 21 DEVELOPMENT OF THE SITE
1 *Barnet Times* 22 September 1988
2 *Daily Telegraph* 23 September 1996. Page 29

CHAPTER 22 PRINCESS PARK MANOR
1 Barnet Council C/03069/BC
2 *Barnet Times* 27 June 1996
3 *The Times* 5 February 2000. Page 2
4 Royal Free Hospital Archives ACC 4/99
5 Land Registry Register of Title NGL735132
6 *Barnet Press* 19 August 2010

INDEX

Abbott, Pete 81,167
Adams, Sergeant 23
AEGIS 124
Alberge, Hyman 45
Albert, Prince Consort 22,26
Alderson, William 5
Alexandra Palace 105,106,108,150
Allen, Keith 162
Allom & Crosse 9
Anderson, Lindsay 160
Ariff, Zeba 138
Armstrong-Jones, Sir Robert 60
Arnos West Community Association 156
Attfield, John 22
Auxiliary Fire Service 107

Baker, George 106
Bal, Dr Subir 51
Banstead Asylum 26,75,99
Barnet Council 142,143,144,149,151
Barnet General Hospital 51,104
Barnet Union 24
Barnwell, Deave 7
Barratt, Nick 163
Battie, William 2
Bazalgette, Sir Joseph 31
Beadles, Cecil F 46
Beagles, Mary 164
Bellway Homes 146
Bensley Thomas 5
Berridge, Robert 90,91
Bethlem (and Bedlam) 4,17,62,160,162
Betstyle 7
Bexley 107
Beyond Bedlam (film) 162
Bloomfield, Dr, Bishop of London 24
Bloomsbury Health Authority 123,133,138
Bolam, John 158,159
Bostle, Eileen 164
Bradley, Dr John 131
Bradley, Thomas 47
Brand, Jo 62
Bridges, James (Duke of Chandos) 7
Britannia Hospital (film) 160
Broadmoor 4
Brooks, Sara 166
Brookstream Corporation 149
Brookwood Hospital 128
Broomfield Park 84
Brown, Gordon 167
Bryant Homes 146

Bulwer Lytton, Edward 56
Bulwer Lytton, Rosina 56

Camden & Islington Area Health Authority 123,131
Campbell, Dr Patrick 138
Carlyle, Janet M 110
Carr, Sofie 108
Carter, Elizabeth 166
Cartwright, Messrs 10
Chase Farm Hospital 119
Chazen, Irving 75
Cherry Tree Inn 28
Cheshunt Cottage Hospital 119
City of London Maternity Hospital 119
Clark, Arthur 106
Claybury 26,75
Clunis, Christopher 134
Cohen, David 47
Cohen, Morris 45
Collins, Hilda 87
Collins, Wilkie 37
Colney Hatch Gas Light & Coke Co 32,33
Colney Hatch Station 24,32,38,108
Comer, Luke 149,154
Commissioners in Lunacy 3,5,9,70,111
Comyns, Mary 63
Conolly, Dr John 56
Cornelius, Richard 153
County Asylums Act 1808 4
Crawshay, George 7,59
Crowden, Graham 160
Cubitt, Lewis 111,157
Cubitt, Thomas 9
Cubitt, William 5
Curtis, Sir William 7

Daly, Allen 59
Dalzell, Dr A C 160
Daukes, Samuel William 9,22,27,157,
Davey, Dr J G 58,59
de Audley, Henry 7
de Morton, William 7
Dickins, Charles Albert 106
Dobson, Anita 162
Doudan, Catherine 37
Duchess of Kent 119
Dunthorne, Ken 96
Dyke, Olive 121

Earlswood 160
East London Union 25
Edmonton Board 27,29

Edmonton Union 24
Edwards, Thomas 88,89
Ellis, Dr William Charles 5
Emsley, Tony 162
Emergency Medical Hospitals 107
English Heritage 150
Essex County Asylum, Brentwood 22
Esporta 150
Euston Station 136

Fairbrass, Craig 162
Fairview Estates 142
Family Life (film) 130
Finchley Society, The 156
Fox, Colonel 99,100
Frayn, Rebecca 163
Friends of Friern Hospital 80
Friern Barnet & Whetstone Residents' Association 156
Friern Hospital Management Committee 158
Friern Village Residents' Association 155

Gallants Farm 41
George III 2
George IV 7
Gibbs, Michael 7
Gibbs, Wilfrid C 110
Gladding, Dave 165
Goodmayes Hospital 133
Gordon, Peter K 110
Great Exhibition 1851 26,57
Great Northern Cemetery 38,98
Great Northern Railway 6,8,24,32,33
Great North Road 5

Hackney Union 25
Hadley Wood 84
Halliwick Estate 7
Halliwick Hospital 68, 119,143,146
Hampstead Health Authority 104,122,139
Hanwell Asylum 5,16,26,56,70,99,111,160
Harris & Godwin 9
Harris, James 158
Haslemere Estates 144
Hawkins, Henry 70,71
Henderson, William Richard 106
Hendon 5
Henry III 7
Henry VIII 1
Hill, Robert Gardiner 56
Holborn Union 25
Holcombe, Charles Thomas 7
Holly Park School 155

Hollickwood 6,7
Holloway Prison 119
Holmes, Doreen 167
Holy Time, The (film) 162
Hood, W Charles 16,17,45,58,67
Hopkins, Ben 162
Hornsey Central Hospital 119
Hornsey House Tavern 6
Horton 75
Hume, Cardinal Basil 74
Humphreys, Maxwell Mark 106
Hurley, Elizabeth 162

Imperial War Museum 4
Inman, Betty 163,167
Inner London Education Authority 115

Jack the Ripper 47
Jean, Vadim 162
Jeffries, Peter 160
Jewish Care 142

Karton, Emma 135
Kessock-Philip, Dr 160
King's Cross Station 136,158
King's Fund 119
Klyberg, Rt Rev 138
Knight, Harry Adam 162
Kosminski, Aaron 47

Lamont, John 106
Lawrence, Dorothy 47,48
Lawrence, Sir Thomas 7
League of Jewish Friends 138
Lee Valley Water 139
Lewis, Ray 165
Leibbrandt, Margaret
Lincoln Lunatic Asylum 56
Lines, G J & Sons 8
Lipman, Maureen 79
Lister Hospital 119
LNER 115
Loach, Ken 130
London County Council 43,98,99,115,122,130
London Fire Brigade 104
Love Hurts III (TV programme) 162
Luck, Andolie 123
Lunacy Act 4
Lunacy Commission 4

Macaulay, Gilbert 46
Macnaughton, Sir Neville 47
Manninger Foundation 73

Marquis of Salisbury 22
Marr, David 107
Marshall, Dr W G 58
Martin, Alan 162
Marylebone Workhouse 45
McArthur, Emily 110
McCann, Mrs 46
McDowell, Malcolm 160
Mental After Care Association 71
Mental Health Acts 51,127,131,135
Mental Treatment Act 1930 119,122
Metal Box Co Ltd 68
Metropolitan Board of Works 31
Middlesex County Asylum, Banstead 26,75
Middlesex County Asylum, Claybury 26,60,62,75
Middlesex County Asylum Hanwell *see Hanwell*
Middlesex County Council 112, 115,122
Middlesex population 5
Middlesex Justices 5,6,7,9
Minchenden School 83
Mind 133
Moore, Thomas 7
Moorfields 4
Morris, Robert 39
Muller, Vernon 72,84,85,136,164,166
Murdoch, Clare 139
Myers, George 22

Napsbury 76
National Association for Mental Health 130
National Schizophrenic Fellowship 133
New Southgate Cemetery 102
Nicholas, Rev Vincent 138
Nicholl, Margaret 7
North Camden District Health Authority 136
North Circular Road 107,115,116,142,144,145
North East Thames Regional Health Authority 122,133,134
North Middlesex Hospital 119
North West Thames Regional Health Authority 146

O'Donoghue, John 86
One Flew Over the Cuckoo's Nest (film)130
Orange Tree inn 22

Parkinson Report 131
Parkside Asylum, Macclesfield 106
Passmore Edwards Hospital 63
Pentonville Prison 119
Perkins, Charles 7
Peter Bedford Trust 132
Phillips, Henry 5
Philpott, John 165

Pinkham, Sir Charles 115
Plancey, Rabbi Alan 138
Plowright, Joan 160
Poplar Union 25
Powell, Enoch 130
Pownall, Henry 22
Price, Margaret 164
Price, Ralph Charles 7
Princess Park Manor Residents' Association 155
Pymmes Brook 30

Queen Mary's Hospital 119
Quinton & Sherlaw, Messrs 78

Rampton 134
Rawlings, Henry 45
Rayner, Claire 137
Reid, Dr 107
Reynolds, John 106
Ridley, Nicholas 143
RMS Lusitania 106
Robinson, Kenneth 125
Rossiter, Leonard 160,162
Rotch, Benjamin 22,23
Royal Earlswood Asylum for Idiots 26
Royal Free Hospital 150
Royal Northern Hospital 119
Ruddom, David 164
Runwell 75

St Ann's Hospital 119,136
St Bartholomew's 62,63,107
St Bernard's 51
St James the Great, Friern Barnet 5
St John's Ambulance Corps 107
St Luke's Asylum 2
St Pancras Station 136
Schreber, Paul 162
Seaward, Dr 45, 46
Sheppard, Dr Edgar 60
Shoppee, C J 22
Signy, Dennis 79
Skaife, John 29,30
Smith, Geoff 79,118,132
Smith, George Knights 8
Smith, Katie C 110
Smith, W H 78
Smith, Peter 150
Southgtae & Colney Hatch Gas Light & Coke Company 32,33
Southgate & District Gas Company 34
Southwwod Hospital 119
Spurgeon, Derek 167

SS Sindoro 106
Standard Telephones & Cables 68,107
Staple, Rev David 138
Staples, Messrs 24
Statute of Labourers 2
Stepney Union 25
Sterile Supplies Unit 139
Sterland, Robert 46
Swain, George 110

Talbot, John Chetwynd 7
Tarmac Construction 144
Testar, Richard 166
Thatcher, Margaret 121,122,136
Thomas, Danford 45
Thomas, Danford 45
Thomas, Rev Pat 82
Thompson, Rev J 23
Thornbury 9
Timen, Andrew 158
Tisard, Dr H J 46
Together 71
Toombs, Ken 68
Tottenham Board 27,29,30
Try Construction 144,146
Tyerman, Dr D F 58,59,61

Umbrella 133
Up the Road to Colney Hatch (radio programme) 162

Warwick, Irene 109
Weller, Dr Malcolm 131,134
Westall, Jerry 133
Westfield, Dr Stephanie 136
Whetstone Society, The 156
White, Dorothy C 110
Whitley Council 128
Whitechapel Union 25
Whittington Hospital 9,119, 131
Winslow, L Forbes 56
Wittingham Asylum, Lancashire 106
Woburn Abbey 84
World of Their Own (TV programme) 162
Wright, Carol 120
WVRS 138

Zito, Jonathan 134